PAEDIATRICS IN THE REICHSUNIVERSITÄT STRAßBURG

PAEDIATRICS IN THE REICHSUNIVERSITÄT STRAßBURG

Children's Medicine at a Bastion of Nazi Ideology

AISLING SHALVEY

UNIVERSITY
of
EXETER
PRESS

First published in 2023 by
University of Exeter Press
Reed Hall, Streatham Drive
Exeter EX4 4QR
UK

www.exeterpress.co.uk

British Library Cataloguing in Publication Data
A catalogue record for this book is available from the British Library.

https://doi.org/10.47788/HUGC9927

ISBN 978-1-80413-089-6 Hardback
ISBN 978-1-80413-090-2 ePub
ISBN 978-1-80413-091-9 PDF

Cover image: 'Protect your Child, Trust the Doctor! Come to the Mothers' Consultation Hours' (original Schütze dein Kind. Vertraue dem Arzt. Komm zu Mütterberatungsstunde). Reichsuniversität Straßburg, 1942.

Typeset in Baskerville MT Std by S4Carlisle Publishing Services Chennai, India

Do mo Sheanmhathair 'Granny', le grá

Contents

Figures

Cover: 'Protect your Child, Trust the Doctor! Come to the Mothers' Consultation Hours' (original Schütze dein Kind. Vertraue dem Arzt. Komm zu Mütterberatungsstunde). Reichsuniversität Straßburg, 1942.

This is the only extant image of paediatric treatment in the Reichsuniversität Straßburg. It was intended to advertise the clinic, particularly the mothers' consultation hours where infants could be brought, free of charge, to check their weight and development, administer vaccines and medications, and to give the parents advice. This was also propaganda material for the NSV, a Nazi organisation, as by encouraging the parents to come to these conultations they could also advise them on eugenics and racial hygiene, as well as ensuring that they were engaging with National Socialist organizations.

The doctors and nurses depicted are unknown, but it is very likely that they were all staff of the children's clinic. The exact date of this photograph is not specified, but it is estimated to have been taken in 1942, and was published by a printer in Straßburg for the local NSDAP (Gau Baden-Elsaß) department of public welfare, training, and education.

This image is reproduced on the cover in part as it is the only image of paediatric treatment in this era for the hospital, but also because it is a symbol of the duality of the Reichsuniversität Straßburg. On one hand, it provided medical care to the population and advertised itself as such, but this care came with the condition of population surveillance and incorporation of occupation politics into daily life, along with indoctrinating the populace by making their healthcare dependent on adherence to Nazi ideology.

Acknowledgements

I am extraordinarily lucky to have so many people who have supported me throughout the process of writing this book, so this list is by no means complete. The first thank you goes to the Fondation pour la Mémoire de la Shoah, and the University of Strasbourg, who have funded this research, and without whom this project could not have come to fruition.

Thank you to Exeter University Press, and in particular Nigel Massen and David Hawkins, my editors, for making wonderful suggestions, catching my mistakes, and bearing with me through redrafts.

Thank you to the Historical Commission of the Reichsuniversität Straßburg for supporting my work. This book is based in large part on my work in Strasbourg that was prompted, inspired, and encouraged by the work of this commission. Thank you to Paul Weindling and Florian Schmaltz, the presidents of the commission, who have given me a platform to share my research and given me the tools to do so. It has been an honour to work with such inspiring academics, but I feel Gabriele Moser, Sabine Hildebrandt, and Christian Bonah require particular thanks; for reading my work, for encouraging me throughout the process, and for providing advice on how to transform my thesis into a book. Thank you also to Catherine Maurer for her encouragement, and to Loïc Lutz and Thérèse Vicent for their help.

To the archivists at the Archives Départementales du Bas-Rhin, Archives de la Ville et de l'Eurométropole, Bundesarchiv Berlin, Humboldt Universität Archiv, Archives Nationales de France at Pierrefitte, Staatsarchiv Sigmaringen, Archiv Universität Wien, Archives du Stephansfeld, Archives de la Faculté du Médecine, Landesarchiv Stuttgart, and the Amies des Hôpitaux Universitaires, for being so helpful with finding aids, inquiries, and access to archival sources. Thank you to Bridgeman Images Berlin and Paris for their help with image licensing and access. I am grateful to the librarians at the Bibliothèque de médecine et odontologie, Bibliothèque nationale et universitaire de Strasbourg, and the Bibliothèque d'Histoire de Médecine for their help in ordering books from often obscure places, and for being so accommodating. Thank you also to the librarians at the German National Academy of Sciences Leopoldina for accommodating me.

Thank you to my family, especially my parents and my sister, for listening to this project for so long, for encouraging me, and for all their support. A particular thank you to Jack Kavanagh, Neale Rooney, and Caoimhe Burke, along with my other friends. The biggest thank you, though, goes to my granny, for inspiring me with her love of history, for all her help with proof-reading, and for regularly calling to keep me on track: this book is dedicated to her.

Preface

This book concerns the 'normal' treatment of patients in a hospital under German occupation during the Second World War. There are a number of medical terms that are used that would not be considered appropriate in today's parlance, such as 'idiocy'. These terms are used in order to convey the meaning of the original documents, because it would not be appropriate to guess at what precise modern diagnosis a given instance of such a term might entail. Other terms such as 'uneducable' and 'unclean' are used to show the stigmatizing language that is recorded in the original document, which reflects how medical professionals viewed their patients, but the use of these terms in this book is not intended to replicate this stigma.

Concerning the naming of patients, this work is informed by the Historical Commission for the Reichsuniversität Straßburg, along with other ethics documents that debate the use of patient names. While this is a complicated issue, at the most basic level, the regulation of the use of patient names is based on the country in which their records are currently kept. Therefore, this work follows French, and sometimes German, regulations on this topic. In this case, as the patients were not victims of unethical experimentation, nor were they victims of the Holocaust, for which the IHRA recommends naming victims, their names are not released in full. Furthermore, as some of them may be still alive, or their family members may be alive, identifying information has been altered slightly to preserve privacy. That being said, if you recognize the description of a person, or have any memories of treatment at the hospital, please do get in contact. For a more detailed discussion on the choice to identify victims in this circumstance, please consult Paul Weindling, 'Données personnelles et protection: nommer les victimes', in *Commission historique pour l'histoire de la faculté de médecine de la Reichsuniversität Straßburg*.

This book is in some ways a microhistory, in that it works with records that have not been previously analysed from one single institution. They form the core of this volume, but I am aware that the Reichsuniversität Straßburg is not a representative sample of how paediatrics worked everywhere in Germany during the Second World War. Nor should this work be read in a vacuum without understanding the broader context, that for reasons of brevity cannot be elaborated upon within the limits of this book. As a result, other themes such as so-called euthanasia, forced sterilization, concentration camps and forced labour camps, occupation politics, and the university system in general are not detailed here. Further information on these issues is included in footnotes that suggest further reading where one might find more in-depth research that can enhance the contextual understanding of this work.

Author's Note

The spellings Strasbourg and Straßburg both appear in this book, but they are not used interchangeably. The reasoning behind this is helpful for the reader in conducting further archival research, but also in understanding the author's decision to help distinguish two different eras more clearly in the text.

Strasbourg is the French name of the city, and so this spelling is the one currently familiar. This spelling is also used to refer to the city prior to German occupation, as well as referring to the place in the present day. Straßburg (sometimes transliterated as Strassburg), on the other hand, is the old German name for the city, and is not used in the present day. It is employed in this text to indicate the city during German occupation.

While the distinction might initially seem unnecessary, this is particularly important in relation to the university—as the Université de Strasbourg and the Reichsuniversität Straßburg are entirely different institutions in very different eras.

One exception to this choice applies in relation to archival documents. Many primary sources that have been consulted for this work are located in French archives, but were originally made during German occupation, using the German form Straßburg. In compiling French finding aids, titles and terms from the document are translated into French to make it searchable. Therefore, where a source is referred to by its French title in a finding aid, the French title is used exactly as it is presented in the archive in order to ensure the reader can find the material.

Glossary of Terms

Abstammungsnachweis: Ancestry certificate, like a family tree detailing the racial characteristics and health of a person's relatives.

Alter Kämpfer: 'Old fighter', meaning that they were one of the earliest members of the Nazi party, joining before it became beneficial for securing employment, indicating an ideological belief in Nazism.

Ariernachweis: Certification of a person's Aryan heritage, usually required for employment under the National Socialist regime.

Blut und Boden: 'Blood and soil', a Nazi slogan uniting the idea of a racially uniform national group with the settlement of land.

Deutsche Forschungsgemeinschaft: German Research Organization.

Deaccession: This refers to the formal and routine removal of material from a collection, in this instance, an archive. This is done particularly in the case of medical records, where the standard is to retain the records for a number of years in case of readmission, then to deaccession them to make space for new records.

Dozent: German term for lecturer, but it can sometimes vary based on context.

Fremdvölkischer: 'Foreign peoples' but could also refer to those of non-Aryan race as well as those of foreign nationality.

Gauleiter: The governor of a province (known as a Gau, as in Gau Baden Elsass), under Nazi rule.

Habilitation: An extra qualification in Germany which is required to lecture in a university, become a head of department, or become a professor. It requires a postdoctoral thesis of original research in the individual's subject area.

Heil- und Pflegeanstalt: 'Hospital and care home', a medical clinic for convalescence and curative treatment.

Hilfsschulen: Schools for special education of children who could not participate in mainstream education.

Hilfsschüler: Pupils who required extra help in schooling, usually provided in a separate institution. An industrial school is an example.

Kaiserreich: The 1871–1918 German Empire under Bismarck as Chancellor and Emperor Wilhelm II.

Kinderfachabteilung: 'Special children's department'; these were constructed to care for children certified as physically or mentally disabled and later were used in the T4 campaign.

Kinderlandverschickungslager: Camp for children away from cities and in the countryside to avoid bombing raids and provide respite during the war. Some of these camps were organized by the Hitler Youth, but many functioned independently.

Kinderreich: 'Child rich'; this was not originally a National Socialist term. It referred to families with a large number of children. During the Nazi era, it became used for families of Aryan blood who had many children, as they were seen as being in service to the Third Reich through increasing the population.

Kreisleiter: A Nazi electoral district officer, a political rank one level below Gauleiter.

Länder: Approximately means German county or local administrative district.

Lebensborn-Heime: Homes established under the plan of Heinrich Himmler to care for 'racially pure' mothers and their children, organized by the SS.

Lebenslauf: Curriculum Vitae that also contains the person's family history, their parents' professions, and their nationality.

Lebensunwertes Leben: 'Lives unworthy of living', a phrase used to justify the killing of the mentally and physically disabled in the context of the T4 campaign.

Minderwertig: 'Inferior'; used in relation to individuals who did not fulfil racial characteristics, also used in relation to those who were disabled and subsequently sent to Kinderfachabteilungen.

Mutterberatungsstunde: 'Mothers' consultation hours'; usually these took place in a poliklinik of a hospital, but sometimes also in community centres. These were managed by nurses with the intention of monitoring the health of children and infants, providing vaccinations and advice to mothers, but also encouraging 'racial hygiene' in the population.

Mutterschulung: 'Mother schooling', again provided by nurses; they taught mothercraft, how to feed infants, and how to take care of children.

Patientenklasse: 'Patient class'; does not correspond exactly with social class, but indicates to what degree the patient's care is provided by medical insurance.

Poliklinik: A clinic that sees patients on an outpatient basis for a variety of illnesses. Often separate from a hospital, but in the case of the Reichsuniversität Straßburg, this poliklinik operated within the hospital as a referral for outpatient care.

Reichsdeutscher: This term was used to mean those who were 'native Germans', but this did not necessarily just extend to those who had German parents. This was integral to the expansion of the German Volk through classifying people in the occupied territories as German based on racial, medical, and social categories, and this was considered a privileged position. Those with French parents born in Alsace could be re-designated as Reichsdeutscher based on these determinants, thus incorporating them to the Volk.

Reichsgesundheitsführung: 'Reich health management'.

Reichsminister für Wissenschaft Erziehung und Volksbildung: Minister for Scientific Training and People's Education.

Reichsmütterdienst: The Reich Mothers' Service; this group organized training courses for mothers.

Sippe: A National Socialist eugenic-based term, roughly meaning ethnic group or 'race'.

Sippentafel: A medical examination indicating physical measurements of the body as well as typology, including information on the patient's family tree, in order to determine their 'Sippe'.

Staatliche Medizinal-Untersuchungsanstalt: State medical examination department. Testing for blood samples, and so on, was often outsourced to this organization by the Reichsuniversität Straßburg.

Staatsangehörigkeit: Nationality. Refers to regional belonging also, such as Saar or Alsace. In the context of Nazi ideology, nationality was determined by blood (*ius sanguinis*), so nationality was often based on ethnic groups.

Sturmabteilung: Paramilitary wing of the Nazi party.

Umsiedlungslager: A camp in which those who were forcibly relocated could be indoctrinated to German customs and National Socialist ideology before integration into the German Reich.

Verfolgungsideen: Persecution complex, used in a diminutive way to dismiss political awareness of Nazi persecution.

Volk: 'People', meaning the German people (including all German-speaking peoples), associated with an ethnic group.

Volksgemeinschaft: 'People's community', meaning the community of German people who were considered native Germans.

Volkskörper: 'The people's body', meant in an ideological sense as in the body politic, but often used to justify physical belonging in a medicalized sense.

Vorlesungsverzeichnis: A course catalogue of all available modules, as well as all relevant examination authorities, lecturers, information on administration and student organizations, compiled at the start of each term and distributed to students.

Westforschung: Western European research. The Reichsuniversität Straßburg was established to be a centre for this kind of research in the Third Reich, focusing on German history, literature, culture, and science as primary in Western Europe.

Archive Abbreviations

ADBR	Archives Départementale du Bas-Rhin, Strasbourg
ADHVS Path.	Archives du Département d'Histoire de la Vie et de la Santé, l'Ancien Bâtiment d'Anatomie, Hôpital Civil, Université de Strasbourg. Pathology collection
ADHVS Psych.	Archives du Département d'Histoire de la Vie et de la Santé, l'Ancien Bâtiment d'Anatomie, Hôpital Civil, Université de Strasbourg. Psychiatric Collection
ADHVS Spec.	Archives du Département d'Histoire de la Vie et de la Santé, Reichsuniversität Straßburg Specimen Collection Archives de l'Ancien Bâtiment d'Anatomie, Hôpital Civile, Université de Strasbourg
AEPSANS	Archives de l'Etablissement Public de Santé Alsace Nord, Stephansfeld (now relocated to Archives Départementales du Bas-Rhin)
AFMS	Archives de la Faculté du Médecine, Université de Strasbourg, Strasbourg. Thesis Archive
AHUS	Archives du Département d'Histoire de la Vie et de la Santé, l'Ancien Bâtiment d'Anatomie, Hôpital Civile, Université de Strasbourg. Paediatric Collection; Amies des Hôpitaux Universitaires Association
AN	Archives Nationales de France, Pierrefitte-sur-Seine

AN-CAD	Archives du Ministère des Affaires Etrangères, Archives Dekanat
AVES	Archives de la Ville et de l'Eurométropole, Strasbourg
BArch	Bundesarchiv Berlin
BIAB	Bridgeman Images Archive, Berlin
BNU	Bibliothèque Nationale et Universitaire de Strasbourg
ITS	International Tracing Service Digital Archive, Bad Arolsen
LA-BW GLA	Landesarchiv Baden-Württemberg, Abt. Generallandesarchiv Karlsruhe
LA-BW HStA	Landesarchiv Baden-Württemberg, Abt. Hauptstaatsarchiv Stuttgart
LA-BW StAS	Landesarchiv Baden-Württemberg, Abt. Staatsarchiv Siegmaringen
UAH	Humboldt Universität Archiv, Kaiserin Auguste Victoria Haus Bestand, Berlin
UAW	Archiv der Universität Wien

Terminology Abbreviations

BKK: Betriebskrankenkasse, company health insurance.
DP: Displaced Persons, the term used for refugees and displaced people in the postwar era.
KdF: Kanzlei des Führers, Hitler's Chancellery.
NSDB: Nazi university lecturers' union.
NSDAP: Nationalsozialistische Deutsche Arbeiterpartei, Nazi party.
NSKK: Nationalsozialistisches Kraftfahrkorps, National Socialist Motor Corps. A paramilitary organization of the Nazi party established in 1931.
NSDStB: Nationalsozialistischer Deutscher Studentenbund, or National Socialist German Students Union, which was an organization of university students integrated into the Nazi party.
HJ: Hitler Youth (boys' youth group).
NSLB: National Socialist Teachers Union.
NSV: Nationalsozialistische Volkswohlfahrt, National Socialist People's Welfare organization.
OKK: Ortskrankenkasse, local health insurance.
SA: Sturmabteilung, a paramilitary division of the Nazi party, established in 1921.
SD: Sicherheitsdienst, security service and intelligence agency of the Nazi party, established in 1931.
SS: Schutzstaffel, a paramilitary division of the Nazi party, established in 1925, with Heinrich Himmler as leader, generally tasked with enforcing 'racial purity'.
UNRRA: United Nations Relief and Rehabilitation Administration, which organized camps and administration for displaced persons in the aftermath of the Second World War.
Waffen-SS: Military branch of the SS.

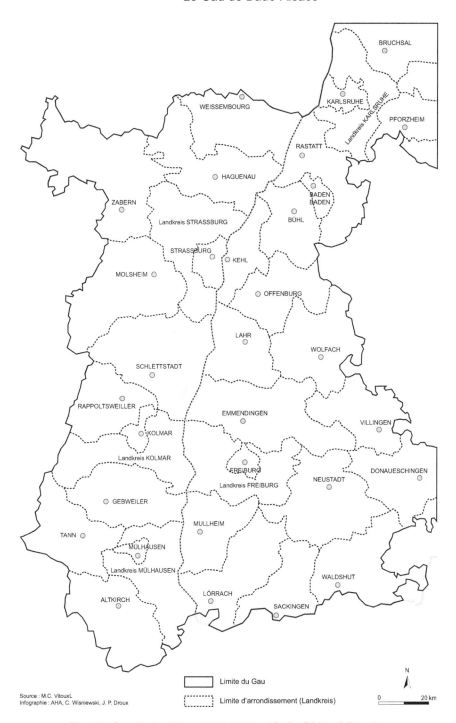

Fig. 1.1. Gau Baden Elsass 1940–1945, with the Rhine delineating the current border of France and Germany.[1]

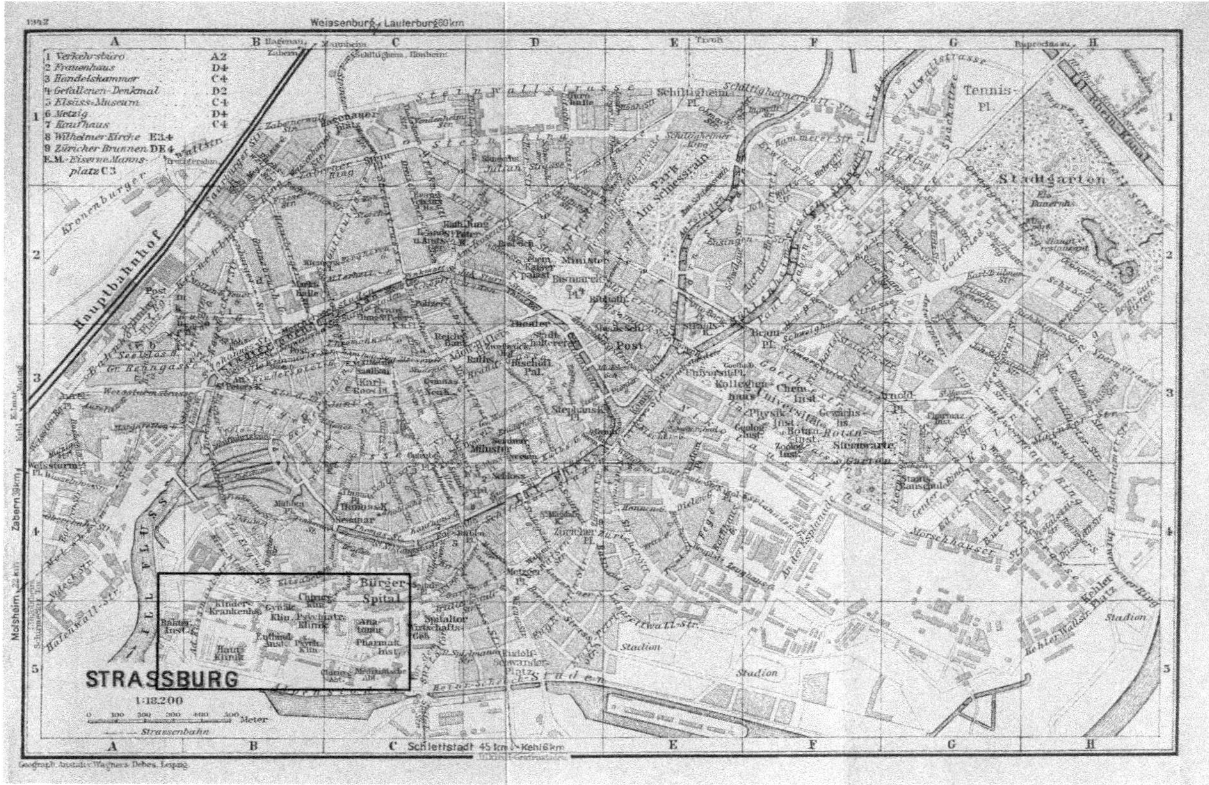

Fig. 1.2. Map of the City of Straßburg, 1942. Box indicating the hospital.[2]

CHAPTER 1

Introduction

> This history was marked in 1941 by the creation of the Reichsuniversität Straßburg, and in particular its medical faculty. Those who ran it were involved in a system of health care and research based on a delusional ideology that flouted the most basic ethics. This painful period continues to cast a form of suspicion on the Strasbourg medical and academic community, which resounds like a guilt-inducing myth.[3]

> The focus ought to be not only on *cure* but also on *care*; not only on doctors' achievements but also on the whole range of patient experience.[4]

Paediatrics is a peculiar medical speciality in that it emerged not from working with a particular condition or organ, but with a demographic group of patients due to their susceptibility to illness at an important phase of life.[5] As a result, this medical speciality was contested until the first decade of the twentieth century, when foundling hospitals and polikliniks developed into specialist children's clinics.[6] Healthy children were seen as a national resource and the speciality of paediatrics placed importance on protecting future citizens by ensuring their health from an early age.[7] While there was a considerable focus on the ideological importance of childhood and paediatric care in the Nazi era, less attention was drawn to the actual experience of routine childhood illness during this time.[8]

This book explores the experience of childhood ill health in Nazi-occupied Strasbourg, in the ideologically significant location that was the Reichsuniversität Straßburg. It will examine the founding principles of the clinic and the hospital as a whole, the staff that worked there, the medical students who conducted their research on the patients, and most importantly, the patients themselves and how they experienced illness during wartime. The book presents a

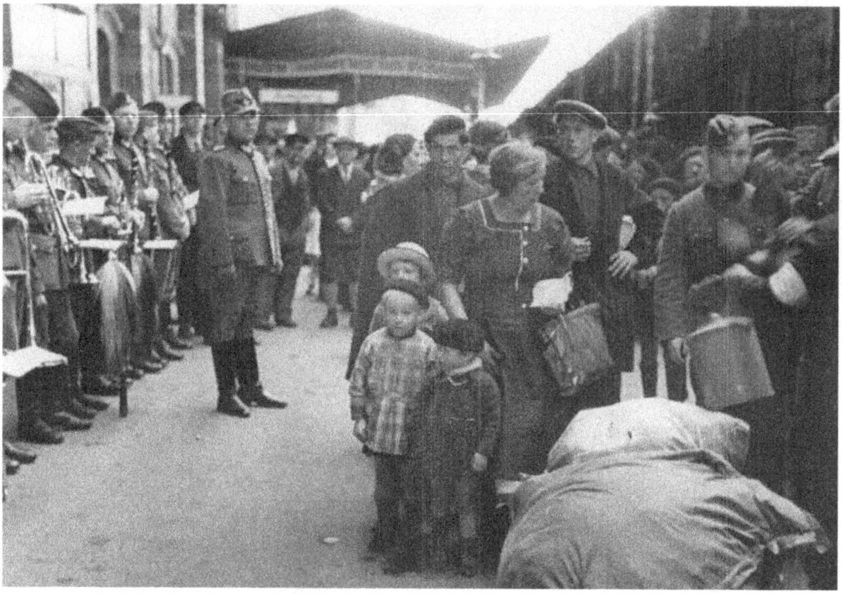

Fig. 1.3. Children at the train station in Straßburg in 1940, waiting to be resettled. The banner under the roof behind them reads 'Alsatians, speak your mother tongue!' in German while a welcome band in military uniform stands to the left.[9]

microhistory of a hospital in the occupied city of Strasbourg from the years 1941 to 1944, and focuses only on one small demographic group: children. While German forces took Alsace in mid-June 1940 and soon began resettling it, this book shall concern itself primarily with the years following the formal inauguration of the Reichsuniversität Straßburg from November 1941.

Despite this concerted focus on a particular time and place, the findings will be of broader importance. Medical treatment in this children's clinic was not all that different from treatment in England, France, or America at the time. While the system was similar, the Reichsuniversität Straßburg hospital was situated in a political and ideological atmosphere where some lives were considered worthless and expendable, while others were of utmost importance. Children got sick, were hospitalized, and recovered. Their parents came to visit, they drew pictures, and wished to go home while they were being treated in the Reichsuniversität Straßburg. This 'normal' treatment coexisted with mistreatment; daily-update letters were written to some parents, while other parents were not considered trustworthy enough—on social and racial grounds—to get news about their children. This 'normal' treatment was influenced by and based in National Socialist ideas of 'worth' and was impacted by the ongoing conflict, both in terms of civilian casualties and supply-chain problems. That these two disparate experiences happened side by side in the same institution provides a lens through which the extent of medical harm in other contexts can be fully understood. This highlights that criminal and inhumane medical experimentation existed in parallel with everyday, and seemingly banal, medical treatment. It also shows how such regimes operate within pre-existing structures that come to form an integral part of the functioning of that regime; this is the case with the treatment of children in this showcase National Socialist university, where this ordinary structure of the hospital became an essential part of the Germanization of the population through determining a person's 'worth' to the regime from childhood. This book argues that ideological signals towards the devaluation and dehumanization of certain members of the population can be traced back to the basic medical care provided in hospitals, particularly in the Reichsuniversität Straßburg—a hospital founded with the intention to promote and foster National Socialist ideology.

The book will not focus on the political turning points of the Second World War, nor will it detail the broader legislative changes in Germany or the regional upheaval in Alsace as a result of National Socialism. Despite this, the Nazi political system, in particular its central idea that people are not equal, is at the core of the discussion and should remain in the reader's mind to help contextualize the following chapters. Due to time constraints and page limitations, I do not provide a broader comparative with other hospitals, or indeed a statistical analysis of all paediatric clinic documents. Furthermore, the intention is to follow a qualitative rather than quantitative approach, focusing on the individual people rather than the numbers. However, do note that there has been extensive statistical analysis and tables completed, so if the reader wishes to consult a more statistical approach, there is a full detailed appendix of paediatric files to compare in Aisling Shalvey, 'History of Paediatric Treatment in the Reichsuniversität Straßburg 1941–1944', PhD thesis, Université de Strasbourg (2021).[10]

The research in this book is informed and presented considering three main historiographic trends: *Alltagsgeschichte*, social history, and a patient-centric reading of medical files. *Alltagsgeschichte*, or the study of everyday history, tends to focus on individuals and social movements, but does not usually look at everyday medical experience.[11] My research incorporates a social history of the population under occupation, focusing not on battles or political treaties, but on how they impacted daily life. The study of a patient group often focuses on Nazi experimentation and research, but this book will also look at the ordinary patient experience, thus bridging this gap between victim narrative, medical history from below, and everyday history.

Methodology

As noted above, this book takes a qualitative rather than quantitative approach—so any statistics mentioned are there to give context, rather than intended as a detailed quantitative overview. This book is based on 2,022 patient files, of which 869 are from the children's clinic, 127 are from the psychiatric clinic, and 1,026 are from the internal medicine clinic—far too many to accurately and concisely detail in a book. Therefore, certain files were chosen to illustrate broader themes and issues that have emerged throughout reading all of these files. These broader themes are nationality, wealth, social inclusion, diagnoses, and the impact of the war. It is important to note, though, that looking at outliers can often provide a better indication of how a place functioned, and hence many of these outliers are included. By this I mean that a number of children of forced labourers, or children who were from Eastern Europe, are included in this analysis, not because they are the norm or because there are many of these cases, but because they are the exception. Through examining these files, we can further contextualize the so-called normal daily treatment of patients in contrasting it with how patients from marginalized populations were treated.

A further note on choosing patient files from such a great number of records is that a considerable number of them look exactly like modern medical records: with very little description as to the individual situation, containing very little information, and mostly detailing routine tests and their results. When given a record with just two pages inside, one detailing a routine blood test and an X-ray, the other being admission and discharge documents, one can glean very little quantitative information. Therefore, the cases that were chosen contained the most information from which one can extrapolate the kind of treatment they received in the hospital. Cases were also chosen so as to represent the whole; hence, this book contains examples from Alsatian, French, German, Eastern European, Western European, male, and female, as well as a variety of socioeconomic backgrounds and ages. This was done intentionally to reflect the broader population found in these files. It must also be noted that as a result of the recent rediscovery of these documents, this analysis is but one aspect that has been uncovered. The patient records are by no means complete or comprehensive, with many gaps for certain months due to routine deaccession of medical documents through the years. Therefore, the conclusions made in this work based on such files may change with time as more documents are uncovered.

As this work details all documents currently known, albeit these documents have considerable gaps, this is, by its nature, to some degree making assumptions. As far as is currently known, no children were subject to forced sterilization, none were sent to Kinderfachabteilungen (nor was the clinic in Straßburg a Kinderfachabteilung), and none were victims of so-called euthanasia. These topics will be broached purely to provide a point of reference to how other clinics operated at the time, and it must be reiterated that this did not happen to children in the Reichsuniversität Straßburg. This fact alone is one of the reasons why this book was written; when forced sterilizations, unethical experiments, and so-called euthanasia occurred across Germany and German-occupied zones, why did this not happen to children in Straßburg? This hospital, and the patient records from it, illustrate how 'normal' treatment coexisted with sterilization, 'euthanasia', and experiments under the same National Socialist system. It provides evidence that not all hospitals and clinics went so far as to kill their patients. It also further contextualizes, through using these files, that there was a choice to be made under this totalitarian regime, and that such unethical treatment and cruelty exists not as diametrically opposite to normal treatment, but on a spectrum. Through these files, we can see that although these children were not killed if they had disabilities, as was the case in other hospitals, they were still described in insulting and demeaning terms, indicating that the medical professionals in the Reichsuniversität Straßburg did adhere to and believe in the central idea that certain children are 'worth more' than others. This treatment cannot then be seen as the opposite of so-called euthanasia, but as part of a continuum, involving the systematic dehumanization of those with disabilities and illnesses, and the eugenicist artificial construction of 'perfection' via indoctrination and exclusion of children within an occupied population.

Note on Sources

A distinct historiographic shift has occurred over time in relation to the study of medical history. C.R. King states: 'Modern writing of medical history began as the history of "great men," then became historicism, and recently has emphasised social and intellectual interpretations of history.'[12] While an older form of medical history focused solely on the individuals who practised medicine, a more current method looks at society, the patient, and their treatment, as well as doctors. This book aims to follow such sociopolitical interpretations of patient treatment, but also of the sources themselves.

The majority of the sources discussed in this book were 'rediscovered' in 2019; this study presents the first in-depth account of previously unknown patient files from paediatric cases in the Reichsuniversität Straßburg. These patient records had been rescued from routine destruction by Professor Storck, Dr Jean-Marc Lévy, and Gérard Schossig in 2008 but had not been analysed subsequent to their rescue. As the former children's clinic was demolished for the construction of the Nouvel Hôpital Civil, a clear-out of old medical files, administrative documents, and other materials occurred as the building was razed in 2008. These retrieved documents had been all but forgotten, and following the request of the Historical Commission for the Reichsuniversität Straßburg, access was granted to these documents.

On 14 May 2019, Christian Bonah, Lea Münch, and Aisling Shalvey went to the pharmacy building to consult with the Amies des Hôpitaux Universitaires on the retrieval of documents and their subsequent study. A full inventory of what records existed at the cold storage basement, and where they were found, was completed. All the records were categorized and analysed, leading to the following case studies and statistical analyses. These records dated from 1941 to 1944, with some extant records from 1945. The records that were recovered are not consecutive, and contain a number of gaps with incomplete months and years. Of the 900 children's clinic patient files recovered, only 869 are legible due to poor conservation over the years. The bed capacity of the children's clinic was over 400 patients at once, so from this we know that the majority of paediatric patient files were destroyed. Despite this, we can garner a broad understanding of the processes of the clinic, of the hospital, and of individual treatment from these 869 records that up to now was only based on assumptions rather than patient files and their individual experiences.

One hundred and twenty-seven paediatric psychiatry records were recovered, but they reflect a more systematic retrieval, as these were formally donated to the DHVS archives as a complete collection. The 5,704 patient files from the internal medicine clinic were also retrieved from routine destruction in the absence of a hospital archive, and were also found in the former cold storage room in the pharmacy building. Although this is a large number of files, it is estimated that this is only half the original number of patient records based on bed capacity. Of these 5,704 records, only approximately 15% relate to patients under eighteen years of age. Therefore, while this book will detail the current state of these sources, it must be remembered

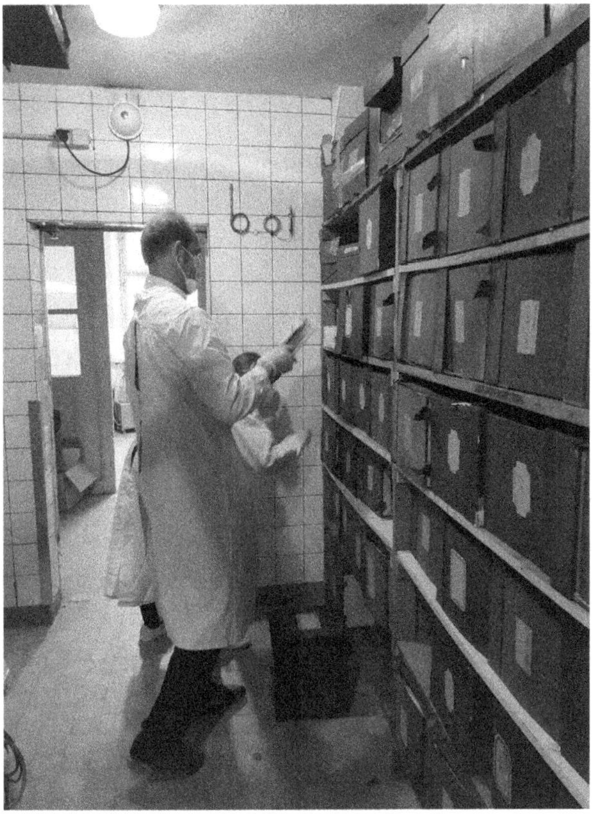

Fig. 1.4. Image of discovering patient files in the cold storage room of the pharmacy building, 2018.

that they are not complete records, and it is entirely possible that further material might emerge with time.

The patient files themselves, for all clinics, follow a similar pattern, and the admission documentation is recorded as follows. The patient's name is noted, along with important determinants of healthcare, such as class, nationality, place and date of birth, diagnosis, as well as referral information. There is a section to record the expected diagnosis on admission, but this may change throughout treatment. Insurance providers, the type of insurance cover, as well as the parents or next of kin information and the family doctor are recorded on the admission register. These key factors will form the core analysis of this book. Within the patient file, one gets a clear indication of the ideology of the era, as 'Sippentafeln', or a chart of hereditary and family disease, is included, along with information on social cohesion such as marriage loans and involvement with the Hitler Youth or other youth groups.

A history of the patient's illness is often presented, along with vaccination information and previous diseases, as well as medication that they are treated with while in hospital. In these records, we frequently have information on the family—from fathers working for the Wehrmacht to mothers who were forced labourers—sometimes letters from parents, and occasional drawings by the patients themselves. We also see intelligence tests, with demeaning and degrading language referring to physical and mental abilities, while other patients are referred to by their pet names as if they were family members. This clear divergence between treatment of those who fit into ideas of the 'Volk' and those who did not will be a central point of this book.

It must also be remembered that while these records often provide some glimpses into the patient's experience through quotes, drawings, or letters, the documents were intended to categorize the patients, and were used by the Nazi occupiers to control the population. While an open call was made for former patients to come forward to share their experiences, good or bad, very few people were willing to speak about their time at the Reichsuniversität Straßburg. This could be for several reasons; first, the experience of going to get a check-up or getting routine vaccinations is not particularly memorable for most people, both during the Second World War and now. Second, many former child patients may not even remember that they were in the Reichsuniversität Straßburg hospital, as a considerable number were under the age of four or five when they were admitted, and those who were old enough to remember may no longer be alive. Therefore, it is primarily family members of those who had a negative experience who came forward with information. Despite this lack of input from the patient perspective, these patient records can be read against the grain, while acknowledging archival silences, to ascertain a better view of how paediatric treatment worked, not only in a hospital occupied during wartime, but in a hospital that aimed to embody National Socialist ideals in both research and day-to-day clinical practice.

Evacuation of Strasbourg, Resettlement of Straßburg, and Germanization of Alsace

On 24 August 1939, the French military issued an evacuation order to the population of Alsace and Moselle, intending the population to be behind the Maginot line, the French defensive perimeter with Germany, by September.[13] Approximately 600,000 people from Alsace were evacuated, carrying their possessions on foot, by bike, and sometimes by car. There were also special trains that took people from the cities and into the French countryside with their belongings.[14] As Ute and Wolfgang Benz noted, this evacuation from their homes left lasting psychological repercussions on many children that impacted their development.[15] While the process of evacuation was difficult for all individuals, for children with a limited understanding of underlying political issues, this was particularly problematic.[16] By 3 September 1939, Strasbourg had been completely deserted for a number of weeks.[17] Olivier Forcade states that the reason for the evacuation was largely due to France being underprepared for invasion, leaving no other viable option but to evacuate the population.[18] By 2 August 1940, the region was occupied by Germany and Robert Wagner was appointed as Gauleiter for Alsace.[19] The Elsässisches Hilfsdienst was established to repatriate Alsatians back to their homes, and resulted in the resettlement of 8,000 people in German-occupied Alsace.[20] The first train of repatriated refugees arrived at the central station in Strasbourg on 6 August 1940 with 780 people. As Figures 1.3 and 1.5 demonstrate, by 2 September 1940, 73,818 people were resettled in Straßburg, with a grand welcome of music and swastika flags for their arrival.[21] As Nichols states, this pomp and ceremony was constructed so as to present a welcoming atmosphere initially; however, the practicalities of how long this welcome lasted varied based on individual territories.[22] The resettled populations were often viewed in a liminal way by the German administration, neither 'us' nor 'them', despite Heinrich Himmler's insistence that they should be treated as the German people would be treated.[23] It is important to note that the individual reception and perception of this process of Germanization was often based on dynamics of social class and financial circumstances, as the experience of those who resettled varied widely.[24]

Prior to the war in 1936, a census of Strasbourg shows that the population of the city was 193,119 inhabitants, establishing a baseline population prior to the conflict. The city was completely evacuated in 1939 due to the approaching war front, and resettled under German occupation. By 1941, the population of Strasbourg was 138,793. While this shows a decrease in population, it is notable how many people returned, but also how many new German settlers came to the city. Despite its complete evacuation, the population regenerated and settled in a remarkably short amount of time, illustrating the ideological importance of occupying the city.[25] Robert Wagner, the Gauleiter of Strasbourg, began the process of Germanizing the population of Alsace following their return.[26]

Grandhomme notes that the reasons for the population returning are numerous. For example, it appealed to the evacuees' sense of 'heimweh', or a sense of belonging to an area and homesickness, to return to Strasbourg.[27]

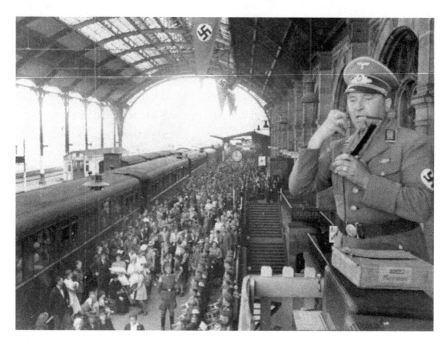

Fig. 1.5. Kreisleiter Hermann Bickler speaking at the central train station in Straßburg, 1940, on the arrival of people to the city.[28]

Strasbourg had been German in an era known as the Kaiserreich, which lasted from 1871 to 1918, when it was returned to France after the First World War. Therefore, particularly for many of the older inhabitants who were German speakers, this mindset of being German prevailed.[29] From personal testimonies, others stated that their parents had fond memories of the Kaiserreich and so saw no problem with returning to their home, without realizing how different life under National Socialism would be.[30] Others felt more strongly German and considered themselves to be part of the regime and so returned out of loyalty. It must be noted, however, that this self-identification was only part of the equation, as Bradley J. Nichols explains. Former German territories, such as Alsace, were subject to Germanization based on the idea of 'recovering' lost German territories, alluding to, as Nichols states, 'an alleged Germanic ancestry [...] [Germanization] epitomized the Nazis' obsession with biological rejuvenation'.[31] The aim was not only to administratively determine the population as German, but to immerse them in German language and culture, and educate them on Nazi racial laws in a process known as 'ethnic reclamation'.[32] This biological rejuvenation then naturally focused on indoctrination and changing the national identity of young children to create a revitalized and loyal German population.

The inhabitants who did return were subject to numerous laws, including a ban on berets, and any publication of French material.[33] This was intended to eliminate any trace of Alsatian or French culture and create a loyal ethnically and culturally German population. As Anne-Ségolène Verneret notes, cooperation with Germanization and resistance to it went together; both existed side by side. There were many degrees of conformity that Verneret details.[34] Broadly, these can be categorized into five types; the non-conformists, who occasionally spoke French in certain groups, but adhered to other rules externally; the refusers, who more openly rejected the regime, such as refusing to send their children to Hitler Youth organizations; the protesters, who openly practised their religion and their bilingualism; and the resisters, who actively participated in resistance organizations and sought to bring down the regime and the system.[35] Those who did not conform to these rules were subject to compulsory re-education camps, or Umschulungslagern, but certain degrees of more private resistance were sometimes tolerated. For example, the case of Henri Henripierre, who was subject to re-education for his supposed communist sympathies.[36] He went on to work as an assistant for August Hirt in the Anatomical Institute at the Reichsuniversität medical faculty. He was ordered to destroy all evidence of the skeleton collection that Hirt was creating with the bodies of Jewish victims from Auschwitz, but instead of destroying the evidence, he recorded the tattooed numbers on their arms, as he recognized that the corpses were not acquired following a natural death.[37] Henripierre's record keeping led to the possibility to identify the victims and classify this experiment as criminal research.[38]

The process of Germanization involved both physical change to the surroundings and a symbolic change. Physical symbols such as removing French flags and replacing them with the swastika occurred, along with the renaming of streets and towns to sound more German; for example, Place Broglie became Adolf Hitler Platz.[39] This process of renaming also occurred with people's names, with French-sounding names changed; René Mehl became Renatus Mehl to fit the process of Germanization.[40] The enforcement of military service and public works service for the population of Alsace functions as both symbolic integration to the German community, and physical battle for the German Reich. As Catherine Maurer notes, Alsace was a particularly important region in terms of concepts of nationhood, as it

> had to suffer from all the ensuing geopolitical effects, changing hands three times within a quarter of a century: in 1919, it came back to France after forty years during which it had belonged to

> Germany; in 1940, it was annexed by the National-Socialist Reich, before being handed back to France in 1944–5. The region thus lies at the meeting point between two powerful states and two distinct linguistic, cultural and legislative areas.[41]

Julien Fuchs noted that the young population in the region were most affected by these changes.[42] Analysing patient files by nationality is complicated by the translation of 'Staatsangehörigkeit', which technically means nationality, but in this case refers more to a regional belonging. The term can refer to categories of resistance, protest, or conforming to the occupying forces, and thus may not necessarily be a personal determinant of national belonging. Indeed, determining nationality could sometimes be a form of covert opposition to the regime, as in the Innere Medizin II Klinik of the Reichsuniversität Straßburg, where nationality was intentionally left blank for some time.[43] It also reflects administrative ideals of who could and could not be considered German, as well as who could be admitted to the Volksgemeinschaft.[44] The medical students training at the Reichsuniversität Straßburg also considered nationality to be an important differentiating factor in medical care, as Hellmuth Will compared the health of Alsatian and German patients,[45] and Edith Schneider compared fingerprints of Alsatian schoolchildren to determine their criminality and racial characteristics.[46] These two highly tendentious avenues of research indicate that it was considered important to biologically determine those who could be considered part of the Volksgemeinschaft. This regional belonging, as Machteld Venken notes, intersected with concepts of racial groups and hereditary difference.[47] So, while nationality is a complex term in this era, examining nationality in the demographic group of those treated in the Reichsuniversität Straßburg is particularly pertinent, in as far as the available sources allow. The Reichsuniversität Straßburg hospital cared for this large population in the city, and even attracted patients from farther afield.

Three-Era Structure of the Reichsuniversität Straßburg

Although the Reichsuniversität Straßburg only existed from 1941 to 1944, its operation can be divided into three distinct eras, which can help to further situate and explain the different focuses and aims as the occupation of Alsace progressed. The first era, from August 1940 to October 1941, can be characterized as focusing on the reopening of the civil hospital and the reintegration and Germanization of the local population. This period is referred to by Christian Bonah as a time of 'an illusion of Alsatian autonomy' in the face of the Nazi regime, during which the majority of doctors and patients were Alsatian.[48] In this era, the population at large as well as the staff of the hospital were subject to a plan of civil reorganization and professional re-education according to National Socialist principles. This included making former staff members swear an oath of allegiance, as well as the ousting of doctors who were not loyal to the regime, for example Dr Charles Apffel in the children's clinic.[49] He was the former chair of paediatrics in Strasbourg, but when Dr Kurt Hofmeier was appointed to the role in 1941, this forced him out. Hofmeier then offered Apffel a lower-ranking position in the children's clinic, which he refused, as he had previously been director. As a result, he refused to attend the inauguration, and entered private practice in Strasbourg, having been effectively pushed out of his job without warning.[50] The first era came to an end with the formal inauguration of the Reichsuniversität Straßburg on 23 November 1941.

The second era runs from November 1941 to June 1943, marking a time of increased investment in the ideal of the Reichsuniversität Straßburg clinics and institutes as a showcase university for National Socialist 'Westforschung'. In this era, the Reichsuniversität Straßburg hierarchy was exclusively German and subject to National Socialist administration. University clinics began to operate at full capacity, and were fully equipped, with the highest occupancy rates of the clinics in this era. Until June 1943, the Alsatian population that remained in Strasbourg engaged in these administrative and hierarchical processes, including joining the party to retain their jobs, but otherwise withdrawing into private activities or exile. Alsatians who remained had to adjust to an entirely German school system, military organization, and social system. Bonah notes that 'the euphoria and atmosphere of renewal that characterised the Reichsuniversität and its clinics' in this second phase gave way, however, to increasing demands and a radicalization of the situation, illustrating how this period of relative stability did not last.[51]

The third and final era, from August 1943 to November 1944, is characterized by increased repression, instability, and radicalization. It is in this era that we see medical files of forced labourers, or Ostarbeitern, appear, as their presence is both increasingly relied upon, but also increasingly marginalized. The special barracks for sick foreign workers in the hospital is constructed, allowing for the provision of medical care for forced labourers, but also for their continued exploitation. This period of radicalization is when August Hirt, Eugen Haagen, and Otto Bickenbach, the three staff members who were tried for war crimes, conduct their criminal medical experiments, some of which take place within the walls of the Reichsuniversität Straßburg. These experiments were facilitated by the radicalization of the military and political situation. This era also places further pressure on the hospital, as increased Allied aerial bombing raids impact medical studies, lead to more civilian casualties, and reveal the extent of material shortages within the clinics, thus leading to a reduced bed capacity but also fewer treatment options available for those that do come to the hospital.

Comparative Between Other Reichsuniversitäten and the Reichsuniversität Straßburg

As mentioned above, this research is primarily a microhistory, focusing on just one demographic group within an institution and how this functioned in wartime, particularly under strong ideological influence. Therefore, a more in-depth analysis and comparison between other universities in Germany is outside the scope of this study. However, it is important to note that the Reichsuniversität Straßburg was not the only university of its kind. It was one of three Reichsuniversitäten; the Reichsuniversität Posen was founded in Poznan in Poland in 1941, the Reichsuniversität Prag was founded in Prague in Czechoslovakia in 1939, and finally the Reichsuniversität Straßburg was founded in Strasbourg in France in 1941.[52] The universities in Prague and Poznan were intended to be centres for 'Ostforschung', or Eastern research, and were instrumental to the expansionist policies in Eastern Europe.[53] These universities were established to be bastions of German innovation and research in the annexed territories, with Strasbourg being the centre for 'Westforschung'.[54]

Tania Elias notes that the date 23 November 1941 was particularly symbolic for the inauguration ceremony of the Reichsuniversität Straßburg, as this was the anniversary of the date that the university had become French again in 1918.[55] Choosing this date was a symbolic retrieval of a former German university, known as the Kaiser Wilhelm Universität during the Kaiserreich from 1877 to 1918.[56] Furthermore, Elias details the ideological stance that was taken in the establishment of the Reichsuniversität Straßburg. She notes that Ernst Anrich intended for the Reichsuniversität Straßburg to 'dethrone the Sorbonne' as a centre for innovative research.[57] All three Reichsuniversitäten were intended to solidify Germanization efforts in these occupied regions.[58] Historical links to Germany were highlighted, appealing to the German expatriate population in these regions, and a strong emphasis was placed on German as the mother tongue (Muttersprache) and on eliminating the local language.[59]

Although Adolf Hitler was not at the inauguration, he sent Robert Wagner a telegram issuing his congratulations and best wishes for the new university,

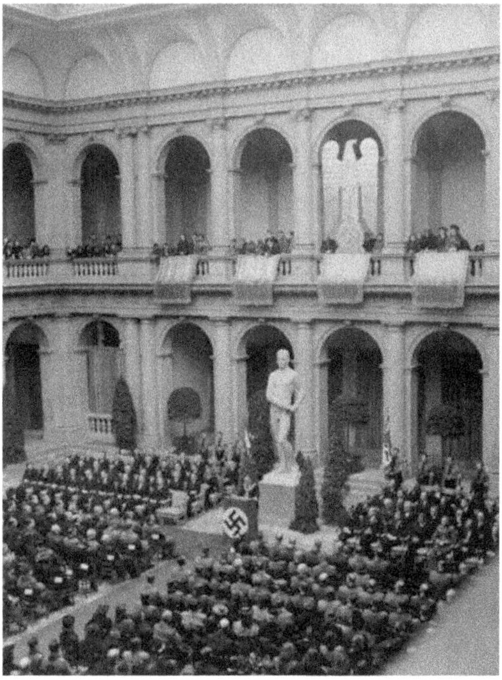

Fig. 1.6. Inauguration ceremony of the Reichsuniversität Straßburg in 1941 at Palais Universitaire.[60]

and donated 250,000 RM toward research at the Reichsuniversität Straßburg.[61] When Adolf Hitler visited Straßburg on 28 June 1940, he described it as an ancient German city and outlined the importance of Alsace as a region of Germany, ignoring both the local language and customs, as well as dismissing the deep-rooted influence of French culture in the region.[62] Prior to the inauguration, staff and professors had been chosen so the ceremony was full of students and staff in what Elias determined to be a pseudo-religious ceremony.[63] Just as the university itself was founded on National Socialist principles, the teaching of students in the medical faculty also followed this ideology. From the Vorlesungsverzeichnissen, a student orientation guide and course catalogue book, we can see the lectures that were offered to students.[64] They included the study of racial biology, wherein students were taught biological determinism and that certain races were inferior.[65] As this university was intended to showcase the forefront of research, this included medical research.

The medical students of the Reichsuniversität Straßburg were taught in multiple fields, and all the lectures on offer to them were outlined in the Vorlesungsverzeichnisse for each semester. Lectures available included anatomy, obstetrics and gynaecology, dentistry, ophthalmology, surgery, orthopaedics, and dermatology. Other courses on newer disciplines included hygiene, bacteriology and serology, racial biology, and neurology. Further courses were also detailed in the Vorlesungsverzeichnissen, as well as the professors in charge of each area.[66] Faculty members were hired in 1940 and 1941 and were subject to the same regulations as that of the general population in Alsace. They had to provide an Ariernachweis and an Abstammungsnachweis (administrative documents pertaining to racial heritage and adherence to the Nazi party), as well as certification from the Nazi party that they were politically reliable.[67] The medical faculties of the Reichsuniversitäten appear to have the most Nazi party members compared to other universities. Part of the reason for this increased percentage of Nazi party faculty members was the ongoing 'aryanization' of medical faculties, as evidenced in Prague.[68]

Comparison between the Kinderklinik in the Reichsuniversität Prag and the Reichsuniversität Straßburg is particularly important, as both were in annexed territories in which a university was newly established. These universities were slightly different to other university clinics in the German Reich as they were founded during the era of National Socialism in a contested geographical region. In the Kinderklinik at the Reichsuniversität Prag, the director of the children's clinic, Dr Carl Gottlieb Bennholdt-Thomsen, extensively studied the question of constitution in contributing to childhood diseases and also the issue of rickets and its prevention through nutritional means.[69] These concerns were shared by Dr Hofmeier in the Reichsuniversität Straßburg, so these areas of research in paediatrics were standard for this era. Dr Bennholdt-Thomsen joined the NS Dozetenbund in 1935, along with the Nazi medical association in 1936 and the NSDAP in 1937, which was considerably later than Hofmeier.[70] He also had a considerable interest in the Hitler Youth, working as their district doctor for Hessen-Nassau, as well as an advisory doctor for the Reich Youth Leadership in Bohemia and Moravia.[71] In 1940, he took over the provisional management of the children's clinic in Prague, and in 1942 was appointed associate professor in paediatrics, as the successor to Dr Hermann Mai. Unlike Hofmeier, Bennholdt-Thomsen retained university positions in the postwar era and did not return to private practice, indicating that his reputation was not compromised because of denazification.[72] He received membership of the Leopoldina (German National Academy of Sciences) in 1952 for his contribution to paediatrics, which illustrates that his reputation remained intact following his involvement with the Reichsuniversität Prag.[73]

Bennholdt-Thomson's predecessor, Dr Hermann Mai, was a considerably more devout Nazi than Hofmeier or Bennholdt-Thomson. He joined the Sturmabteilung (SA) in 1933 and joined the SS, NSDB, NSDAP, NSV, and the National Socialist German Medical Association in 1937.[74] He became an SS Untersturmführer in April 1940. He was appointed as chair of the Reichsuniversität Prag in 1939 but was quite amenable to his Czech colleagues. He volunteered with the hereditary health court in Munich, in which he ordered the forced sterilization of at least twelve women and men.[75] In the postwar era, he was well received for quite some time, having a foundation named after him by the German Society for Child and Adolescent Medicine in 1983, which was renamed in 2017.[76] Mai received the Paracelsus Medal in 1978.[77] He also retained a university position after the war, going on to a full professorship in paediatrics in Münster in 1954.[78]

From the examples of these Reichsuniversitäten, we can extrapolate that membership and participation in one of these ideologically important universities was not enough to hinder a postwar career in paediatrics. One can also ascertain that the Alte Kämpfer, some of the first members of the Nazi party, ideally with military experience, were sought out for the position of clinic director in this climate, particularly given the importance of incorporating annexed territories.

Criminal Research at the Reichsuniversität Straßburg: An Overview of Hirt, Haagen, and Bickenbach

Prior research on the Reichsuniversität Straßburg has focused on the three better-known medical faculty members who were subsequently tried for war crimes due to their research; August Hirt, Eugen Haagen, and Otto Bickenbach.[79] While similar research did not occur at the children's clinic, it is important to examine their work, both as a basis for understanding previous historiography on the topic, but also to examine how the Reichsuniversität Straßburg provided institutional backing without which this research could not have been facilitated. This section details just a fraction of the current state of research on the Reichsuniversität Straßburg; for further information on this, please consult Aisling Shalvey, 'History of Paediatric Treatment in the Reichsuniversität Straßburg 1941–1944', PhD thesis, Université de Strasbourg (2021).

Dr August Hirt fought in the First World War, for which he was awarded the Iron Cross. He developed a fluorescence microscope while in Heidelberg with Dr Philipp Ellinger, whom he later discredited because he was Jewish.

This invention was revolutionary in microscopy. In 1932, Hirt was appointed Professor of Anatomy in Düsseldorf, and in the same year he joined the Kampfbund für deutsche Kultur (League for the Defence of German Culture), a nationalist and anti-Semitic movement, then he became a member of the SS on 1 April 1933, before joining the NSDAP on 1 May 1937.[80] He then worked at Greifswald as the chair of anatomy, and retained a private research collection there, which he brought with him when he came to Straßburg. Hirt was appointed as head of the anatomical institute in the Reichsuniversität Straßburg in 1941. The theses of students in the Reichsuniversität Straßburg studied this fluorescence microscopy technique with the intention of creating a map of fluorescence for the whole human body. While the anatomy institute shared a building with pathology, they were considerably different, as pathology was more integrated into the clinical operation of the hospital, being focused primarily on diagnostics, while anatomy was more centred on research. Hirt became involved with the Ahnenerbe, an organization of the SS which was focused on conducting research that would prove the cultural, historic, and racial supremacy of Germany. Wolfram Sievers was the head of this organization, and as anatomy (as well as archaeology and anthropology) was central to this, Hirt conducted his research on skeletons of Jewish concentration camp victims with the backing of this organization. He requested that Jewish prisoners in Auschwitz concentration camp be sent to Natzweiler-Struthof concentration camp, closer to Straßburg, to be killed there.[81] They would be examined and then their bodies would be macerated to create a skeleton collection that would compare Jewish bodies to Aryans. There were eighty-six victims of this experiment.[82] In 1952, Hirt was tried for war crimes, but he committed suicide in the Black Forest after the evacuation of the Reichsuniversität Straßburg and so never faced prosecution.

Concurrent to this analysis of Professor Hirt, similar analysis has been conducted on Professor Otto Bickenbach, who was the director of the institute of internal medicine at Reichsuniversität Straßburg. He initially began experimenting with phosgene gas at the University of Heidelberg in connection with the damage this gas had caused to the lungs of soldiers during the First World War.[83] In 1940, he began to test chemicals that would reduce the harm caused by phosgene gas, as up until that point the only treatments were bloodletting and administering oxygen. He began to investigate the effects of Urotropin on animals, which made them resistant to phosgene damage.[84] In 1942, Bickenbach began to collaborate with the Institut für Wehrwissenschaftliche Zweckforschung of the SS-Ahnenerbe, and he showed his results of animal experimentation to a conference in

Straßburg. As a result of this, he was allowed to conduct research at Natzweiler-Struthof concentration camp from 1943.[85] Bickenbach argued in a postwar testimony that he conducted the experiments to save civilians from expected gas warfare.[86] He was tried for human experimentation and poisoning with phosgene gas which killed four people; these experiments were conducted in the Natzweiler camp, where a gas chamber was built specifically for this purpose in August 1943.[87] He was also tried for war crimes in 1952 as a result of his research on concentration camp prisoners; he appealed in 1954 and was sentenced to twenty years' hard labour following trial in Lyon.[88]

Prior to his employment at the Reichsuniversität Straßburg, Eugen Haagen was a scientist of considerable renown, as he had worked at the Rockefeller Foundation for Medical Research on the yellow fever virus in 1932.[89] He was appointed as the professor of hygiene and the director of the Hygiene Institute of the Reichsuniversität Straßburg in 1941. While in Strasbourg, he researched influenza, typhus, penicillin, sulfonamides, epidemic hepatitis, and yellow fever (1941–1943).[90] He developed a live vaccine and experimented on inmates of the Natzweiler-Struthof concentration camp from 1943 to 1944.[91] Most notably, Haagen 'ordered' Roma victims from Auschwitz specifically for vaccine testing in Natzweiler.[92] In his notebook, which was provided as evidence by the French prosecution, Haagen's assistant noted his request for healthy inmates, thus proving these experiments were conducted on his own initiative and did not have therapeutic intent. Despite this, the Nuremberg Medical Trial did not ascertain the number of victims involved to these experiments, and left the question open for further prosecution at the French Military Tribunal in Metz from 1947 to 1954.[93] Haagen was employed at the Federal German Research Centre for Viral Animal Diseases from 1955 until he retired in 1965.[94] While individuals conducted criminal research at the university, it appears that such research coexisted with a 'normal' teaching hospital.[95]

Scope of this Book

The following chapters present the history of paediatric care in the Reichsuniversität Straßburg, encompassing the children's clinic, psychiatric clinic, internal medicine clinic, and their presentation in student research. The background of the clinic director, Dr Kurt Hofmeier, as well as the fellow staff members of the clinic, will be briefly outlined. The dissolution of the clinic, and the Reichsuniversität Straßburg as a whole, will be discussed. The aim of the research presented in the following chapters is to highlight the grey area; with the background of criminal research being conducted by Hirt, Haagen, and Bickenbach in the Reichsuniversität Straßburg, there was also fairly standard medical research being conducted. While people were being killed in Natzweiler-Struthof, not far from the hospital, others were undergoing seemingly innocuous medical examination in the clinic to ascertain their 'belonging' to the German Volk. While some patients, based on this medicalized judgement of belonging, were being given any and all treatments available, other patients were being killed due to a doctor's diagnosis. While some staff members took National Socialism as an opportunity to progress in their career and embraced its racist ideology, their co-workers were actively resisting the regime.[96] This research then highlights that while there is a dichotomy within medicine in this era, there is also an insidious middle ground, of passive collaboration, of grouping people based on their nationality, race, and class and attributing resources based on this judgement, of publishing and replicating exclusionary ideas, and of encouraging students to do the same. And of course, behind all of this, which this research seeks to highlight, are the individual families and individual patients this affected most.

Explaining all this research as 'pseudoscience' has the effect of distancing modern researchers from the legacy of Nazi research. By being able to dismiss it as not real science, one does not hold it to the same standard, expecting that all of their work was unethical. The reality was quite different. Informed consent was sought from parents, medical standards and protocols were followed, and patients were treated in a timely manner with appropriate medication. As Sabine Hildebrandt notes, science did not go 'mad' in this era, and to claim that it did is an easy way to avoid questioning their research practices and the extent of ethical violations. Scientists understood quite clearly the scientific norms and were able to provide appropriate treatment. That they then withheld this treatment, or intentionally harmed individuals, in accordance with their ideological stance, foregrounds how ideology can influence and distort medical care. This 'normal' treatment and research is evident in the Reichsuniversität Straßburg children's clinic, and provides a lens through which the extent of medical harm can be properly understood.

CHAPTER 2

Staff of the Children's Clinic of the Reichsuniversität Straßburg

> One thought of one doctor as head of the infant department and another as head of the children's clinic and polyclinic. With my vocation to Straßburg, the division of paediatrics into infant care and into children's health was no longer necessary [...] Anyone who has followed the development of paediatrics in the last decennia in Germany will regard it with me as a joyous achievement that such a division of paediatrics has been prevented in Straßburg.[1]

Paediatrics as a separate medical discipline became legitimized through the adoption of university professorships and specialized departments focused on health in childhood, in Germany, Europe, and the US in the late 1800s.[2] Paediatric practice was considerably impacted during the era of National Socialism as more than 400 Jewish paediatricians were dismissed from 1933 to 1939.[3] As the Reichsuniversität Straßburg was founded to be a bastion of Nazi ideology, the selection of staff based on their ideological stance had a considerable influence on individual departments, and on the treatment of patients.

Paediatric care was initially focused on reducing infant mortality, through provision of adequate nutrition, and improvements in environment and cleanliness, as well as vaccination. This eventually led to improvements in midwifery and encouraging higher breastfeeding rates to improve infant health.[4] The specialization in paediatrics from the 1870s is linked to the rise of public health and the concern with biologically based social hygiene.[5] The specialization of doctors, and the establishment of university professors for paediatrics such as Adalbert Czerny, as well as the concern with infant mortality rates, were instrumental in the firm establishment of paediatrics.[6] By 1883 in Germany, the professional association of child health had ninety-eight members, but by 1910 this had risen to 295 members, illustrating the rise in specialization of paediatric care. Philipp Osten, Wolfgang Eckart, and Georg Hoffmann note the significance that up to 1910 in Germany, the words 'poor' and 'sick' were synonymous, as infant mortality in poor industrial areas was over 30%.[7] Therefore, a large amount of paediatric healthcare in the late nineteenth and early twentieth centuries was dispensed by charitable organizations in order to address this disparity in infant mortality between rich and poor.[8]

Angelika Lautenschlager has remarked on the fact that the speciality of paediatrics grew with the establishment of more children's clinics, and with it grew the realization that 'children are not small adults to whom conventional therapies can be transferred. Children have their own disesases, they react differently to medication [...] and therefore need their own medicine.'[9] So, the new speciality of paediatrics focused not only on infant mortality rates or poor children but on illnesses that particularly impacted children, such as polio, diphtheria, and the prevention of disease through breastfeeding, nutrition research, improvements in environment, and vaccination.[10]

As Paul Weindling notes, motherhood was idealized in campaigns to raise the birth rate through the encouragement of large families, as Germany was said to be 'a nation without youth' due to the high casualties from the First World War.[11] At the beginning of the twentieth century, children came to be seen as a state resource that had to be carefully managed, thus legitimizing a focus on collective societal rights over individual parental rights.[12] The innocent child motif had considerable power in moving individuals to support ideological positions, such as Nazism.[13] Paediatrics was an integral part of National Socialism; Michael Buddrus notes the militaristic tones employed by the Reichsjugendführer in 1933 that 'the youth of today is the worker and soldier of tomorrow. Keeping German youth healthy must therefore be considered a priority.'[14]

Due to the links with eugenics, paediatrics soon became one of the medical disciplines with the most zealous adherents of Nazi ideology.[15] Eduard Seidler notes that paediatrics initially focused on providing for the future of a race or population through the preservation of their health, but also states that these ideas were present long before National Socialism.[16]

History of the Children's Clinic in Strasbourg

Strasbourg Bürgerspital children's clinic began as a single room for sick infants in 1738.[17] By 1839, the children's clinic had expanded to fill an entire building and boasted a capacity of forty-five beds.[18] When Professor William Welch

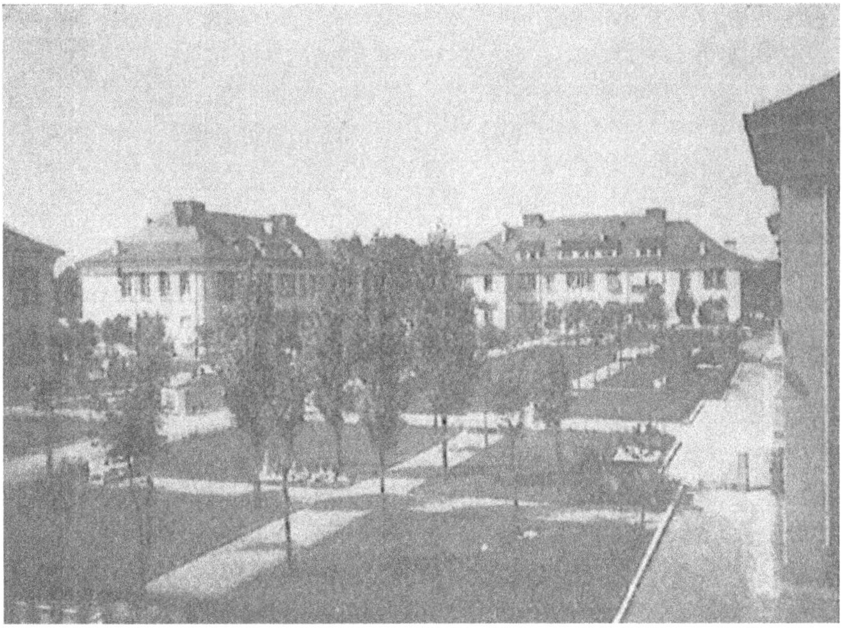

Fig. 2.1. Image of the Kinderklinik from Adalbert Czerny, 1911, illustrating the pavilion structure.[19]

of Johns Hopkins University Hospital came to visit in 1871, he stated that the Strasbourg hospital had some of the most advanced facilities he had ever seen.[20] Soon the clinic outgrew its original location, and so Paul Bonatz was hired as an architect to design a purpose-built new children's clinic in 1910, and the construction was completed two years later.[21] It was considered to be revolutionary, given that it comprised six separate buildings, each in a pavilion style, intended for the segregation of different illnesses.[22] These six buildings were almost identical and were situated around a rectangular garden.[23] Originally these pavilions contained patients with different diseases in separate sections to prevent the spread of contagious childhood illnesses like measles. The main building was for the neonatal unit, the polyclinic, and an amphitheatre for lectures to medical students.[24] The main building managed access to the rest of the buildings, making it easier to control the spread of disease. The inclusion of a central rectangular garden, paths, and terraces was considered essential as it allowed air to circulate and gave children access to sun and the outdoors to speed up recovery.[25]

In 1919, Professor Paul Rohmer became the director of the children's clinic under the new French administration.[26] Modern laboratories had been built in the main building, along with a classroom and a library.[27] Rohmer also established a centre for tuberculosis and a special pavilion for contagious diseases with twenty-seven beds, and an isolation house for premature infants.[28] A special department for dehydrating illnesses was established and each room was climate controlled through heating and large windows. The fifth building became a quarantine section, and the sixth was the private children's clinic.[29] The adoption of autopsies and histological testing in paediatric cases was again revolutionary and drastically improved diagnostics. The clinic was adapted to accommodate radiology and physiotherapy, improving the diagnostic and treatment options for children.

In total, the clinic could accommodate 441 children, which made it the largest single clinic in the hospital.[30] It is unclear if this number of admissions was ever reached, as the occupancy rate was less than 84%.[31] In 1939, the staff and patients of the Strasbourg children's clinic were evacuated to l'Hôpital Parrot in Périgueux.[32] When the city of Strasbourg was occupied by the German army in 1940, the former building of the French 'clinique infantile' became the German 'Kinderklinik'. Following the evacuation of the clinic, it appears that almost everything had to be bought to replace materials taken by the French administration to the clinic in Périgueux. In 1940, Dr Ernst wrote an extensive inventory of the clinics and what material was required; the children's clinic seems to have required the most equipment to return to functioning order, with a full-page list of laboratory equipment and basic materials.[33] Despite this, the clinic, and the hospital in general, were quite well stocked by 1941, indicating its key ideological position as a 'showcase university' for a new Germany.[34]

The new director of the children's clinic was Dr Kurt Hofmeier, who was born in Königsberg in 1896 and came from a Prussian military family.[35] He served as a lieutenant of the field artillery from 1914 to 1918 and was awarded the first- and second-class Iron Cross.[36] As a result of his early enlistment, and his birth in the 1890s, Hofmeier was part of the 'junge Frontgeneration'—a group who were actively involved in student politics before the war started, had an idealistic vision of Germany which led them to enlist early in the war, and served as a foundation for their response to the Second World War.[37] Consequently, this group were also the most disillusioned with the results of the Treaty of Versailles, and became more engaged with Nazi politics in the aftermath of the Weimar Republic. They also engaged in conservative student groups—Hofmeier joined the Corps Hasso-Nassovia Marburg, a right-wing student group, which influenced his political views.[38] These individuals, who had fought in the war from 1914, were those who would be selected as teaching staff for the Reichsuniversität Straßburg.[39]

In October 1922, Hofmeier finished his medical training and became a civilian as well as a military doctor. In 1931, he joined the NSDAP, and in 1932 he joined the National Socialist Motor Corps and became a member of the Nazi Doctors Organization.[40] As a result of this early involvement in the Nazi party, he is classified as an Alte Kämpfer, and a dedicated National Socialist. In August 1940, Ernst Anrich noted the criteria for selecting the clinic directors for the Reichsuniversität Straßburg included 'lively National Socialism [...] willingness to comradeship' with a preference for those who were Alte Kämpfer.[41] This preference for Alte Kämpfer was shown in the Reichsuniversität Prag.

While Hofmeier worked in other positions prior to Strasbourg, namely as director of the Kaiserin Auguste Viktoria Haus (a hospital complex in Berlin founded to reduce infant mortality), he was not the first choice for the role of director of the children's clinic.[42] It does appear that his Nazi connections, rather than the quality of his research, led to his appointment as director of the children's clinic in 1941.[43] One considerable example is the recommendation letter he received for his appointment to Strasbourg from Fritz Lenz, an influential eugenicist who endorsed the German occupation of Eastern Europe. Lenz believed this was justified due to the racial hierarchy, and served as an expert on the committee for population and racial policy. He noted that Hofmeier's monograph entitled 'The Importance of Heredity for Paediatrics' filled a noticeable gap in the research on the question of heredity in children and contributed to expertise in the field of immunity research and neuropathic diathesis as well as bacteriology in children.[44] In this work, he referenced Otmar von Verschuer, Eugen Fischer, Erwin Bauer, and Fritz Lenz, giving the latter a special thanks in the introduction.[45] All of these figures were well-known eugenicists who were instrumental in the development of a Nazi policy on racial hygiene and 'euthanasia', and as Hofmeier referenced them frequently, he saw value in their ideas. Hofmeier also stated that an in-depth knowledge of racial hygiene practices were essential for the paediatrician in order to be able to eliminate disease:

> The incidence of mortality [...] and premature births are to a considerable extent caused by environmental and hereditary factors. In the early death of these individuals, who are to be regarded as inferior due to their heredity, a selection process is to be welcomed from the perspective of race hygiene.

This quote illustrates that while he aimed to reduce infant mortality, this was through the lens of racial hygiene and a belief that certain individuals were inferior.[46]

Hofmeier's publications focused on assimilation to the German Volk, a theme which would be integral to the incorporation of Alsace. He spoke about the issue of adoption, and the confirmation of racial worth of children in the absence of their family tree. He stated that 'The children who experience birth trauma are generally those with inferior hereditary facilities. The normally developed child generally recovers from the physiological birthing process without any disturbances', which gives an indication of his views on the weakened health of premature children.[47]

Hofmeier went on to say that the participation of the paediatrician in the *Gesetz zur Verhütung Erbkranken Nachwuchses* (the Law for the Prevention of Hereditary Diseases, which subsequently led to the T4 'euthanasia' campaign) was essential for the health of the population.[48] He noted that the success of the law for the prevention of hereditary diseases was predicated on the cooperation of paediatricians in notifying the authorities for every case of developmental problems, insanity, and congenital problems:

> In order to successfully implement the law for the prevention of hereditary infantile offspring, a notification requirement has been introduced for every case of congenital feeble-mindedness. The exogenous causes of feeble-mindedness are listed as obstetric trauma, meningitis, encephalitis, and other inflammatory processes [...] The cooperation of paediatricians in the early detection of congenital mental retardation is urgently needed. In many cases it is not done in the necessary manner because the discussion of the possibility of its occurrence in a family may not be a pleasant part of the medical profession.[49]

Hofmeier completed his habilitation in Berlin in 1938 and helped to organize a conference which aimed to bring together the Hitler Youth and paediatricians to highlight the central importance of German children.[50] He highlighted the importance of children engaging with the Hitler Youth in his edited book, *Physical and Spiritual Education of Children and Young People* (1939).[51] This adherence to Nazi ideas of the Hitler Youth and the importance of hereditary health influenced his time at the Reichsuniversität Straßburg.

Staff in the Children's Clinic

Staff in the children's clinic in Strasbourg were expected to follow Nazi ideology, and former staff members mentioned how National Socialist rituals were incorporated in the daily functioning of the clinic. This is particularly evident in the attendance of paediatric staff from the Reichsuniversität Straßburg at the Alt Rehse Führerschule from 13 March to 5 April 1941.[52] Alt Rehse was a six-week camp for doctors, nurses, and midwives to study racial ideology, genetics, and eugenics with the intention of renewing their Nazi ideology, which they would then bring to their daily medical practice.[53] René Burgun's private photo album from this course at Alt Rehse includes René Mehl, the paediatrician. It is unknown how many other staff members from the paediatric clinic attended, but it is evident that the staff of the children's clinic were subject to indoctrination if they were not already loyal party members.

Marlène Link, a former doctor in the children's clinic, stated in an interview that Hofmeier wore his Wehrmacht uniform with high leather boots under his white doctor's coat daily, illustrating his strong nationalist and

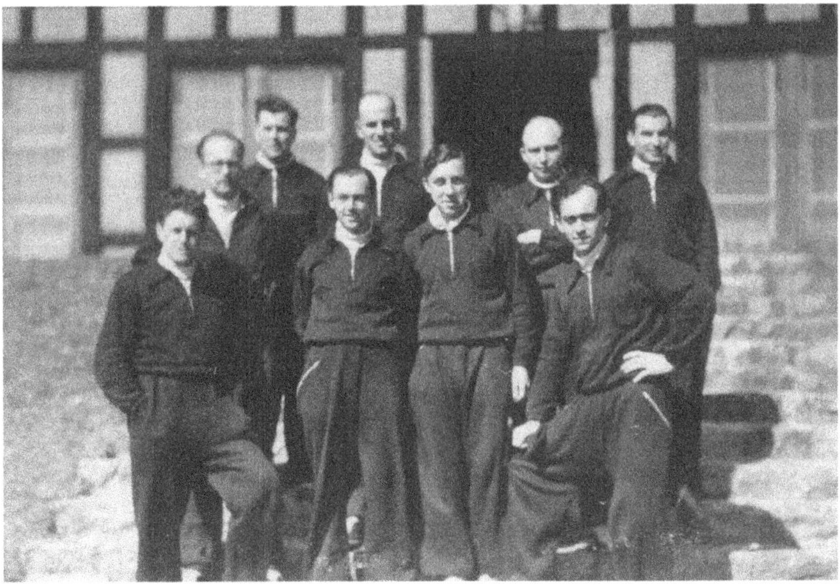

Fig. 2.2. Reichsuniversität Straßburg doctors at Alt Rehse, 1941. Front row (l–r): René Mehl (paediatrician), Erwin Wiest (surgeon), René Burgun (dermatologist), and Frédéric Froehlich (surgeon). Back row (l–r): Paul Steimlé (surgeon), Charles Heinz (internist), René Piffert (internist), Auguste Lieber (internist), and Paul Claer (gynaecologist).[54]

militarist sentiments; however, she does not state if he wore a Nazi armband at work.[55] She noted that his daily greeting was 'Heil Hitler, ladies and gentlemen' but also stated that this greeting was not widely practised by all professors, illustrating that Hofmeier fostered Nazi customs even where it was not compulsory.[56] While Hofmeier took on the majority of lecturing and supervision of students, a core lecturer for paediatrics was the Austrian Dr Hansjörg Steinmaurer.

Hansjörg Steinmaurer became a member of the NSDAP in 1933—similarly to Professor Hofmeier—which was illegal in pre-Anschluss Austria.[57] He studied medicine at the University of Innsbruck and the University of Vienna. Under the supervision of Dr Hamburger, he experimented with the diphtheria toxin in patients' blood at the children's clinic of the University of Vienna and published on this topic in 1938.[58] In July 1940, he habilitated in paediatrics, and in March 1941 he became a dozent (senior lecturer) for paediatrics in the University of Vienna children's clinic.[59] Dr Hamburger was a dedicated National Socialist, and had worked previously with Dr Hofmeier in the construction of a Kinderkundliche Woche in Vienna.[60] Steinmaurer also completed research on the topic of serotherapeutics, pathological anatomy, and vaccine research in animals. In 1940, Dr Chiari and Dr Hamburger wrote to the Professorenkollegium of the medical faculty at the University of Vienna to state that he had been a loyal member of the NSDAP with a good character, and so he was given the title of Dr Med Habil.[61] As part of Steinmaurer's application process to the Reichsuniversität Straßburg, the NSDAP had to attest to his political reliability, which was approved in February 1942.[62] Steinmaurer was employed as a Dozent Dr Med Habil Oberarzt for the paediatric clinic at the Reichsuniversität Straßburg from 1 February 1942.[63] In March 1942, the Reichsminister für Wissenschaft, Erziehung und Volksbildung attested to his appointment in Strasbourg in both clinical practice in the children's clinic, and also teaching in the clinic.[64] Steinmaurer was requested to conduct military service, but despite this request, the President of the Reichsuniversität Straßburg stated that

> [Steinmaurer] is absolutely necessary as a specialist for the children's clinic, especially since there is an extraordinary shortage of specialists. The conscription of Dr Steinmaurer to military service would have an extremely unfavourable effect with regard to the medical care of the 250 children currently accommodated in the children's clinic.[65]

This letter indicates the considerable disruptions to clinical practice and care that resulted from the military involvement of doctors and students at the Reichsuniversität Straßburg, as well as attempts to retain staff at the hospital.[66] Steinmaurer taught infectious diseases in childhood (1941–1942),[67] introduction to paediatric practice (1942),[68] a course on vaccination, and a paediatricians' seminar (1943).[69] However, he was marked as Zur Zeit im Feld (At the Front) from the Vorlesungsverzeichnis in 1943–1944, and the lectures he formerly taught were divided between Dr Hofmeier and Dr Kiehl.[70]

Dr Karl Willer was born in Strasbourg in 1903 and served as a lieutenant in the French army.[71] Despite his involvement with the French army, the NSDAP stated that he had no political affiliation.[72] The Kreispersonalamt of the NSDAP informed the Dekan of the medical faculty that Karl Willer should join a Nazi organization.[73] On presentation of a certificate to state that he had joined, then his case would be considered to be employed at the children's clinic.[74] While this certificate is not included in the file, Professor Stein wrote to the Chef der Zivilverwaltung in August that Willer had registered to work with the Hitler Youth and had reported to the district doctor, Dr Frank.[75] It is unknown in what capacity Willer worked with the Hitler Youth, but paediatricians routinely aided the Hitler Youth in medical screenings.[76] In the postwar era, individuals claimed that they were not really engaged in the party even though they had membership; therefore the specific organizations an individual joined can determine the degree of engagement with Nazi policies; without information on what specific group they joined, it is difficult to ascertain their personal thoughts on Nazism. Dr Willer joined a Nazi organization, despite seemingly having no political inclinations. His reasons for doing so are unknown, but it is possible that this 'recommendation' to join a Nazi organization was enough to persuade him to join the Hitler Youth in a medical capacity. This is in contrast to Renatus Mehl, who retained his job for several months despite not joining a Nazi organization and the external pressure to do so.

Dr Renatus Mehl was born in Hagenau in 1910, but was never a Francophile according to the investigation by the Kreisleitung der NSDAP in August 1941.[77] Despite his participation in the war from September 1939 to August 1940 in the French army, and the medal he received for his war effort, the Kreisleiter of the NSDAP declared that he had no strong political affiliations. The dean of the medical faculty replied to this report in September 1941, stating that 'It is hoped that he will soon find his way to the NSDAP or one of its branches. There are no fundamental concerns about his use as an assistant in the children's clinic.'[78]

In 1943, the NSDAP noted that Mehl held no known views against Germanization but was still politically inhibited.[79] Despite this, the Chef der Zivilverwaltung in Strasbourg stated that he had 'only now agreed to join an NS organization', though it is not mentioned which specific organization he became a member of.[80] It is likely this was as a result of external pressure rather than personal convictions, as they note that they would 'wait and see' regarding his political affiliations. Through the actions of the staff, the three-era structure can be seen more clearly; as Steinmaurer is sent to the front, there is an increased pressure on the staff members that remain to conform. This is indicative of the political pressure on individuals to join the Nazi cause, not necessarily due to personal conviction but in order to secure employment. This is in contrast to the zealous adherents of Nazism as seen in Dr Kiehl, Dr Steinmaurer, and Dr Hofmeier; it appears they all worked together in the clinic, indicating differing degrees of compromise and collaboration among the staff.

Paediatric Nursing

The question of who exactly provided nursing care in the Reichsuniversität Straßburg children's clinic is a complex one. While the Diaconesses de Strasbourg, a Protestant community of women (comparable to a Catholic order of nuns), had been nursing sick children in Strasbourg since 1842, it is unlikely that they were present in the clinic between 1940 and 1944.[81] The Sisters of Charity signed a contract in 1942 with the Reichsministerium für Wissenschaft, Erziehung und Volksbildung to specify the clinics in which they would work, but the children's clinic is not on that list.[82] These sisters had been present at the children's clinic since 1811, so it is possible that there were Sisters of Charity present after the signing of this contract in 1942.[83] A list of nurses dating to approximately 1941 has been found. This list was part of an archival source entitled 'DRK-Schwestern', but as the majority of the listed nurses were present before 1940, their specific status in the organization was not mentioned.[84] It is likely that they were members of the German Red Cross, due to the title on the record, and as this was one of the largest medical organizations in Germany, with 1.4 million members.[85] On 9 December 1937, 'The Law on the German Red Cross' was signed, which marked the full incorporation of the German Red Cross into the Nazi state.[86] This meant that the members of the German Red Cross had to swear allegiance to Adolf Hitler and had to identify with the Nazi regime; therefore, all nurses at the Reichsuniversität Straßburg had to declare their allegiance to the Nazi state.[87] This ideological affiliation is reflected upon in Hilde Steppe's book *Krankenpflege im Nationalsozialismus*, in which she notes that the nurse was considered the linchpin in terms of National Socialist health policy.[88] This was because, in providing community-based care, they could monitor the population and ensure their adherence to racial health policies, reporting families that did not conform. Steppe also notes that while they were hierarchically under the doctors of the clinic, they did operate semi-independently, taking on tasks like counselling, supervision, and education for keeping the population healthy, particularly through racial and hereditary healthcare provided at the mother consultation service.[89]

Paediatric nursing in this era was predominantly a profession for women due to the convergence of childcare and motherhood with the management of sick children.[90] Nursing care was organized hierarchically, with nursing sisters at the top who largely organized the nurses rather than actually caring for patients. The next stage comprised fully qualified nurses who did the majority of the work, while there were also trainee nurses who shadowed the nurses before completing their examinations. In the children's clinic, one fully trained nurse could take charge of four paediatric patients. In principle, there were to be eight trainee nurses for every ten sisters and six nurses, indicating the considerable number of trainee nurses.[91] In the first term in 1942, there were twelve trainee nurses, but by 1944, there were twenty-five, illustrating the growth of the clinic, but also the capacity for teaching and examining student nurses.[92] It also speaks to the ongoing impact of war, as there was a further reliance on trainee nurses during wartime as fully qualified nurses were required for caring for soldiers, as evidenced in the three-era structure of the Reichsuniversität Straßburg.

The Poliklinik was an extension of the children's clinic, established to provide outpatient care to children who did not require overnight admission to the hospital.[93] It was administratively a part of the children's clinic, and so it shared staff and resources with the rest of the children's clinic; hence, there are no separate records for admissions there, as it was in the same clinic, just a different ward. The Poliklinik could be used to monitor patients who had left the formal inpatient setting of the children's clinic and was also a more open treatment facility attached to the clinic.[94] This facility pre-dated the Reichsuniversität Straßburg, but its function and structure remained the same. It was located on the ground floor of the main building of the children's clinic and consisted of a number of separate rooms. It had a large waiting room, with a separate entrance and exit for suspected contagious cases. Rohmer noted that the seats in the waiting room were specifically

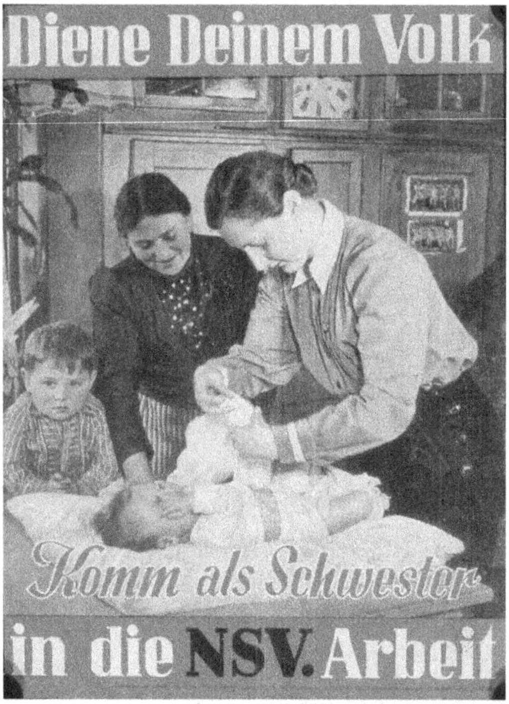
Diene Deinem Volk
Komm als Schwester
in die NSV. Arbeit

Fig. 2.3. Propaganda image reading 'Serve your people: Come work as a nurse (sister) for the NSV'. This image highlights the centrality of paediatric care to the idealized German Volk, and how racial hygiene was part of that, with 'Volk' here referring to Aryan children that would be part of the German people.[95]

placed separately, rather than one single waiting bench, in order to separate those who might be contagious.[96] The Poliklinik contained a room for physical examinations like hearing and sight tests, as well as three individual consultation rooms, and an administrative room where admission files were prepared. The Mutterberatungsstunde, or mothers' consultation hours, were held in the Poliklinik so that new mothers could bring their children for short check-ups and health screenings as well as vaccinations.[97] These consultations taught new mothers how to take care of children, but they also played an integral role in the monitoring of the local population, for their integration into the National Socialist system, but also for determining if the children had any signs of hereditary diseases. As Steppe notes, these check-ups were important as nurses were taught that the only way to keep the population healthy was to remove 'diseased elements' at the earliest possible opportunity, largely through health monitoring at the Mutterberatungsstunden.[98] This check-up sometimes revealed concerns that led to admission to the children's clinic. This was the case with Hedwig H., a five-month-old Alsatian child, of whom a routine examination in the Poliklinik during a Mutterberatungsstunde led to admission to the children's clinic for a skin disorder called lichen rubra planum.[99]

While the patient records from this aspect of the children's clinic no longer exist for the Poliklinik under the Reichsuniversität Straßburg, the size of this clinic and the number of children that were treated can be garnered from the records of the nursing service. Nurses were also responsible for maintaining a breast milk bank which was integral to the health of premature and underweight infants. It was backed by Hofmeier to the dean of the medical faculty, Professor Stein, wherein he emphasized the importance of adequate nutrition in the prevention of disease in children and infants. This scheme accounted for approximately 200 litres of milk a day used in the children's clinic.[100] As Kravetz notes, breast milk was viewed as a national resource in the Nazi era, as reproduction was politicized and breast milk collection centres reinforced the ideology that healthy children were central to the war effort.[101] The Reichsmütterdienst and the Mutterschulung taught women that their position in feeding and caring for German babies was their obligation to the German Volk, and this was achieved through extensive breastfeeding propaganda as well as incentivized breast milk donation.[102] Kravetz also notes that nurses were seen as integral to the success of the breastfeeding campaigns, as they could take time with mothers to encourage them to breastfeed or also to donate excess milk. This appears to be foregrounded in the *Richtlinien für Säuglingsschwestern in der nachgehenden Säuglingsfürsorge*, which was distributed by the Chef der Zivilverwaltung in June 1941. The Richtlinien highlighted the specific roles that nurses had in relation to clinical work as well as their contribution to public health campaigns:

> For this purpose, Säuglingsschwestern der Reichsbund der freien Schwestern und Pflegerinnen are employed by the NSV to help the family with baby care and nutrition. It means that they show the mothers how the child is properly bathed and directed and how the food is prepared. Their task is also to inform the mother about the necessity of breastfeeding, and if necessary, to give practical instruction.[103]

The nursing students in Strasbourg were taught about these campaigns, and were tested on this in their final exams.[104] The collection of breast milk for these banks also appears to have been constructed along racial lines, as Kravetz states that those who wished to donate breast milk had to first come to the clinic to have a racial exam, and only then would they be admitted as a donor.[105] Furthermore, doctors reprimanded women who could not, or chose not to, breastfeed as being selfish and contributing to higher infant mortality.[106] By the end of 1944, there were forty-four breast milk banks in the Reich, one of which was in Strasbourg.[107]

The majority of nurses had been part of the staff prior to the transfer of the clinic to German administration (twenty-four joined prior to 1940, with only three joining post-1940), indicating a considerable amount of retention of staff from the French period. Therefore, the question of their organizational affiliation remains, as they entered the service before 1940.

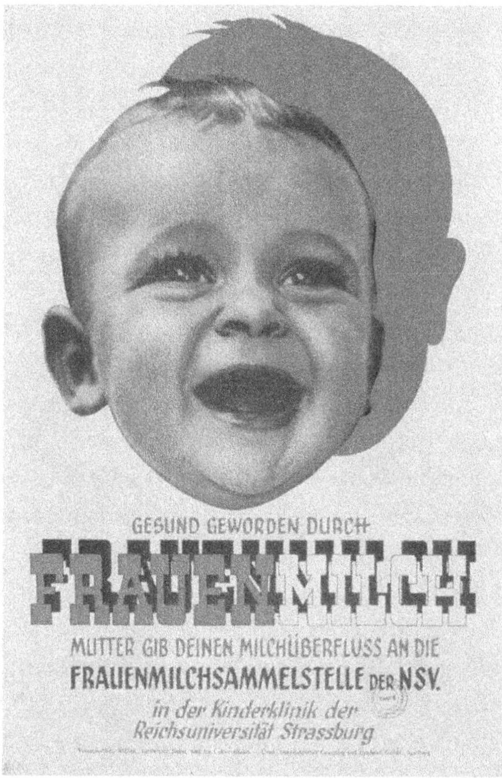

Fig. 2.4. Propaganda poster for the Straßburg children's clinic, urging new mothers to give their excess breast milk to the clinic. Message states: '[Infants] Get healthy through breast milk: Mother give your excess milk to the breast milk collection point of the NSV in the children's clinic of the Reichsuniversität Straßburg.'[108]

The same political background checks were required of nurses as well as doctors.[109] In order to facilitate a larger number of nurses, and continuity of staff, they allowed the registration of full-time nurses with French diplomas providing they passed a racial examination to determine that they were of German blood.[110] The degree of continuity of staff is indicated in Table 2.1 illustrating the fully qualified nursing staff and their backgrounds.

In total, there were nine neonatal nurses, one X-ray assistant, four general nurses, and fourteen specialist paediatric nurses, with eight of the twenty-eight nurses employed as temporary staff. One possible reason for this considerable number of nurses is that children required more one-on-one attention. This is clear when the staffing level in paediatrics, of one nurse for every four patients, is compared to other clinics. An example is the surgical clinic with one nurse per seven patients, one nurse per six patients in the medical clinics, one nurse per five patients in the gynaecology clinic, and one nurse per eight patients in dermatology. The number of nurses, excluding nursing sisters, was quite large and indicates the capacity for paediatric treatment, both within the clinic proper and in the Poliklinik.[111]

Much like the doctors, the nurses utilized the teaching environment of the hospital to train and supervise new nurses. On 22 November 1941, the *Straßburger Neueste Nachrichten* reported the opening of the paediatric nursing school at the Reichsuniversität Straßburg.[112] Representatives of the Wehrmacht were in attendance, and a ceremony was held in the festival hall at the clinic as thirty-six nurses were awarded the brooch of the *Reichsbund der Freien Schwestern und Pflegerinnen*. From 1936 onwards, the *Reichsbund der Freien Schwestern und Pflegerinnen* was the only professional organization of nurses that was allowed to exist in Nazi Germany; Catholic, Protestant, and Red Cross Nurses all had to be members of this organization in order to practise.[113] This further complicates ascertaining which organization the nurses were originally part of. The article in the *Straßburger Neueste Nachrichten* also notes that Professor Hofmeier would manage their education, while Oberin Reiter would be the head matron.[114] Their training was extensively detailed, including theoretical instruction on the biological structure of the body, practical lessons on bedside manner and treatments, physical exercise, and ideological training with the NSV. As the clinic already had 260 patients, this was an ample opportunity for the forty new trainee nurses to study here during the eighteen-month course. It also noted the symbolic importance of training nurses in a Nazi worldview west of the Rhine and stated that twenty-five of these new student nurses were from Alsace.[115] Throughout the nurses' training, they had to pass practical and written examinations, and the specific skills that were recorded

Table 2.1. Paediatric nursing personnel in the Reichsuniversität Straßburg children's clinic. Estimated date, 1941; precise date not provided in archive original.[116]

Paediatric Nursing Staff in the Reichsuniversität Straßburg				
Name	**Birthplace**	**Contract type**	**Role**	**Entry year**
Mathilde Meisch	Strassburg	Permanent	X-ray assistant	1910
Mathilde Bohnert	Strassburg	Permanent	Paediatric nurse	1919
Elizabeth Huth	Niederbronn	Permanent	Neonatal nurse	1921
Karoline Michel	Pfaffenhofen	Permanent	General nurse	1922
Maria Kniesel	Ruffach	Permanent	Neonatal nurse	1923
Anna M Fuchs	Strassburg	Permanent	General nurse	1924
Rosalie Muller	Strassburg	Permanent	Neonatal nurse	1924
Emilie Richert	Brumath	Permanent	Neonatal nurse	1926
Marianne Christ	Strassburg	Permanent	Paediatric nurse	1927
Alice Crozer	Stoztheim	Permanent	Paediatric nurse	1927
Bertha Jaeckle	Strassburg	Permanent	Neonatal nurse	1928
Elizabeth Braun	Diedenhof	Permanent	Paediatric nurse	1929
Mariette Richter	Kolmar	Permanent	Neonatal nurse	1930
Leonie Spiess	Sultzmatt	Permanent	Neonatal nurse	1931

Margarete Ruh	Strassburg	Temporary	Paediatric nurse	1932
Elizabeth Christ	Strassburg	Permanent	Paediatric nurse	1932
Adrienne Flory	Saaralben	Permanent	General nurse	1934
Johanna Spiess	Sultzmatt	Permanent	Neonatal nurse	1934
Luiza Strohl	Bischweiler	Permanent	Neonatal nurse	1934
Elizabeth Munch	Molsheim	Permanent	General nurse	1935
Sylvia Ehlinger	Mulhausen	Permanent	Paediatric nurse	1936
Gabrielle Krebs	Mulhausen	Temporary	Paediatric nurse	1937
Melanie Mary	Sufflenheim	Temporary	Paediatric nurse	1937
Luise Jemoli	Munster	Temporary	Paediatric nurse	1939
Maria Kohler	Niederhaslach	Temporary	Paediatric nurse	1939
Heiter Johanna	Kingersheim	Temporary	Paediatric nurse	1940
Elizabeth Rue	Diemeringen	Temporary	Paediatric nurse	1940
Erna Schirck	Strassburg	Temporary	Paediatric nurse	1940

by Oberin Reiter and sent to Dr Sprauer in 1944 illustrate what they were expected to know. These include vaccinations, urine examination, intubation, blood transfusions, tuberculin reaction tests, pleural puncture techniques, tracheotomy, catheterization, recognizing sepsis and encephalitis, care of premature infants, eczema, diphtheria, measles, whooping cough, rickets, and seizures, among further descriptions of care for illnesses and breastfeeding awareness campaigns.[117]

Children's Clinic Staff Involvement with the Lebensbornheim 'Schwarzwald' in Nordrach

Lebensborn e.V. was an SS organization established by Heinrich Himmler with the aim of offering welfare assistance to those having 'racially valuable' children, and also to provide improved maternity and infant welfare to those who were considered 'racially valuable'.[118] Himmler hoped to increase the birth rate, especially among young SS soldiers; 61% of the SS were bachelors in 1939, and those who were married had an average of 1.1 children per family, rising to 1.5 children for the officer class.[119] Therefore, couples who would ordinarily have married before having children but had been prevented from doing so by the war, or mothers whose SS partners had died in combat, were encouraged to increase the size of their families and were assured that they would be given the best of care. With this goal in mind, Lebensborn homes opened to provide maternity care to pregnant women who could prove their 'racial purity', providing ideological training such as mothercraft classes, and assistance to achieve an expected 100% breastfeeding rate.[120] Women would then give birth in these homes, and their children would be cared for up to their first year of life. Mothers who could then prove their ability to take care of these 'racially pure' children would be allowed to take them home, while other mothers, if they were unable to provide for the child, could leave their children there to be adopted by a family who passed racial tests.[121] These 'racially pure' children in Lebensborn homes were given the best of nutrition and care in order to ensure their health.[122] As the war progressed, and it became evident that these homes were not as fruitful as expected, children who were considered 'racially pure' were taken from their families in Eastern Europe, to be 'Germanized' and then adopted by a 'racially suitable' German family.[123] The importance of adoption along racial lines was highlighted by Hofmeier in his work *Heredity and Adoption: The Significance of Pathological Heredity and Hereditary Diseases in Adoptive Parents and Adoptive Children*, published in 1942, while he was director of the children's clinic.[124]

It was claimed by Lebensborn officials that only 700 people were employees of the organization; the approximate number of births as a result of the Lebensborn project is 12,000 children.[125] This illustrates that the cooperation of external medical professionals was essential to the fulfilment of their goals of maternal health and ensuring the development of racially 'pure' children. The Lebensborn home 'Schwarzwald' in the town of Nordrach in Baden-Württemberg was established in 1942 at the former Rothschild tuberculosis sanatorium.[126] This hospital formerly catered for Jewish patients, who were deported to Theresienstadt ghetto, and subsequently Auschwitz, in order to use the building as a Lebensborn home.[127] As it was a former Jewish hospital, the building and its contents were 'Aryanized' by throwing out equipment and books from the library that were not deemed adherent to the Nazi ideology.[128] While the Schwarzwald home had a target occupancy rate of sixty-five children, this number was not achieved in their first year, as in 1942 only five births were certified.[129] The numbers did increase in subsequent years, as 1943 saw ninety-seven births, and in 1944 there was a record of 110 births, far higher than the initial target occupancy. In 1945, only twenty-eight children were born there, leading to a total of 240 children born at Schwarzwald Lebensborn home, with an infant mortality rate of 1.25%.[130]

There were five nurses, one head nurse, one secretary, a house doctor, a deputy doctor, and maintenance staff working in this home. While it had a house doctor, Dr August Hagenmeier, it also required an external consultant to write reports and check on the children at regular intervals to ensure they were developing as expected. Dr Georg Ebner of the Lebensborn home asked Dr Hofmeier if he could suggest a suitable doctor from the Reichsuniversität Straßburg children's clinic who could dedicate some time every six to eight weeks to come to Nordrach and check the health of the Lebensborn children.[131] Hofmeier responded in May 1943, stating that he would be happy to help at the Lebensborn home, and that he would drive himself and an assistant to the home in the near future as he was 'very interested in the establishment of the institution'.[132] They arranged a meeting on a Saturday after the Pentecost holiday in 1943 for the first visit, and Hofmeier brought Dr Wolfgang Kiehl with him as an assistant.

Thereafter, Dr Kiehl became the consultant doctor for the Lebensborn home in Nordrach, with occasional referrals to Hofmeier. Kiehl was reimbursed 50RM for each visit, and Dr Ebner arranged transport for him from the train station and reimbursement for travel expenses.[133] Despite the request of Dr Ebner to visit every six to eight weeks, Kiehl visited Schwarzwald every four weeks.[134] Only two of Dr Kiehl's reports into the home are extant; in July 1943, on his first trip as a solo medical consultant, he noted that the home 'makes an exceptionally well-kept and clean impression'.[135] He also praised the 100% breastfeeding rate, and examined all children for vitamin D and rickets as well as other ailments. As a result of these examinations, he ordered vitamin D supplementation and viagntol to be given to each child as a prophylaxis measure.[136] In his second report from December 1943, he noted that despite the cold weather, children should spend more time outside on the veranda, criticizing the lack of a rainproof shelter there to enable year-round use of the air cure.[137] As the children born in Lebensborn homes had to be mentally and physically developed, any delays were concerning; Kiehl stated that two children were 'somewhat striking' to him in terms of mental and physical development, and he would be monitoring them closely.[138] Kiehl also stated that should any child become unwell, they should be transferred to the children's clinic in Strasbourg.[139]

Children that were born in Lebensborn homes were not immune from the ideology that imperfect children were a threat to the national body. Indeed, national belonging was somewhat medicalized, with physical and mental examinations conducted on children in Eastern Europe before they were considered 'Germanizeable' then taken to Lebensborn homes and forced to assimilate. The medical consultant was also in charge of medical examinations of these 'stolen children' (*Raubkinder*) in the Lebensborn home.[140] In other Lebensborn homes, children with mental or physical developmental problems were referred by the medical consultants to Kinderfachabteilungen, where they would be killed. While this did not occur in Nordrach, if a child was born that was considered 'imperfect', it was the role of the medical consultant to refer them outside of the Lebensborn home to be killed. This can be seen in the case of Brigitte Schmidt, who was born in the Wienerwald Lebensborn home in 1941 near Vienna.[141] She was transferred to the Kinderfachabteilung in Spiegelgrund in Vienna as a result of the orders of Dr Gasser, the consultant for the Lebensborn home, who declared her 'psychologically underdeveloped'.[142] In the letter from Dr Schwab, the director of the home in 1942, he stated that 'the child is to be taken to the clinic mentioned above, which, as far as I know, is also active in the sense of eradication'.[143] It is clear then that the consultant was aware of what would happen to her after his decision to transfer her. She was killed in the Kinderfachabteilung on 9 November 1942 at just one year old, and her body was used for medical studies after her death.[144]

It is evident that Hofmeier's consultant position for Lebensborn was intended to control and assimilate the occupied population, which was crucial for the success of the next generation, as they believed 'the youth of today is the soldier of tomorrow'.[145] This role included medical management of individual children, provision for preventative healthcare such as the prescribed vitamin D supplement for all Lebensborn children, but also the responsibility that if any births led to less than 'perfect' children, then the consultant would have the duty of sending these children to an institution that would ensure their death.

Conclusion

Paediatrics was a popular specialism at the Reichsuniversität Straßburg, as the clinic expanded its staff and its remit for teaching new medical students. However, the clinic was considerably impacted by the war, as members of staff left their teaching and research behind to serve at the front.[146] Paediatrics had one of the highest numbers of student theses, and many courses on offer. While Hofmeier continued to write in this era, he published significantly less than prior to his arrival in the Reichsuniversität Straßburg, and the material did not deal with research specific to Strasbourg but instead addressed more general questions. These seem to be geared toward incorporation of the local population into the German Volk, through studying questions of hereditary worth, the illnesses present in the clinic, and the issue of adoption. It is clear that the clinic was in some ways limited by its own success. With such a large number of students being supervised, monographs still being published, as well as the majority of teaching being conducted by the director of the clinic, Hofmeier did not pursue research projects as staff in other departments did. It must also be remembered that this department was not intended as a research institute, but as a practical clinic. In the final period of the Reichsuniversität Straßburg from 1943 to 1944, other departments increased their emphasis on research and this was when criminal experiments were undertaken in the absence of such an emphasis on teaching and supervision.[147] It appears that in this final period, consolidation of student theses and continuation of lecturing capacity, as well as the treatment of patients, were the priorities for the staff of the children's clinic. Hofmeier was approached to contribute to medical care in the Lebensborn home Schwarzwald in Nordrach, but he contributed voluntarily, as did Kiehl. Kiehl far exceeded his duties in visiting every four weeks instead of the recommended six to eight weeks. Postwar legitimization of their role, and the denial of their contribution to the Lebensborn programme, will be further examined in later chapters. The next chapter focuses on patient treatment in the children's clinic, and examines how this adherence to ensuring the health of the Volk was evident in patient care.

CHAPTER 3

Paediatric Treatment at the Children's Clinic of the Reichsuniversität Straßburg

> In order to successfully implement the *Law for the Prevention of Hereditary Diseases*, the obligation to notify is introduced for every case of congenital insanity, already the suspicion is notifiable according to Bessau and Catel the role of the obstetric trauma is overestimated here. In general, the exogenous factors are probably strongly in the background. The cooperation of the paediatrician for early detection of congenital insanity is urgently needed.[1]

This chapter asks: who were the children that were treated in the clinic? To interrogate this thoroughly, we also need to ask how this clinic functioned in an environment founded on Nazi ideology. What was the process of being admitted to the hospital, and what provision for follow-up outpatient care was provided? What diagnoses, ages, nationalities, and classes were represented in the patient demographic? What were their treatments, and how did the process of hospitalization impact them? The patient files from the children's clinic will form the basis of case studies, examining themes such as infectious disease, nationality, class, multiple births, and heredity, as well as living conditions, infant mortality, and so-called illegitimacy. This methodology of using patient case studies to illustrate the conditions of a particular institution has been used with great success in work such as that of Flora Graefe and Isabelle von Bueltzingsloewen.[2] As Florian Steger states, examining patient case records can act as a tool of historical research, but the wording used in such patient records can also illustrate how medical practitioners thought about their patients. As mentioned in the introduction, medical care for the next generation was of considerable importance during

National Socialism; however, this was predicated on multiple factors, one of which was economic justification. Hilde Steppe noted in *Krankenpflege im Nationalsozialismus* that there was a clear economic element to the provision of medical care, particularly in justifying who could contribute economically in the future, and those who would be considered a drain on the system.[3] This ideology then is compounded in terms of paediatric care, sorting children into those who could later provide for and contribute to the National Socialist system, in contrast to those who could not financially subsidize their care.

Class and Financial Circumstances

Class in this instance refers to Patientenklassen, rather than social class, although the two are closely related. Each patient file has a section denoting Patientenklasse, which corresponded with what class of care they were to receive. The division into classes relates to the classification of the payment for hospital services which had been established in the Kaiserreich era (1871–1918) and was retained into the Nazi era. For first-class patients, the services rendered (medical treatment, accommodation, food quality) were the most expensive, second class was less expensive, and the third class was the cheapest. The costs of medical treatment in first class, including laboratory costs and medications, were usually paid by the patient without the involvement of insurance. Second-class patients had private health insurance and paid the cost of their treatment themselves.

Following negotiation between the second-class patient health insurance company and the doctors, the individual applied for reimbursement from their insurance company; however, this did not always cover the entire cost, so they could be subject to financial risk. Costs for patients in third class were paid by a health insurance company or the community welfare association. The majority of patients were classified as third class, as people would receive a certain amount of health care through their employment contracts.[4] This third-class level of care even extended to forced labourers and those in Umsiedlungslagern, which were resettlement camps for those considered to be 'Germanizeable' who had been relocated from Eastern Europe. The poor and unemployed also received a similar type of insurance through public welfare support and so were also designated as third class. The important differentiation in patient class emerges as the Reichsuniversität Straßburg was a teaching hospital. Under the 1914 statutes of the Heidelberg Hospital, which continued up to the Nazi era, only third-class patients were allowed to be used for medical teaching purposes.[5] As a result of this, third-class patients could be transferred to special departments or individual doctors in accordance with the medical practitioner's desire for teaching and research.[6] It is unclear whether this differentiation between wealth and class was more pronounced under National Socialism.

Class and personal associations with the doctors seems to have had a notable impact on the treatment of the child, or at least communication about their treatment with their parents. It also may have had an impact on the length of their hospital stay, as indicated in the case of Francine L., the daughter of a business manager, who entered the hospital on 18 September 1943 and was almost one year old. Francine was admitted as a French second-class patient, and diagnosed with hypernephroma, a kidney tumour.[7] Her doctor referred her because of a suspected kidney malformation that caused her to be in a 'very miserable condition'.[8] Extensive testing included urine and blood glucose levels, which were normal, although she appeared undernourished. On 24 September, Dr Zukschwerdt recommended that as her condition was not too serious, surgery was not urgently required, and so Dr Hofmeier devised a nutritional plan for Francine to see if this could alleviate her symptoms.[9] She was given extra food, which was selected and detailed by Hofmeier in accordance with his research on vitamins and childhood nutrition.[10] After this, Francine 'rose very quickly and was cheerful and happy before being released' on 11 October 1944.[11] It appears that her mother was an acquaintance of Dr Hofmeier, as he personally wrote to her to update her about her child. He listed what she had been eating for every meal, and further observations as to her mood and general condition.[12] Her mother appeared to have been in contact with Francine, as she complained of the cold in the clinic, which Hofmeier stated could not be avoided given the weather. When the child returned home, the hospital received further updates, as Francine's mother expressed gratitude that, following treatment, 'she [is] so lively and jumps all day long at the lattice of the bed'.[13] It appears in certain cases there was considerable follow-up contact and further examinations, as, following her release, Hofmeier expressed his concern that there were not adequate paediatric facilities to deal with her kidney problems closer to their home in Metz. This emphasizes both that outpatient care was central to paediatric treatment and patients' discharge from hospital, but also that patient class was one of the determinants of how valuable their parents' opinion of their treatment was, and indeed how the doctors perceived their ability to care for their own children. This can be interpreted as an extension of the Nazi concept of preserving the Volk above all else, including above individual parental rights; the importance of nationality and parental rights will be elaborated upon later in the chapter.

Patient class played an important part in the care of children in Strasbourg, particularly when one considers practices of patient transfer from other paediatric clinics in hospitals. Doctors were obliged to register any children that were born with, or displayed signs after birth of, a particular list of illnesses as outlined in the Law for the Prevention of Hereditary Diseases. Some of the illnesses mentioned in this list occur in Strasbourg: epilepsy, Little's disease, schizophrenia, physical defects, 'idiocy', and Down's syndrome, among other illnesses, illustrating that the population should technically have been subject to transfers.[14] The consequences of this law could lead to sterilization, as ordered by the hereditary health courts, or so-called euthanasia at another institution. However, as Volker Roelcke outlines, whether doctors actually fulfilled this legal obligation is another question, as it appears there were no consequences for refusing to refer children.[15] In fact, he specifies that two-thirds of private practice doctors in the Schwalbach district of Franconia did not submit a single report to the hereditary health court.[16] There are a number of reasons for the lack of reporting: a doctor might be a secret opponent of the regime and so refuse to participate in this registration; doctors depended on their patients to keep their practice going; and—the reason that appears the most prominent in Strasbourg—a financial one. Ultimately, if you transfer all your chronically ill patients, then you cannot financially claim for the medical treatment and length of hospital stay provided. As well as this, there had been open opposition from certain communities when child 'euthanasia' was discovered, and it is reasonable to assume that such patient transfers would have elicited a similarly vocal response in Alsace.[17] In the interest then of financial benefit, as well as appeasing and attracting the occupied population, it seems that patient class significantly influenced patient care. It is important to note that although this reporting was obligatory, Strasbourg was not alone in not completing these reports. This obligation was not routinely policed, but depended on the individual practitioners taking the initiative to fill these in; however, this does not mean that it was voluntary.

Nationality and Staatsangehörigkeit

The region of Alsace, and particularly the city of Strasbourg, is notable in the plurality of national identity of its citizens. This issue of nationality politics and the problematic categorization of nationality has been further detailed in the introduction. Most patients in the children's clinic were Alsatian (555), or German (90), while patients were also admitted from Belgium, Italy, Luxembourg, Switzerland, and France.[18] However, Reichsdeutscher, the second largest category of patient, with 127 patients, is important to note, as this designation was not based on place of birth, or even on parents' birthplace, but was used as a German ethnic identifier. Therefore, we see an increase in people being designated as Reichsdeutscher as the occupation progresses, illustrating the Germanization of the people. Given the geographical proximity of Belgium, Luxembourg, and Switzerland, along with other Western European regions, it is understandable that they are featured in the patient demographics. Eastern European children were also admitted, illustrating the integral role that Strasbourg played in the relocation and Germanization of the population, particularly as the war progressed.

One example of an Alsatian patient is that of Ernst Z., who was admitted as a third-class patient in February 1942 at two months old. Dr Lévy wrote a referral note in February for the child to be admitted to hospital, stating that due to conspicuous umbilical hernia, oedema, and convulsions, the child was requested to undergo tests and observation to discover the cause

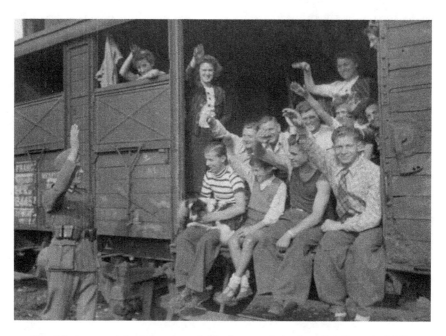

Fig. 3.1. Image of the relocation of Alsatian people back to Straßburg in 1940, giving the Nazi salute.[19]

of his illness.[20] On admission, a record was made of the child's family and living situation. Although Ernst's sibling had died six months earlier, his parents were healthy and no hereditary conditions were listed. Their living situation was considered good as they lived in a modern building, Ernst had his own bedroom, and was exclusively breastfed. Having ruled out hereditary or environmental factors, a pneumoencephalography was performed in order to view the ventricles inside the brain to determine the cause of the seizures; his ventricles were considerably enlarged.[21] His cerebrospinal fluid was also tested, revealing increased pressure on the brain. Ophthalmological testing was then conducted to see if this increased pressure had damaged his eyesight, but it was found to be normal. Ernst's blood was also tested and findings all returned as negative for common infections. On 5 March, he was sent home, and Dr Hofmeier requested that Dr Levy send him back to get a check-up in six months.[22] Hofmeier did not expect a good prognosis, as they suspected these problems were caused by difficulties at birth. Leucoplast bandages, chloralhydrate, and drawing of spinal fluid were recommended, as well as luminal for Ernst's convulsions. From this case, we get an indication of the normal course of treatment for patients of Alsatian origin. This also illustrates the management of illnesses at the clinic, as well as the variety of tests and treatments available. It also shows that follow-up care through check-ups was standard to ensure the health of the population.

Irmgard D. is an example of a patient who was in a relatively privileged position due to her family's adherence to the regime. She was admitted to the children's clinic in March 1944, aged four.[23] Her family were noted to be Reichsdeutscher, and her parents received a marriage loan for setting up their family. These marriage loans were distributed from 1938 with the intention of filling a gap in social service provision, and increasing the number of children born to 'racially valuable' parents; that Irmgard's parents could avail of such a loan illustrates their privileged position.[24] As a result of the marriage loan, they had four children, which was considered 'Kinderreiche' or child rich, a highly prized position.[25] Her father was in the Wehrmacht; the notes do not specify what role he held, but regardless, his involvement was of considerable benefit. Irmgard was admitted with tuberculous meningitis and a fever. It was noted that due to the good condition of the house, where each child had their own bed, only the patient was unwell, and her siblings had no signs of illness. This shows the importance that was placed on seemingly 'appropriate' conditions, as well as the emphasis placed on environment for healthcare outcomes. Irmgard's spinal fluid was tested, along with standard blood tests. Her developmental milestones were checked, such as the age when she began to walk and talk, and she was considered to be of a good standard for her age. Poliomyelitis was suspected, given that she had some spinal paralysis, but this was ruled out following further culture tests on the spinal fluid, and the constantly elevated temperature. On 15 March 1944, her parents requested that she return home, and Hofmeier agreed, giving a prescription of Albucid tablets (a sulfonamide antibiotic) and plenty of fluids. Her parents had some degree of agency over the fate of their child, as they were able to formally request her return home. That her parents could advocate for her return home with a prescription indicated their higher status because of their adherence to the Nazi system, and the value placed on their judgement as parents.

A number of paediatric patients were admitted from Eastern Europe, which begs the question of how they arrived, and—even more pertinent—whether their treatment was markedly different from the Alsatian and German patients. As Strasbourg was part of the broader administration of the German Reich, the patients reflect the demographics of the local area, including the presence of forced labourers and people who were forcibly resettled. One child came from an Umsiedlungslager—in this instance, from Yugoslavia.[26] 'Germanization' involved forcing them to abandon their native language and adopt German, as well as an in-depth medical examination to determine their fitness to be a member of the German 'Volk'.[27] Once this was complete, their nationality could be changed in their file to German, which illustrates the fragility of the concept of nationality in relation to the occupied region; it could be changed pending social approval of a medical professional.

Johann B. was three years old when he was admitted to the children's clinic at the Reichsuniversität Straßburg, with a diagnosis of 'mental retardation'.[28] The reasoning for this appears to be his behaviour rather than a lack of developmental abilities for his age. As Florian Steger notes, the description of behaviour and productivity could play a significant role in provision—or lack—of treatment.[29] Johann's parents, who were Polish, worked at an unspecified labour camp in Germany. The only letters concerning Johann were from Dr Hofmeier to Dr Hans in Brumath, who referred him to the clinic, and were not addressed to his parents.[30] They explained that the child could stand, and walk, but would not speak German. It was initially thought that he had hearing problems, but it was found that he simply did not understand German. When the staff spoke to Johann in German, he would raise his hands above his head and cry. The staff of the clinic also noted that he was very withdrawn and would refuse to play with other children, and would instead make repetitive stereotyped movements to calm himself down. There does appear to have been some contact with the parents in person, as a full family history was taken wherein the mother stated that her labour was prolonged and difficult in giving birth to him. They also stated that she could understand German, and when their observations of the child led to no improvement in his condition, he was discharged from the clinic. While this account appears to indicate what could be described as an autistic spectrum disorder, it is also notable that Johann's responses to traumatic stimuli were well reasoned. His raising his hands above his head and crying when encountering German is indicative of the evident trauma experienced, and his withdrawal from playing with the other children can also be explained in that their games were largely in German, thus prompting his isolation. The stereotyped movements he exhibits indicate an attempt at self-soothing in the absence of parents to console him. This case was dismissed as 'mental retardation' with 'mental backwardness', with no therapeutic prospects, and so he was discharged on 7 October 1941 after a week in the clinic.[31] As Steger notes, pejorative and stigmatizing language used such as the description of 'mental backwardness' was not unique to the Nazi era, but it illustrates the prevalence of dehumanizing ideas, as patients are reduced to discriminatory descriptions of their abilities.[32] This sort of language is found most often in records of Eastern European children, or those not considered 'Germanizeable'. Such a judgement could also rule out longer-term care in an outpatient capacity, which was an integral part of medical care.

Management of Chronic Conditions and Outpatient Care

Illnesses such as polio, diphtheria, meningitis, tuberculosis, and scarlet fever, among others, were particularly prevalent in this era, and as a result, children required well-rounded treatment in order to overcome illnesses like poliomyelitis. The most prevalent diagnoses seen in the children's clinic of the Reichsuniversität Straßburg were consistent with this era in that contagious diseases were the majority of admissions. Chief among these was scarlet fever (eighty-one cases), pneumonia (sixty-four cases), and diphtheria (fifty-seven cases).[33]

One example of patient care during such an outbreak is Margarete, who was admitted to the hospital during the polio epidemic of July 1944, at two years old.[34] She was listed as a third-class Alsatian patient, and by the time of her admission had developed considerable paralysis in her left leg, and a weak right leg, with completely absent reflexes in both legs. Her history of illness was noted, and it was recorded that she had suffered from scarlet fever

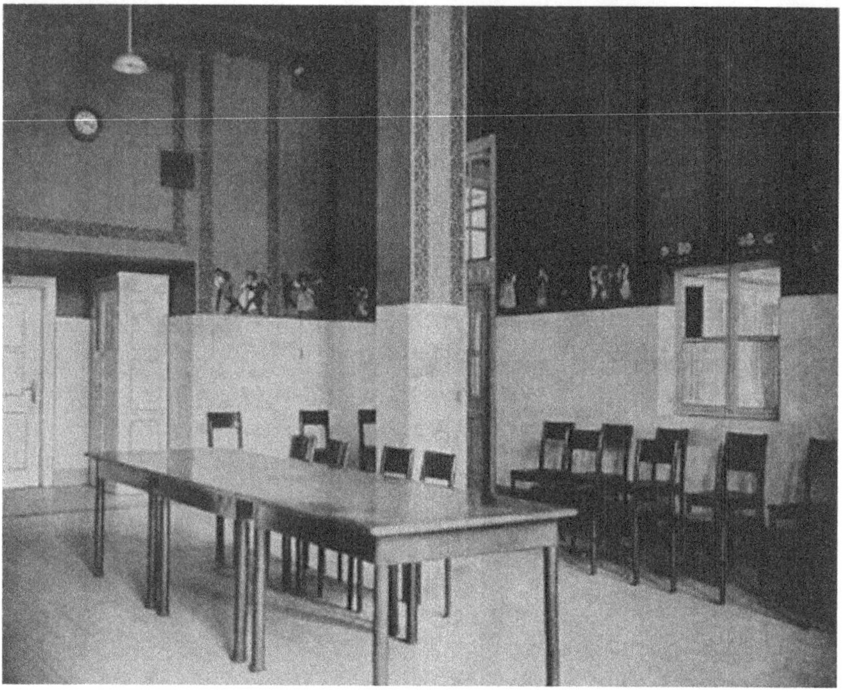

Fig. 3.2. The outpatient poliklinik. This image was taken in 1932, but the structure and appearance remained the same in the Nazi era.[35]

and an ear infection. A family history was taken, noting that both her parents and her one sibling were healthy, and each had their own rooms. On admission, she was subject to routine blood tests, all of which came back negative for other illnesses.[36] As noted in Abraham's work, polio diagnosis and treatment was heavily dependent on an integrated network of precision laboratory testing and follow-up treatment.[37] Czerny explains that this combination of laboratories and patient wards was a particular advantage in the children's clinic in Strasbourg, and this system was retained into the Reichsuniversität era.[38] The practical application of this integrated system and its benefits are shown in Margarete's case. Dr Schubert recommended that Margarete should receive fresh air, and daily massages to reduce muscle atrophy. Regular physiotherapy was recommended at the hospital, as well as a leg brace for night-time use.[39] Symptomatol was prescribed, as well as hot compresses to relieve her pain. After more than two months of intensive treatment at the clinic, she was discharged to continue the treatment regimen at home. From Margarete's case, we can see that third-class treatment did not necessarily deprive a patient of decent medical care, provided the person was considered

'Germanizeable'. This provides an insight into how patients with chronic conditions were treated on an ongoing basis, as well as how patients in Strasbourg dealt with epidemic illnesses of the era.

Congenital and acquired heart problems also feature heavily in the data, requiring consistent monitoring and treatment. The data reveals the technology available in Strasbourg to conduct this kind of ongoing treatment, as they used an ECG machine, which only became routine in 1939.[40] This required admission to a hospital and monitoring with medication in conjunction with an ECG machine. Although the children's clinic could conduct such examinations, the internal medicine clinic (which will be covered in more detail in Chapter 6) had extended provision for ECG machines, as well as other diagnostic technologies, so several children were transferred there for treatment. One patient who availed of this treatment was Klaus D., who was admitted to the children's clinic in June 1943, aged eight.[41] He was listed as a second-class Reichsdeutscher patient with impaired growth and was described as very pale. He was brought to the Poliklinik by his mother, who was concerned at his weak constitution, and an abnormality in his pulse was detected.[42] Klaus was treated with digitalis for 'weakness'; a common side effect was slowing of the heart rate, and he was put on bed rest.[43] He had an ECG, which showed arrhythmia perpetua, and a heartbeat of 150 beats per minute. Dr Dieker at the X-ray department took some images of his

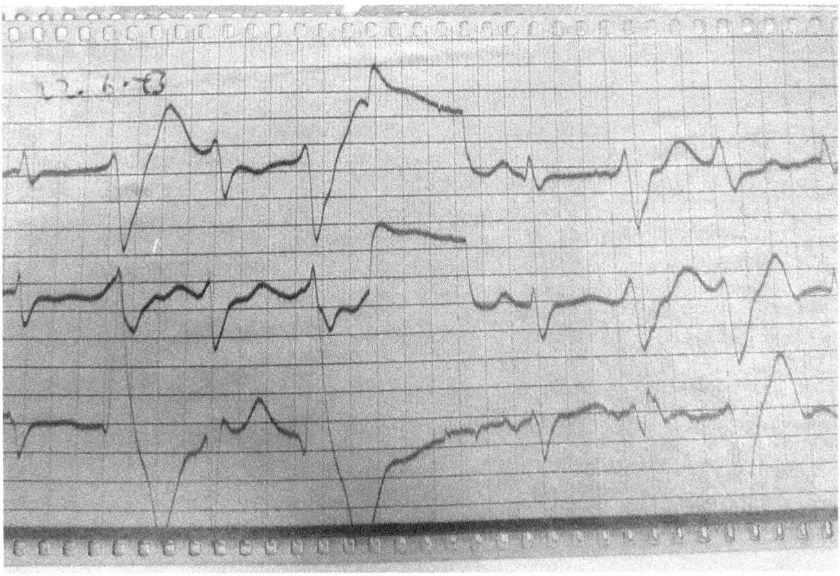

Fig. 3.3. Excerpt from the three-lead ECG of Klaus D., taken 22 June 1943.[44]

heart and stated that the retrocardial space was considerably narrowed and the heart was more spherical in shape, leading him to suspect myocarditis as a complicating factor. After one month in the clinic, Klaus showed very little improvement. He was sent home on the condition his treatment with digitalis was continued and that he return for check-ups regularly.

Epidemic illnesses such as scarlet fever, diphtheria, and measles contributed to a significant number of hospital admissions. While this data records only admissions to hospital, such illnesses could often strike not just the child who was sent to hospital, but many members of the same family. The impact of epidemic illnesses on the entire family is evidenced in the case of nine-year-old Peter G., who was admitted to the children's clinic in May 1942. He was listed as a third-class Alsatian patient, but importantly, he was from a Kinderreiche family, which indicates the importance of large families.[45] Dr Albert Bury, the general practitioner to the family, wrote a letter to the children's clinic, affectionately calling the child 'little G', indicating the more informal nature of the relationship with a general practitioner than a hospital doctor. He suspected diphtheria and ordered tests to be conducted. He stated: 'it seems to me that there is a large family and the danger for the environment is high'.[46] Therefore, the main aim in hospitalizing Peter, as listed in the admission records, was to prevent the further spread of suspected diphtheria to the other children in the household. A patient history was taken, and it was discovered that he had previously had measles but had not suffered any complications from this infection. Peter was extensively tested in the clinic, with results coming back positive for diphtheria. He was then given diphtheria serum. On 30 May, he was given a scarlet fever vaccine, and the parents were requested to bring him back for the second dose in July.[47] This highlights that the status of the family and the possible further infection of other children played a role in hospital admissions when little else could be done to restrict outbreaks.

Treatment of Twins

Research on twins was of great interest in this era, not only in Germany but also further afield, as it made some hereditarian principles more evident before the advent of genetic research and testing. One example of this is detailed further by Sheila Faith Weiss, who describes how Otmar Freiherr von Verschuer's research on 4,000 twins was used to illustrate heritability of intelligence and mental disabilities, but also criminal tendencies, as well as physical illnesses like tuberculosis. This research was funded by the Nazi government but also by the New York-based Rockefeller Foundation, highlighting how this focus on twins was not only of interest in Germany.[48] Verschuer presented his research on twins to the Royal Society in London in 1939, and reflected on Francis Galton's twin studies.[49] The Nazi focus on twins was linked not only to the common scientific research of the era, but also focused on how a larger Aryan population could be produced, and how human fecundity could be increased to produce more twins.[50] This culminated in fertility experiments, sterilization, and twin studies conducted in Auschwitz concentration camp.[51] This focus on including hereditary assessment in medical admission files in the Reichsuniversität Straßburg reflects the emphasis on increasing fertility for selected groups. One such example is the cooperation between the children's clinic and the racial hygiene department of the Reichsuniversität Straßburg under the directorship of Dr Wolfgang Lehmann.[52] In the medical thesis of Otto Dahms, conducted at the paediatric clinic under the supervision of Dr Kurt Hofmeier in 1944, he relies heavily on the assistance of Lehmann at the racial hygiene department.[53] His thesis focuses on seven pairs of twins, of whom only one twin was ill with poliomyelitis.[54] The aim of the study appears to trace a heritable cause of polio, as it focuses heavily on family history, Sippentafeln, and physical measurements rather than vectors of infection. This was all conducted on children who were admitted to the children's clinic for treatment, but the extra examinations were conducted using a racial hygiene analysis form from the racial hygiene department under Dr Lehmann. Interestingly, it also follows the patients after their release from hospital, and as one patient refuses to participate in the follow-up on 'religious grounds', it appears that he received consent for this study from the patients' families.[55] The examination sheets contained extensive information on each set of twins, detailing their measurements, anthropological data such as the shape and colour of the eyes, skin, and hair, but also included information on childhood developmental milestones such as when the children first learned to walk and talk. The data also has a section detailing how the mother of the children tells them apart, illustrating that the degree of similarity and difference of the identical twins was of importance to the research. Information concerning their blood groups and history of twins in the family was also discussed, along with the general health of the family, showing the importance of heredity.

One case in Otto Dahm's thesis addresses Brigitte and Christiana, born in December 1943, and it is mentioned that they were strikingly similar in appearance.[56] Their mother believed that Brigitte contracted poliomyelitis from their cousin, and she was admitted to the children's clinic. Brigitte had left-sided facial paralysis and poor reflexes, but few other symptoms. Urine and blood tests were performed, along with a lumbar puncture and tuberculin probe test on both twins to provide a comparison. It is significant that an invasive test, such as a lumbar puncture, was performed on a child with no clinical reason to do so, simply to compare with their twin.[57] This is a direct contravention of the Richtlinien of the time, which prevented such procedures when the patient themselves would not be able to benefit from the procedure. There was no record in the thesis of medications used, but Brigitte was released from the clinic on 10 November with a considerable improvement in movement. Following this initial medical analysis, Dahms follows up with a Sippentafel, indicating that the mother had a history of psychiatric illness, and that there were a number of twins on their father's side of the family. The extent to which the family were aware of the reasons for these questions and this research is unknown, but it is evident that collaboration between the children's clinic and the racial hygiene department was predicated not necessarily on experimental research, but on surveying the population to analyse fertility and multiple births in a racial context.

Helga and Monika were born one month premature on 26 November 1943.[58] While they were delivered at home, they were then brought to the midwifery school for routine check-ups, where it was noted that they were anaemic and had pneumonia. When they were four weeks old, their mother brought them from their home in Kehl to the children's clinic in Straßburg as private patients. On admission, their records first stated that they were Catholic and Reichsdeutsche, then a hereditary health check was performed. No heritable diseases were noted, nor did they mention any history of twins in the family. This indicates the institutional importance of ascertaining heritability of illness, as researched by Hofmeier and his students. Monika was treated for pneumonia and anaemia, as well as prematurity, and was given blood transfusions and eleudron tablets. Helga also had two blood transfusions for anaemia, from which she quickly recovered. On 23 February, Maria T., their mother, wrote to request their transfer to a private ward within the children's clinic, and it appears this request was granted. She also stated in the letter that she was made aware of the obligations associated with this request on her part, which indicates a consultation on medical care, ongoing treatment, and best practice with the doctors present, as well as parental consent.[59] Both infants were breastfed, and tested negative for diphtheria bacteria with the Staatliche Medizinal-Untersuchungsanstalt. Both twins were released, considerably improved and increased in weight, on 29 January 1944. Their care was followed up by Professor Jacobi at the obstetrics and gynaecology clinic of the Reichsuniversität Straßburg as well as the children's clinic on 11 February 1944. It was noted that both twins were well developed and progressing as expected. This further highlights Paul Weindling's point that severely disabled children, those from marginalized populations such as Roma and Jewish children, and those who were from lower socioeconomic groups were seen as 'legitimate research material' in Nazi medicine, and were seen as disposable once their research aims were fulfilled.[60] However, for those who were from higher socioeconomic groups, those who could assimilate to the Volk and were designated as Reichsdeutscher were given options of paying for private care, given follow-up treatment, and were well informed about their loved ones and their prognosis.

While twin patients who were admitted to the clinic appear to have been exclusively from higher socioeconomic groups, and so were not the subject of research, twin studies were conducted by the clinic director and the students. Hofmeier formerly studied the impact of heredity in disease through his work on twins and poliomyelitis entitled 'Poliomyelitis of the Cerebral Type in Monozygotic Twins', which was published in 1938.[61] He conducted this research with his co-author, K. Dinckler, including full comparative tables on the twins' development, nutrition, blood cultures, lumbar punctures, and comparative X-rays.[62] He suggested that as both twins reacted similarly with encephalitis symptoms as a result of poliomyelitis infection, they had the same gene with the same reaction, which led to their identical symptoms. In this work, he referenced Verschuer's *Erbpathologie*, and referenced the impact of heredity and 'inferior' genes in the development of neuropsychaesthenic symptoms, or physical symptoms of so-called degeneracy.[63] While this study was conducted prior to his appointment at the Reichsuniversität Straßburg, this research indicates the theories he believed in and how they could be used in cases of twins in the children's clinic. This type of research involving twins was also conducted by students and referenced in work by students at the Reichsuniversität Straßburg children's clinic. It appears that while twins were studied in relation to race and heredity theories by Hofmeier and his students, they were not treated differently to other patients in the Reichsuniversität children's clinic beyond this enhanced emphasis on inheritance of traits and illnesses.

Social Issues as a Medical Concern

Social cohesion was a key facet of paediatrics in occupied Alsace. This went from advertising savings banks for children to banning the publication of

French-language material and forbidding the wearing of berets.[64] French culture was suppressed in all forms, from published material to schools and social gatherings, in public and in private. Children were forbidden from speaking French, and all schools were aligned to teaching the Nazi curriculum as found in all other schools in Germany.[65] In 1941, there was an opening ceremony of the Hitler Youth Alsace division and 5,000 children attended; while it was not compulsory until 1942, it was evidently popular due to the social benefits derived from membership.[66]

According to official statistics, by 1 November 1941 there were 91,808 members of the Alsace branch of the Hitler Youth.[67] Conversely, lack of social assimilation in this occupied area was pathologized, wherein children who were perceived to be socially problematic were medicalized. Social cohesion also extended to medical care, in that a robust social healthcare system, complete with follow-up outpatient clinics, would encourage interaction with the new social system in occupied Alsace. Conformity with the National Socialist regime was integral, so social discord was a concern that was medicalized.[68] Given that the Reichsuniversität Straßburg was a teaching hospital, we see this focus on social problems quite clearly in student theses. One such example is that of Helmuth Will's thesis, which examined the prevalence of nervous disorders in children in Strasbourg.[69]

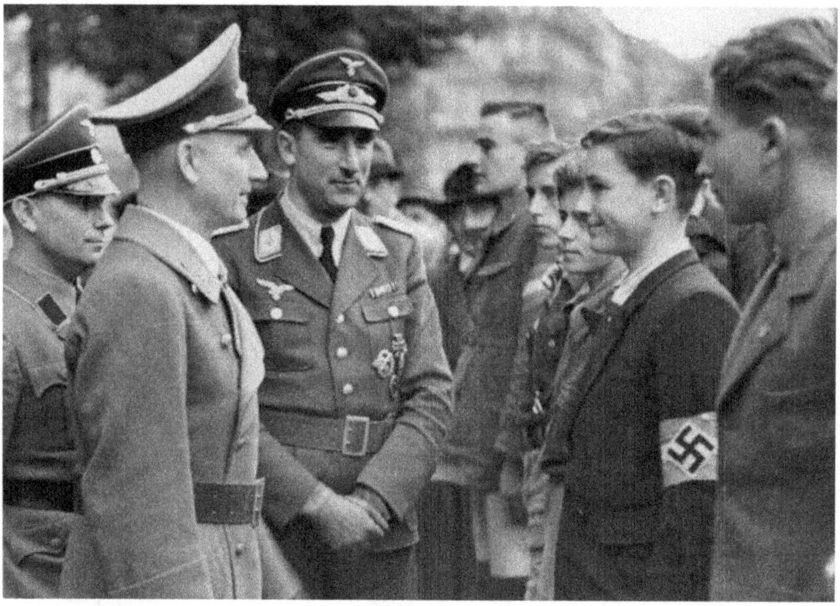

Fig. 3.4. Gauleiter Robert Wagner meeting the Hitler Youth in Straßburg.[70]

This was also examined by Dr Hofmeier in his article, 'On the Hereditary Condition of Infectious Diseases of the Nervous System', published in *Monatsschrift für Kinderheilkunde* in 1938.[71] Will noted that while the prevalence of infectious diseases had reduced in the children's clinic from the time of the old Reich, the current social conditions had a considerable influence on the health of children:

> The children [...] are not any more exposed to infectious diseases than the children in the old Reich. The social conditions, however, seem to have a significant impact against this. In any case, the majority of the children with nervous disorders, such as those in our medical histories, are from the lowest circles of society, many are illegitimate children.[72]

Another student, Werner Hessling, noted that illegitimacy was a risk factor for higher infant mortality that must be monitored.[73] Hofmeier noted that the majority of the children who were placed for adoption were illegitimate and this was of concern given the lack of knowledge about their hereditary disposition.[74] Hofmeier also suggested that the acceptance of the wider social group was necessary before adoption took place as a child had an important part to play in social life, therefore their hereditary disposition should be of considerable importance to the family and community. He also agreed that illegitimacy increased the risk of health-related issues as 'the married mother naturally takes more care in her pregnancy' and illegitimate children were less likely to be breastfed.[75] Hofmeier acknowledged the importance of environment to the development of children, and therefore advocated the adoption of children and their education and integration to the community, in alignment with Nazi ideology, which focused not only on eliminating those not considered to be beneficial to the Volk, but also the development of children who were deemed of worth to the Volk.[76] It is possible that Hofmeier's focus on poor social conditions and 'illegitimate' children in Strasbourg was due to concerns about the integration of occupied Alsace into Germany and the issue of 'selecting' infants for adoption that could be influenced by inadequate early environmental conditions. This clearly links to his involvement in the Lebensborn home across the border in Nordrach, as he was trying to ensure the adopted children were of 'good stock'.

These concerns about illegitimacy and health appear in the Reichsuniversität Straßburg children's clinic patient files. One example is the case of Karl Heinz B., who was admitted to the clinic in June 1943 with congenital syphilis.[77] Although he was almost one year old, he was considered to be underdeveloped, with dirty skin, multiple abscesses, and boils.[78] His parents were young, and unmarried, and his family was listed as Reichsdeutscher. As a result of this combination of social and medical factors, tests were conducted on Karl Heinz for diphtheria bacteria and for syphilis, and his mother was also tested for syphilis.[79] An X-ray examination was conducted and determined that there were no changes to his bones in conjunction with congenital syphilis.[80] He was treated with luminal, a common medication for anxiety and seizures, cibazol, which was a standard antimicrobial medicine, and spirocid, which was prescribed for congenital syphilis. He was then released and told to return in two months for further treatment, which illustrates the capacity for follow-up care and outpatient treatment. Due to his status as Reichsdeutscher, follow-up care and medication was provided, illustrating that they considered him capable of improvement and possible adoption. This is an indication of how, within paediatric care under National Socialism, so-called asocial characteristics could be overlooked providing one could be useful to the Volk, and how both medical care and medicalized exclusion coexisted.[81]

Length of Stay in Hospital and Outpatient Process

Many patients required consistent specialist care for chronic conditions or follow-up examinations that could only be provided in a hospital setting. As a result, a number of patients in the children's clinic received outpatient care as a condition of their release from the clinic. Considering the outbreaks of poliomyelitis and other illnesses such as scarlet fever, it is understandable that many patients had to be accommodated in the children's clinic for a longer term. One hundred and twenty children were treated in the clinic for less than one week, while the majority of children stayed in the clinic between one week and one month (302 patients).[82] Of the 869 legible cases, eighty-nine children died while in the clinic, which was a remarkably low mortality rate for the era, given the prevalence of epidemic diseases and the limited access to antibiotics. There were twenty-six children who stayed at the clinic longer than six months, illustrating the possibility to provide longer-term in-clinic care to certain patients. In the case of nineteen patients, a date of release from the clinic was never recorded. This may indicate that the patient stayed in the hospital until the return of French administration, or they may have been transferred to another clinic.

It appears that the capacity in the Poliklinik of the children's clinic was quite substantial. The nurses from the German Red Cross noted how staffing would work when clinic numbers reached 5,000 per year.[83] Unfortunately, the patient records from the outpatient facility of the Poliklinik have not yet been found, but based on the records of patients who were hospitalized to the wards of the children's clinic, many of those attending the Poliklinik would have been follow-up appointments after their discharge from the hospital ward. This is evident in the case of Irene E., a three-year-old Alsatian patient, who was admitted in May 1943. Her notes state that she had felt unwell for three days and was admitted to hospital.[84] She was extensively tested, and found positive for scarlet fever, but as she was experiencing no complications, she was discharged on 30 June 1943. The condition for her release was her attendance at the Poliklinik in ten days to conduct a follow-up X-ray and further tests.[85] It appears that there was also consideration given to preventing the spread of disease in larger families as an incentive to monitor children as outpatients, and by extension the social cohesion of the family to the new National Socialist regime. This highlights the importance of protecting the future of the regime through the social cohesion of the young generations, while simultaneously ensuring that they were fit, healthy, and free from disease.

Impact of Hospitalization on Children

In the case studies already discussed, most children were admitted for what can be classified as standard paediatric care. The illnesses they present with are those that one would expect in this era, and the medications and treatments used were standard practice at this time. While this is useful to contextualize how patients were treated, this data cannot explain the experience of patients during their hospitalization. This normal paediatric care began to be examined more critically in the 1940s as doctors began to advocate for increased visits from parents to alleviate what would later be considered separation anxiety, particularly in younger children, who could not be prepared for the experience of hospital care.

Medical treatment continued to be provided throughout the war. Based on patient care and parents' reactions to this period of hospitalization, a scientific film produced by Bowlby and Robertson entitled *A Two Year Old Goes to Hospital* highlights the concerns of some parents in this era. The aim of this film was to investigate the behavioural changes in a child as a result of separation from their parents during their stay in hospital.[86] While this film emerged after the war, it was filmed as a result of information garnered from paediatric patients during the war, and can therefore help to examine the patient experience. The film presents time-stamped snapshots of a two-year-old patient named Laura, who appears to withdraw into herself as well as engage in uncharacteristic behaviours. Despite the moving nature of *A Two Year Old Goes to Hospital*, critics suggested that it was a poor representation of childhood distress in hospital.

> [As] it should be said that the value of films as an argument in scientific debates is limited [...] they can only show that a certain phenomenon may take place, not that it generally takes place, and under which specific circumstances. Thus, Robertson's opponents could always argue that Laura, her parents, or the hospital were somehow exceptional and that other children in (other) hospitals were perfectly fine. At any rate, they could argue with some justification that it remained far from proven that her distress was caused by the separation.[87]

It must be noted that the desire for parents to remain with their children during their stay in hospital was not influenced by doctors or research; this push to have access to their children while in the ward pre-dated the investigation into separation anxiety. In the cases of Andreas N. and Erich M., among others, their parents believed their visits to be important to the health and wellbeing of the child.[88] From the letters that remain, it appears that parents had to formally request to visit their child or request their release, illustrating that such visits were not standard practice.[89]

Indeed, parents visiting their children in hospital, and communication with the family about their child's care, was impacted by factors such as nationality, financial status, and social class.[90] That parents wanted to visit their children indicates that the move to include parents was driven by families prior to this scientific film proving the impact of separation on patients. One such example in the context of National Socialism is found in the Kinderfachabteilung Spiegelgrund in Vienna, where Günther K. was admitted to the clinic because his neighbours declared the family to be 'asocial' in 1943.[91] He was not given any definitive diagnosis, but was kept in the clinic because the staff stated that 'it is necessary'. While he was in the clinic, his mother wrote extensively to the staff, demanding to know why he was sent to an institution when he had no psychological problems. His mother wrote: 'I would like to inform you that we want our Günther back [...] We demand our child. It is sad that the child is being made out to be feeble-minded [...] But that you have our child as a guinea pig [...] and make him out to be insane, we won't allow it, he's our flesh and blood. We won't rest until we have the child.'[92] Despite these requests to visit, and to take her son from the clinic, this was repeatedly refused by the doctors, and Günther was killed in June 1944.[93] In this case, it is possible that the determinant of the family as 'asocial' impacted their ability to see their son, as they were not considered a positive influence. This can be viewed in contrast to parents who were granted visitation of their children. In some cases, children were even discharged from hospital by their parents against medical advice, but this was only pending the social status of the parents. It must also be noted that Kinderfachabteilungen operated differently to normal clinics, in that visits could sometimes be abruptly ended or prevented with the intention of killing the patient.

Children admitted to the hospital of the Reichsuniversität Straßburg were impacted by this separation from their parents. As Michael Jeremy Jolley notes, nurses were usually the ones tasked with implementing new medical ideas. One of these ideas was that parents would upset children by their visits, and were generally ignorant of medical practices and so would jeopardize the children's progress.[94] It is unknown if class affected the frequency or amount of visits allowed in the children's clinic in Strasbourg, but more correspondence and information concerning the health and welfare of the child was provided to families of an upper-class background, as in the case of Francine L.[95]

Play is an indicator of the normal hospital conditions that existed in the children's clinic in Strasbourg. It was also used by doctors as an indication as to how the child was feeling; children who were profoundly unwell were of course unable to interact with toys, but approaching their release date, patient files often record their engagement in play. The impact of play on the experience of hospitalization in children is explored by Barnes in his 1995 article. He states that 'play is an essential characteristic of childhood [...] but in hospital it has a very special significance. It is a means of assisting coping strategies, thus reducing anxieties, and offering the child a medium through which information can be given.'[96]

This appears to have been a concern in the Reichsuniversität Straßburg too, as Hofmeier ordered more toys for the children's clinic in time for Christmas.[97] Play as an indicator of improvement in health is also noted in many cases, including that of Francine L., where her mother notes her playing and jumping in bed as an indication of her improved health and mood.[98] Playing was considered important at the Reichsuniversität Straßburg, as this was included in the patient notes as an indicator of improvement. The case of six-year-old Ulof H. illustrates this, as it was noted on his medical chart that on 30 June he had begun to play with his toys again following his admission for scarlet fever.[99] At the children's clinic, playing signalled that the patients were feeling better and could engage with their caregivers at the hospital. Conversely, the lack of interest in play was pathologized in Kinderfachabteilungen, as evidenced in the example of Hans Asperger, where this was thought to indicate a lack of social cohesion.[100] This in turn marked the desire to play with other children, or the lack thereof, as conspicuous, suggesting a child who might not be willing or capable to engage in work for the benefit of the Volk. This often led to such children being diagnosed either as 'asocial', or incapable of work (arbeitsunfähig), either of which could be conspicuous. This can be seen in the case of Johann B., as mentioned earlier, where the lack of interest in toys indicated a lack of social cohesion, which in turn was medicalized. The presence of accounts of children playing with one another and with toys in the Reichsuniversität Straßburg indicates the stability of the clinic in the midst of political upheaval, where it continued to function as a normal paediatric clinic, albeit one that was predicated on National Socialist ideology. Prioritization of providing for the 'worker and soldier of tomorrow' is evident here, as the clinic tried to influence parents to include their children in the regime. German families who engage with the regime are afforded better treatment, so Germanization is incentivized through this hierarchical system based on nationality, the class structure, and principles of racial hygiene.

Conclusion

The Reichsuniversität Straßburg hospital, in the first and second eras of its existence, was in a rather privileged position, as there does not seem to have been a shortage of medical equipment, food, or hospital beds. That being said, the war impacted medical care in other ways, as children were admitted to the hospital (although not the children's clinic) for injuries sustained during bombing raids, although it is not clear that clinical outcomes for routine cases worsened.[101] This chapter has shown that the patients treated at the clinic came from diverse social and national groups, but their medical care was tailored accordingly. Such a hierarchical healthcare and social system pre-existed National Socialism, and helped to justify the stratification of patients, not based solely on health insurance contributions, but on social cohesion, and on racial and regional belonging.

This chapter has also highlighted the impact that the war had on patient care, and has shown that because of its central ideological position, the clinic continued to be supplied well throughout the war. Despite this, issues such as separation from parents and aerial bombing can be seen in patient files, as well as increased Germanization of the population. Who was asked for their consent—and why—has also been a focus here, further solidifying the social and racial structures that dictated patients' ability to determine their own medical care. This issue will be further addressed in relation to forced labourers in Chapter 6, revealing how the directors at the Reichsuniversität Straßburg were selected in part based on how well they could impart this segregation and Germanization of the population through selective medical care.

CHAPTER 4

Paediatric Patients in Psychiatric Care

> Many of the involved and most active psychiatrists were the leading reform-oriented psychiatrists of the time [...] But the reality was different [...] An unfounded therapeutic optimism led to the loss of sight of those where they failed. The most disabled persons, the most difficult patients, should always be in the centre of our attention and care.[1]

The previous chapter established how patient treatment was based on a hierarchy of nationality and social cohesion. This only pertained to the treatment of physical illnesses, as mental illnesses and neurological problems were treated in the psychiatric clinic. In this chapter, the findings from the previous chapter will be used as a lens to examine the treatment of children in psychiatric care. This chapter focuses on an in-depth analysis of the children who were treated in the psychiatric clinic of the Reichsuniversität Straßburg, examining the illnesses they presented with and their treatment. I consider particularly the themes of nationality, duration of hospital stay, patient transfer and advocacy, intelligence testing, and modern therapies in the 127 patient files. Following a statistical overview of the clinic, a number of patient files are examined in case studies. These case studies illustrate different aspects of treatment in the clinic, including patients who travelled large distances (from as far away as South Africa) for treatment at the institution, patients who had extensive medical treatment, those who were readmitted, and those who died in the clinic. Some patients from Eastern European countries, such as Ukraine, Russia, and Poland, are examined through case studies to illustrate how their treatment differed from those who were German citizens or Alsatian. This primary-source analysis is then foregrounded in a discussion of current literature on the topic to help illustrate the findings.

Background of the Psychiatric Clinic

The Reichsuniversität Straßburg had a large psychiatric clinic, with over 400 beds available.[2] From 1941 to 1944, there were 127 children admitted to this clinic; a small proportion of the more than 3,000 patients (the rest of them being adults) who were treated there.[3] Dr August Bostroem was appointed as head of this large psychiatric clinic in October 1942, and served as its chair until his death in February 1944.[4] He was born in Gießen in 1886 and studied in Freiburg and Gießen.[5] He completed his medical studies in 1909, and went on to serve as a doctor in the First World War.[6] He was promoted to professor and practised in Leipzig, Munich, and Königsberg, publishing extensively on psychiatric practice.[7] Bostroem became a member of the NSLB in 1934, and joined the NSDAP in 1937, which was integral to his nomination as chair of psychiatry in Straßburg.[8] His publications focused on the topics of psychosis, mania, syphilis, encephalitis, and catatonia, among other illnesses.[9] Professor Bostroem died of a heart attack while he was the director of the clinic in Straßburg in February 1944, and the position of director passed to Dr Nikolaus Jensch, who had previously worked in the clinic and was its interim director from 1941 until Bostroem's appointment.[10]

Dr Jensch served as the director of the clinic again until it was evacuated in November 1944.[11] He was born in Breslau in 1913 and became a member of the NSDAP and SA in 1933.[12] Dr Jensch was best known for his study on castration, entitled *Investigations into Emasculated Moral Crimes: Collection of Psychiatric and Neurological Individual Presentations*, published in 1944.[13] Both Bostroem and Jensch appear to have been highly regarded in the psychiatric community at the time, judging from both their appointment to the Reichsuniversität Straßburg and by the referral letters of patients. In many cases, the referral of patients from other hospitals made specific reference to being unable to treat the patient any further, but that Jensch or Bostroem would be able to treat them or provide some degree of clarity on the case.[14]

Dr Bostroem wrote a letter to Dr Johannes Stein, dean of the medical faculty, on 25 January 1944, proposing to create a separate psychiatric department exclusively for the care of children, as the current clinic was designed for adults.[15]

> The solution I envisaged would have the advantage that the children and young people in question would not need to be accommodated in the psychiatric clinic, which always causes certain difficulties in view of the known prejudices. The planned

> space in the clinic would then only be used for the observation of strong devious and criminal or other young people, and this separation from the others would prove to be desirable.[16]

From his letter, it is unclear where exactly the institution was planned to be, or what capacity the new facility would have.[17] This may be part of the reason for the transfer of paediatric patients to Stephansfeld Heil-und Pflegeanstalt as a result of a lack of space or due to the intention to move children from the adult psychiatric facility.[18] Dr Stein replied that he approved of Dr Bostroem's solution as it would be an excellent advantage to the city and to the care of children who were more 'difficult'.[19] This letter also highlights that in the third era of the Reichsuniversität Straßburg, heightened suspicion of the population and possible 'devious' elements were to be kept in a more controlled environment, reflecting the increase in National Socialist fervour and the impact this would have on medical care. The care of the 127 children at the adult psychiatric clinic was not the intention, and plans were being made for a more suitable arrangement for paediatric psychiatry.

So-called Euthanasia of the Mentally Ill

As Alsace was part of Germany while the Reichsuniversität psychiatric clinic was operational, it is vital to understand the background of psychiatric care in Germany in this era.[20] In Germany during National Socialism, psychiatric care included two seemingly contradictory facets: on one hand, new therapies such as insulin shock, cardiazol, electroshock therapy, and new methods of imaging such as pneumoencephalography and improvement in barbiturates led to increased capacity to identify and treat some mental illnesses.[21] However, on the other hand, this 'therapeutic optimism' existed alongside the belief that one could only help those who were curable by killing those who could not be cured, thus 'eliminating life unworthy of life'.[22] This process happened in many different stages and methods, some of which overlapped, but they must be considered independently; these are Aktion T4, known as 'decentralized euthanasia' or 'wild euthanasia', and 14f13. This targeted elimination happened in a series of different systemic processes. The first was 'child euthanasia', whereby physically and mentally handicapped children under the age of sixteen were killed from 1939. This began with the Reich Committee for the Scientific Registration of Serious Hereditary and Congenital Diseases organized by the Chancellery of the Führer via a registration form. Questionnaires were voluntarily filled out from 18 August 1939 by doctors and nurses, indicating infants and children under three years old who had mental or physical disabilities, who would then be admitted to a special children's ward for observation. This was later expanded to include those between three and sixteen. At least 5,000 children were murdered in thirty special children's units.[23] These questionnaires would be sent to the Reich Committee for the Scientific Registration of Serious Hereditary and Congenital Illnesses.[24] Karl Brandt, Werner Catel, Hans Heinze, Hellmuth Unger, and Ernst Wentzler, as part of the Kanzlei des Führers (KdF), determined if each child would live or die, with a cross marked on their file if they were to be transferred to an extermination centre.[25] Despite letters to the institution inquiring as to the welfare of their children or requests to see them, the parents often only heard that their children had died after they had been murdered, and even then, the cause of death was always fictitious.[26]

The second form of 'euthanasia' was Aktion T4, which was the decentralized killing of psychiatric patients from 1940 to 1941. This happened in conjunction with 'child euthanasia' but targeted adults, and determined who would live or die based on an external committee. Hitler wrote a letter in 1940, backdated to 1 September 1939, allowing the killing of patients, and phrasing it as 'mercy killing for the incurably ill'.[27] However, this was not open legislation in a decree or law, so it was effectively secret except to the staff of killing centres and hospitals. These murders took place in dedicated killing centres, where patients were transferred, often very far from their original hospitalization location, with the intention that the family members would be unable to trace their loved ones. This officially ended in 1941, in part due to public protest.[28] It must be noted, though, that this idea of 'mercy killing' for those who were ill was not entirely unknown to the public, as popular propaganda films like *Ich Klage An* illustrate.[29] The protagonist in the film had multiple sclerosis, and her husband, who was a doctor, killed her with an overdose of medication. He was put on trial, but the murder was framed as a romantic and merciful act, while her death was framed as a duty because she was an invalid. Crucially, she chose to die, when those who were killed as part of T4 did not get a choice, nor were their families informed. Nonetheless, this film received wide support from the public.

The third form of 'euthanasia' was Sonderbehandlung 14f13, where concentration camp prisoners who were unable to work were gassed to death in the former Aktion T4 killing centres (prior to the construction of gas chambers in concentration camps) between 1941 and 1943.[30] This marked an important change in the purpose of concentration camps, moving from a brutal source of forced labour to dedicated killing centres for entire social groups, based on this Sonderbehandlung 14f13.

The fourth form was 'decentralized euthanasia', sometimes called 'wild euthanasia', which was the killing of psychiatric patients and the physically disabled after Aktion T4 formally ended, via barbiturates, starvation, neglect, and injections of medication from 1942 onwards.[31] This therefore existed simultaneously with many other forms of 'euthanasia', and was not decided by a panel of doctors, but usually by an individual doctor or nurse who knew the patient and treated them personally. This also could happen in any institution, not necessarily in a dedicated killing centre. It is important to consider, though, that although the majority of the victims of these different 'euthanasia' campaigns were psychiatrically ill, or mentally or physically disabled, a large number of people were merely considered social outcasts of the Nazi system, being 'diagnosed' as asocial, or not given a diagnosis at all, but institutionalized and eventually killed.[32]

While this system was implemented across Germany and its occupied territories, it is important to note that there was a considerable degree of regional variety. This can be seen in the Reichsuniversität Straßburg, which did not complete these registration forms for children. As mentioned in the previous chapter, this is possibly due to financial reasons, as doctors received payment based on the treatments provided, but if patients were transferred elsewhere, they would not be paid. This is not entirely unprecedented, as Roelcke illustrates in the example of a district in Franconia, where 75% of doctors were Nazi party members, but two-thirds of them did not submit a single report.[33] Doctors were dependent on patients for their practice, and filling in these forms was entirely voluntary, with no negative consequences for not reporting patients.[34] It appears that this was the case in Straßburg too, where doctors did not report or refer paediatric patients to external institutions due to their diagnosis, apparently for financial reasons and also to encourage assimilation of the population into Germany. Despite this lack of adherence to the 'euthanasia' programmes for children in Straßburg, ideas of supposed 'worth' to the Volk, as well as some patients being considered more curable than others (and thus more worthy of treatment and care), are evident from the patient files. The financial aspect of patient care cannot be underestimated; Hilde Steppe notes that 'ballast existence' was used as a phrase to indicate that the individual could not contribute financially to society, and thus would require care.[35] Diagnoses went hand in hand with economic concerns in terms of how a patient was viewed, as those with more 'curable' illnesses who could pay for their care were often afforded the most modern treatment and therapies possible, while those who could not afford to pay, or those with an 'incurable' diagnosis, would not be provided with the same care.[36]

Diagnoses of Paediatric Patients in the Psychiatric Clinic

Certain diagnoses, as noted by the 1939 Reich Committee for the Scientific Registration of Serious Hereditary and Congenital Illnesses, were recorded and considered incurable, and subsequently targeted as part of the T4 campaign.[37] This specifically concerned congenital malformations, learning disabilities (then called 'mental retardation'), idiocy and mongolism (Down's syndrome), blindness and deafness, microcephaly, hydrocephaly, limb malformations and spinal column malformations, paralysis, and spastic conditions (e.g. Little's disease).[38] Therefore, the question of what diagnoses were found among children admitted to the psychiatric clinic in Straßburg is particularly important.

The most common illnesses were psychopathy (twenty-four cases), followed by epilepsy (twenty cases), and schizophrenia (fifteen cases). There were, however, diagnoses that were not included in the graph due to only occurring once in the 127 cases.[39] The youngest patient admitted to the clinic was two years old, while the case studies included in this chapter are patients up to the age of seventeen; most patients in the clinic were, of course, adults. The age of patients on admission does not appear to have influenced their diagnosis or outcome.

Of the 127 child patients admitted to the psychiatric clinic in Straßburg, four died in the clinic. The number of patients who perished in the clinic is low considering that those cases died from quite severe conditions, such as Sydenham's chorea, and two cases of encephalitis.[40] In Heidelberg children's clinic, even by 1943, children were still dying for no clear reason with seemingly no interventions to prevent death.[41] This was not the case in Straßburg. While four patients died in the clinic in Straßburg, there is no indication that these were not natural deaths. Furthermore, some patients presented with illnesses that would have been targeted either with a lack of treatment in accordance with determinants of behaviour, willingness to work, as well as pejorative descriptors of mental state such as 'stupid' in other hospitals, but they continued to be treated in the clinic in Straßburg.[42]

Duration of Stay for Paediatric Patients

The length of stay in a psychiatric institution, along with capacity to work, as well as behaviour and other factors, was one of the main indications as to whether a patient would be targeted for 'euthanasia'.[43] Examining the patient data for the length of stay in the clinic can help to determine what care they received. The majority of paediatric patients sent to the psychiatric clinic were admitted for a short period: 14.6% of patients stayed less than one week, while 38.7% stayed between one week and one month. One example of a short stay for psychiatric reasons is that of Melitta S. from Mannheim, who was thirteen years old. She was sent to the Kinderlandverschickungslager in Klingenthal by her parents in 1944. Melitta suddenly fell ill while there and was referred to the psychiatric clinic by her teachers at the camp.[44] In their letter on 8 February 1944, they note that she was behaving in a peculiar manner, finding it difficult to write and experiencing weakness in her right arm and leg.[45] These symptoms were worrying enough to write for a referral to the psychiatric clinic in Strasbourg, to which she was admitted and diagnosed with Sydenham's chorea.[46] Dr Jensch noted that on admission, Melitta had uncontrollable movements of her limbs, and despite their treatment, her condition worsened rapidly and could not be improved with medications.[47] A blood test was performed at the Staatliche Medizinal-Untersuchungsanstalt, where Wasserman, Meinicke, and Kahn tests were all negative.[48] On 13 February, Melitta died following extensive treatment with cardiazol, traubenzucker, sympatol, and other medications.[49] Dr Frank from the Hitler Youth wrote to Dr Jensch requesting the autopsy report.[50] In March, Dr Jensch wrote to Dr Holscher in Mannheim, informing him of the findings from the autopsy, stating that endocarditis rheumaticia was found, which may have contributed to her death, although Syndenham's chorea was the official listed cause of death.[51] This case illustrates the capacity for urgent treatment, as telegrams were exchanged to prepare for the immediate transfer of the patient to the clinic from the camp. It also highlights the degree of involvement that Hitler Youth organizations had with children, as well as correspondence between doctors and the Hitler Youth. As the class system and the influence of nationality as mentioned in the previous chapter applied to psychiatric cases too, we see in this case particularly privileged treatment including follow-up diagnostic confirmation, information being sent to the parents via the Kinderlandverschickungslager, and extensive medications.

While the majority (53.3.%) of patients stayed for a short period, many children required longer-term care: 21.9% of patients stayed in the clinic between one month and six months, but 2.2.% of patients remained in the clinic for more than one year. One reason for this is that a number of the longer admission cases did not appear to be curable, or indeed treatable with any degree of improvement.[52] It is possible that the release of some patients was prompted by overcrowding, as many were released without any indication of an improvement in their condition, or a possible ongoing treatment plan or referral general practitioner for their outpatient care.[53]

One example of a longer-term patient is that of seven-year-old Susanna D., who was born in Johannesburg in South Africa.[54] Her father returned to Germany with his daughter following his wife's death, seeking treatment for an unknown psychiatric issue. He believed a mishandling of her birth had led to mental difficulties, including her inability to speak.[55] She was diagnosed with 'idiocy' in the psychiatric hospital in Graz, but they stated that they could do no more for her and transferred her to Straßburg, where they recommended Dr Bostroem for her treatment.[56] This case includes correspondence between Susanna's father and the clinic, including lengthy letters both from the clinic and from her father to Dr Jensch concerning the patient history of his daughter as well as concerns about her welfare. Such letters are an important source in indicating how families were involved in patient care.[57] The issue of social class comes to the fore in the case of Susanna D., as it was noted in correspondence with the clinic that the family were paying privately for her care, and that her father was an engineer.[58] It appears that his status as a well-educated and wealthy man influenced their correspondence about his daughter's treatment, informing him in advance of every step they took, but also possibly influenced the treatment they gave his daughter. In correspondence with her father, the Heil- und Pflegeanstalt für Epileptischen in Kork addressed the patient as 'Susi', which was how her father addressed her.[59] Given that in German, it is standard to use the more formal 'Sie' and the patient's surname, rather than an informal 'Du', or in this instance a patient's nickname, this is particularly significant in showing the social status of the family, and how the doctors treated her. She was treated with thyroxin, indicating that the doctors had diagnosed a thyroid issue that may have been a cause of her slow intellectual development.[60] Such treatment came about as a result of the discovery of phytelkenourea (PKU) in 1934 by Ivar Asbjørn Følling, wherein the enzyme phenylalanine hydroxylase is lacking and so excess phenylalanine cannot be broken down by the body, leading to mental developmental delays.[61] This treatment was based upon contemporary medical practice and therapeutic optimism in their ideas about the influence of nutrition and hormones on mental capacity.[62] The treatment was stopped after some time as it appeared to have no effect on her condition; they described the girl as a 'slightly mongoloid idiot', and determined that there was no more they could do for her.[63] Susanna was not given a definitive release date, so it is unknown how long she remained at the institution—illustrating that if a patient could pay extensively for their care, they were retained in the clinic for a longer stay.

Transfer of Patients

As in other institutions at the time, longer-term care was most often provided in another institution, such as Stephansfeld Heil-und Pflegeanstalt, where sixteen paediatric patients were sent from the Reichsuniversität Straßburg psychiatric clinic. Parents sometimes formally requested a transfer to Stephansfeld, indicating some degree of patient advocacy in the case of children, as evidenced in the case of Karl F. in 1941.[64] Karl was seventeen years old on admission to the psychiatric clinic in November 1941 and was diagnosed with schizophrenia.[65] He was referred by Dr Burckel from the hospital in Hagenau, on the wishes of his parents, who stated that they would cover the costs of his treatment in the psychiatric clinic in Strasbourg.[66] In his patient history, it was noted that he had been sick for a number of weeks with suspected osteomyelitis, and therefore numerous blood tests were performed which all came back clear for syphilis.[67] In March 1942, Dr Frey replied to a letter from Karl's parents stating that 'as to their wishes', he would be sent to Stephansfeld.[68] The reasons for the parents' request to send their child to Stephansfeld are not noted, but they wrote a letter in March stating:

> We agree if they want to take our son there, as we had arranged yesterday. Karl also agreed straight away. He only wants to get out of the clinic, hoping for freedom [...] We hope for the best. Please be so good as to let us know what day you think Karl should be taken away. I would like to be with him, and I still have a bill to pay, so I can take care of everything right away.[69]

It would appear that the parents were informed about the patient's condition and had some degree of influence over the treatment of their son, and indeed that Karl was informed about this change. Weindling, Czech, and Druml discuss the issue of 'informed consent' in relation to patient files and experimentation, noting that while some form of informed consent existed in Germany from 1900, this cannot be considered equivalent to current perceptions of consent, given that the focus was on individual doctors' integrity rather than the patient.[70] Kaelber states that parents were often consulted about the transfer of their children but given false information and hope of a more modern treatment that would never materialize.[71] This led to them actively putting their children into these institutions after the appeal of doctors for them to consent to this 'expert treatment'.[72] In this instance, Karl's parents were convinced that the transfer of their child was the best course of action. In the patient's transfer letter to Stephansfeld Heil-und Pflegeanstalt, Jensch noted that Karl was being transferred for 'hebephrenie', which illustrates the evolution of diagnoses and differing opinions as each patient's case progresses.[73] The issue of visitation was raised in Karl's case, as his mother requested permission to see him on Sundays. This request was granted, but it is evident that this permission was not common practice, as the director replied a day later, stating: 'Exceptionally you get permission with your two sons to visit Karl one Sunday in the month. You will submit this letter to the institution administrator as a passport.'[74]

Visitation was allowed, albeit rarely, as it appears to have been only once a month. Requests for release of patients were also answered in this case, as the family wrote an extensive letter in June asking for their son to be returned home. The letter stated that Karl spoke about missing the garden and wanted to go home, while the family raised their concerns about him being alone.[75] Their request was denied, with the response stating that Karl was 'still irritable at times, generally shows a repellent behaviour and is also often unclean. So we will have to wait a little longer.'[76] On 30 July, Emil F. signed his son Karl out of Stephansfeld Heil-und Pflegeanstalt, declaring that 'I [Emil] undertake to give him [Karl] [...] the necessary supervision in his family', and paid the 3.30 RM per day for his care.[77] It must be noted, however, that this document requesting his release is different to informed consent records prior to patient treatment. It is possible that the level of care given to Karl F. correlated to the wealth of his family and their ability to pay the high cost for his care, as well as their concern for the welfare of their son and their desire for him to return home.

Nationality and Staatsangehörigkeit

Among the 127 paediatric psychiatric cases, their nationality was predominantly German and Alsatian.[78] This information was garnered from the 'Staatsangehörigkeit' column in the patient file, which often listed 'Volksdeutsche' or 'Deutsch' even if they were from another region.[79] There is a marked difference in recording and thus possibly in treatment between those who were considered German or Alsatian versus those who were from Eastern Europe. This difference in treatment or in the amount of detail given in the patient record is not noted in Northern Europeans, which implies a certain degree of difference in treatment in the clinic. Those who were considered foreign, or those who were deemed 'minderweritg' or 'inferior', were given significantly less detailed notes about their treatment and almost non-existent information about medical procedures, consent, or contact with their family.

Emilie G., an Alsatian patient born in Colmar, was admitted to the clinic in March 1942, aged fifteen.[80] Emilie's admission record noted that she enjoyed playing with dolls, had a good appetite and only quietened when she was with her mother.[81] Her care was paid for by the Ortskrankenkasse Straßburg Familienmitglied health insurance, and it was remarked that she suffered some weakness and paralysis due to Little's disease, following an unspecified brain injury early in life. Emilie's reflexes and muscle tone were considered to be very poor, and she was subjected to multiple tests including a blood test and lumbar puncture.[82] A pneumoencephalography was performed, which involved the removal of cerebrospinal fluid and its replacement with air in order to see the brain more clearly.[83] While this method of imaging was more effective than X-ray alone, it was a very painful procedure and often led to side effects such as nausea, vomiting, severe headaches, neck stiffness, and tachycardia.[84] The pneumoencephalography procedure was verbally explained to the parents, as Emilie's father signed permission for this to be done, noting that he understood the procedure.[85] Dr Haessler stated that there was very little air in the subarachnoid area, and noted considerable abnormalities in her brain.[86] This illustrates that there was correspondence between the parents and the clinic, and that they were consulted to some degree as to her treatment and tests performed. On 25 March, the child was noticeably agitated, as she 'has considerable anxiety/fear and cried for her mother even though she had been given half an ampoule of scopolamine Ephetanin and Eukodal. Tolerated everything well. No complaints at all in the evening.'[87]

In March, Emilie was sent home, followed by an admission to an unspecified sick children's home, although it is not evident that any improvement was seen in her symptoms during her stay. She was admitted to the hospital a second time from 18 April to 14 June 1942, but despite this readmission, she was sent home with no apparent improvement in her condition.[88] It is notable that consent from her parents for this painful procedure is present in this case, but absent in cases of foreign patients, indicating that class and nationality may have impacted consultation in medical care.[89]

This discrepancy in the size of patient files between German and Alsatian patients and those from Eastern Europe is especially evident in the case study of Watzlaff Z., a patient who was admitted to the psychiatric ward on 9 March 1944, aged sixteen.[90] His admission form states that he was admitted in order to determine if his condition was genuine epilepsy, or if his seizures were due to a different underlying cause.[91] His Staatsangehörigkeit, or nationality, was Ukrainian but his home was listed as Kork Baden Umsiedlungslager der Volksdeutschen Mittelstelle, a form of resettlement camp for those deemed to be 'Germanizeable'.[92] This illustrates that Watzlaff was part of the resettlement programme under the propaganda campaign of 'Heim ins Reich'.[93] His placement in Kork was organized by the Einwandererzentralstelle, a central office for immigration and resettlement based in Litzmanstadt, who wrote to the Reichsuniversität psychiatric clinic requesting Watzlaff's admission.[94] While Umsiedlungslager camps were organized for the processing of 'Fremdvölkischer' and the Germanization of the population in Alsace, it is unknown why a Ukrainian was moved to an Umsiedlungslager camp so far from his original home.

Watzlaff's record indicated that although his nationality was Ukranian, he was considered 'Aryan'.[95] His psychiatric assessment therefore was part of the process of becoming 'Volksdeutsche', which involved the medical assessment to ascertain if they were of healthy blood and would not pass on any heritable diseases as a new German citizen.[96] While it is the only such case that was found among the children's psychiatric files, it can be ascertained that the Reichsuniversität Straßburg played a role in the certification of people from the East and from Alsace as 'Volksdeutsche' through their medical examinations in the hospital.[97] In Watzlaff's case, he was kept at the hospital for three days, and was not treated with electroshock therapy, or with any psychopharmaceuticals or other medications. He was therefore released three days after admission, back to the Umsiedlungslager, after determination that his seizures were not due to epilepsy. It is not noted what other reason could be given for his seizures, and it is possible he was sent to the hospital for close observation rather than treatment purposes.[98]

In the case of other foreign patients, much less information is provided in their patient record, indicating the prioritization of patients who were ethnically German or those who could pay higher sums for their healthcare.[99] Their files do not include correspondence with parents, and often do not list an address. It is notable that for foreign patients, their duration of stay appears to be quite short, in most cases less than one week. This is in contrast to wealthy German patients, whose stays were considerably longer, possibly for financial reasons, with a more in-depth record and considerable communication with the family about their care.

Modern Therapies

Electroconvulsive therapy was a new technique in the 1940s, with many hospitals employing earlier methods of treatment such as cardiazol, a circulatory stimulant drug that can induce convulsions, and insulin therapies.[100] Cardiazol therapy was considered to be the more modern treatment by the 1937 international congress on cardiazol, insulin coma therapy, and deep sleep treatments at Münsingen.[101] Cardiazol had notable disadvantages, including unpredictable dosages, a feeling of dread in the patient, and alarming seizures, but was claimed to have more potential to cure patients.[102] Conversely, insulin therapy had been in use for longer, but risked irreversible coma.[103] While both of these treatments were in use at the psychiatric clinic at the Reichsuniversität Straßburg, as well as in other psychiatric institutions of this era, it is notable that they also adopted the most modern treatment of electroconvulsive therapy as early as 1942, even in children.[104] A medical thesis entitled 'Disturbances of Thought in the Electroshock Treatment of Manic Depressive Spectrum of Mental Illness' was completed by Rudolf Gross in 1944 in Straßburg on the topic of the therapeutic range in electroconvulsive therapy, but focused solely on the treatment of adults in the psychiatric clinic.[105] Although formal research focused on adults, many children received electroshock treatment in the psychiatric clinic, in conjunction with older therapies such as insulin and cardiazol.

Georg E., a sixteen-year-old boy from Metz, was treated with electroconvulsive therapy following his admission in August 1942 for catatonia.[106] Georg was in a good state of general development, and was able to understand questions to which he gave monosyllabic answers.[107] Dr Loewenbruck sent him to Straßburg from Metz by ambulance due to the severity of his mental illness, which was affecting his ability to work.[108] What is notable about this case is not that he received electroconvulsive therapy, but that during his seven-month stay at the clinic, he was subject to forty-five courses of electroshock treatment, with increasing voltage, often with only one day between courses.[109] This number far exceeds the research done in the clinic by Rudolf Gross in 1944 on the therapeutic range of ECT. Georg's course of ECT began on 4 July in Metz, before he was transferred to Straßburg; he fell into a stupor and was said to be significantly quietened.[110] By 15 August, there was still no noticeable improvement; Georg hallucinated frequently and refused to stay in bed.[111] On 14 December, cardiazol treatment began, electroconvulsive treatment ended, and luminal and asoman were administered.[112] On 8 February 1943, Georg had a seizure, although what type and the duration

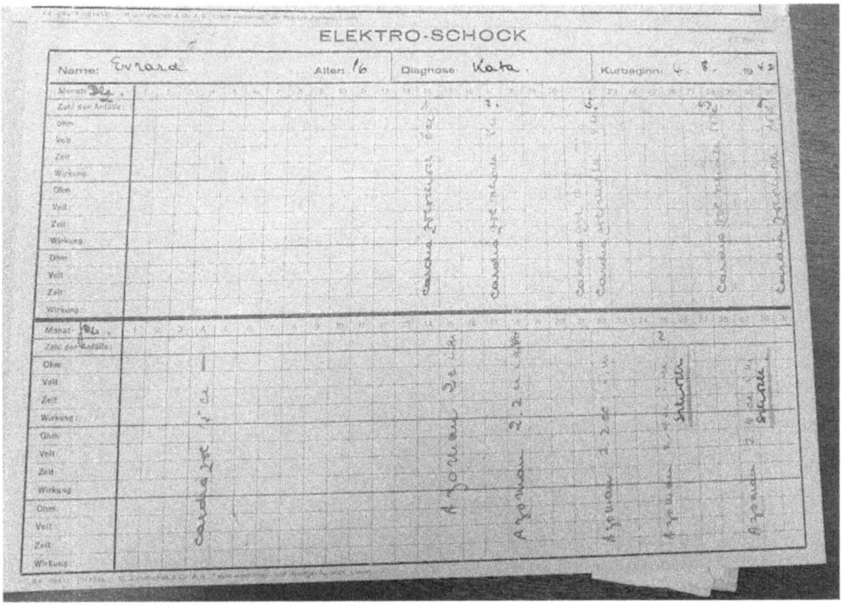

Fig. 4.1. Electroshock chart for Georg E., 1942.[113]

is not listed. By 27 March, Dr Jensch stated that the patient had fully recovered due to the use of electroconvulsive therapy and recommended the use of luminal and abasin to Dr Loewenbruck to manage the condition. This extensive use of electroshock on a young patient, in conjunction with pre-existing psychopharmaceuticals, is notable, as many other patients received similar treatment, though not to the same extent or duration. Despite the seeming severity of his mental health issues, he was not transferred to Stephansfeld or any other Heil-und Pflegeanstalt, but transferred home to be managed, if necessary, through psychopharmaceuticals.[114] Similar releases are shown in many other paediatric psychiatric patients' files, whereby their condition was managed by a local doctor at home through psychopharmaceutical means.

Intelligence Testing

Intelligence tests were used extensively in psychiatric evaluation in the psychiatric clinic in Straßburg, as well as in many other institutions of the time, particularly in children from the 1930s onwards. [115] In 'The Importance of Heredity for Paediatrics', Dr Kurt Hofmeier advocated the use of the Binet Bobertag Norden test to confirm the diagnosis of idiocy in children, and explained that while idiocy could be inherited, it did not necessarily always run in families.[116] Hofmeier also estimated that based on this test, approximately one million people should be admitted to a Hilfsschüle.[117] Valentine Hoffbeck states that under the Nazi regime, the Hilfschulen that were ideologically intended to help care for children who could not keep up with traditional schooling.[118] The focus on the potential of some children with psychiatric illnesses did not detract from the emphasis on educability and reform; if a child was noted to be beyond such reform or was 'uneducable' ('bildungsunfähig'), they were not granted the same treatment and were often simply transferred to other institutions.[119] Crucially, the ability to work, patient behaviour, length of stay in the clinic, and race, along with disability and psychiatric diagnosis combined, determined a patient's treatment (or lack thereof); the perception of their value to the regime and community regarding their hereditary value was important, and informed the kind of treatment they would receive.[120]

Questions included in the Binet Bobertag Norden test in Straßburg went from easier questions on general knowledge such as 'How many days in a year?' and 'How many hours in a day?' to geographical and historical questions such as 'What is the capital of France?' and 'Who was Bismarck?'[121] More difficult questions were included that required verbal reasoning such as 'Explain the phrase "hunger is the best sauce"' and more complex mathematical questions such as '130-58' and '12x13'.[122] There were also a number of more ideological questions, including 'Make a sentence from the following words: "Soldier, War, Fatherland"' and 'What enemies did we have in the World War?'[123] Based on their results in this test, the patient would be assigned an intelligence age and thus diagnosed with idiocy or imbecility or feeblemindedness, which could determine if a child was sent to a Kinderfachabteilung. A.F. Tredgold, a British doctor who analysed mental development and educability, criticized intelligence tests, stating that they require certain basic skills in order for the patient to perform them.[124] This is evidenced in the intelligence test provided from the psychiatric clinic, as it required a good knowledge of German, some degree of literacy, cooperation, and socially defined important facts such as knowing who the 'enemies' were in the First World War.[125]

Renatus T., a ten-year-old Alsatian patient, was subject to Binet Bobertag Norden testing in the clinic during his admission for juvenile psychopathy. Despite his stay of two months at the hospital, there are very few notes on the treatments given to the patient but a considerable number about his general appearance and character. Renatus was described as a 'tender, pale boy with freckles' in good health when he was admitted to the psychiatric clinic on 5 July 1944.[126] His admission file details his home life and this appeared to be the reason why he was admitted. He was deemed small for his age with considerable dark circles under his eyes.[127] The doctors noted that he was an only child whose stepfather had died at the front and was being raised by his mother, who 'was very rough and brutal with [Renatus]'.[128] Renatus had to sleep on a bench three times as she had not returned from her job at the postal depot to open the door to their house, and he regularly had to wake up and go to school by himself without breakfast.[129] On 6 September 1944, he was sent to Stephansfeld, and the reason for his transfer was: 'Summary: a 10-year-old boy from an asocial family who is inadequately looked after by his mother and who has become conspicuous due to a lack of intelligence [...] Admission to Stephansfeld.'[130]

This concern with his 'asocial' family situation is given considerable attention, as this term was used to convey socially disruptive behaviour that was burdensome to the community and could be inherited.[131] His daily routine was detailed along with the contents of his home, which may reflect the consideration of environmental issues contributing to his lower than average mental age (estimated to be between eight and nine years old).[132] Doctors from the psychiatric clinic describe his home: 'in terms of order and cleanliness left much to be desired. The apartment facility is very poor.'[133] This comment highlights the social aspect of the doctor–patient interaction, as doctors observed a living environment that was considerably different to their own. Their concern also emerges from a social hygiene perspective as they believed that environment could negatively influence childhood development. Although his behaviour is described as erratic (he lit a fire under another patient's bed),[134] the doctor noted that 'he has sparkling eyes during his intelligence exam'.[135] In August, following Renatus's intelligence test, Dr Kessler noted:

> This deficiency has a particularly unfavourable effect due to the fact that his intellectual disposition is only moderate [...] In the intelligence test according to Binet Bobertag Norden, he lagged considerably behind the performance that can be expected from normally gifted child of the same age.[136]

That intelligence testing could determine possible educability was of considerable importance, as children who were thought to be 'educable' were often treated with the intention to make them useful to society.[137] In the Reichsuniversität Straßburg psychiatric clinic, the mental age ascertained from Binet Bobertag Norden testing influenced what degree of 'idiocy' was diagnosed.

Glimpses of the Patient Voice

The patient's voice is particularly evident in the file of Josef L., an Alsatian patient, who was admitted in October 1942, aged eleven.[138] His manners are noted, as he appeared to enjoy the clinic, and he thanked everyone for everything there.[139] Blood tests were performed on Josef that were sent to the Staatliche Medizinal-Untersuchungsanstalt where Wassermann, Meinicke, and Kahn tests were all found to be negative. On 21 October, Dr Hagdorn at the ear, nose, and throat (ENT or otolaryngology) clinic in Straßburg examined Josef and noted that he had a significant septum deviation, although Dr Hagdorn stated that Josef was too young to be operated on for this issue.[140] While there are no direct quotes from him, his passions and life outside of the clinic are particularly poignant, as he drew a detailed picture of the gates of the hospital, and of what appears to be a Messerschmitt Bf 109F-4 on the back of a racial purity chart.[141]

In Josef's patient notes, the doctor described him as a talkative child, who was quite good at school, particularly at painting, as he wanted to be a painter when he grew up.[142] Josef had no friends at school and always played alone. In contrast to Johann B., mentioned in the previous chapter, this lack of desire to play with other patients is not pathologized, probably as he is Alsatian, so he is considered 'Germanizeable' and therefore allowed to draw in the anticipation that he will be useful to the Volk. Josef also spoke fondly of his

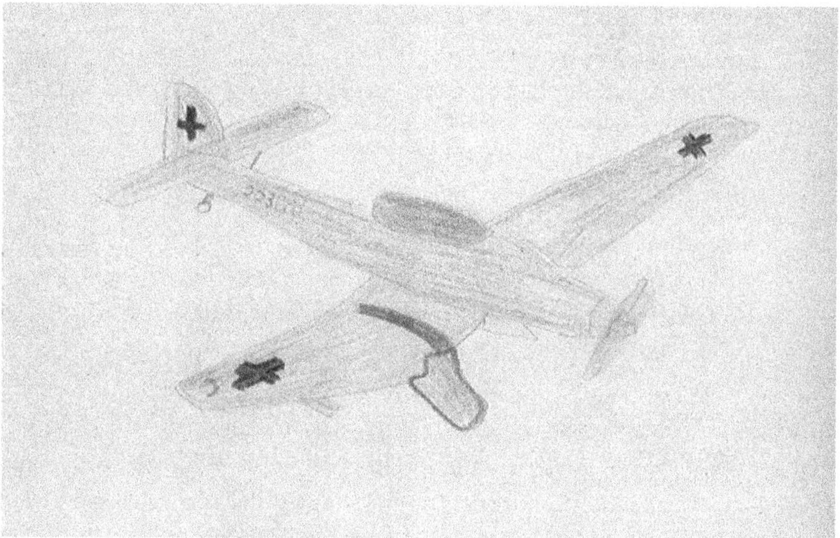

Fig. 4.2. Drawing of a Messerschmitt Bf 109F-4 by Josef L., 1942.[143]

evacuation from Strasbourg to Toulon, as he enjoyed the seaside and the horses there (his favourite animal).[144] These details are notable as they do not convey any medical information, yet they are meticulously recorded in his file, thus giving an insight to the patient voice. His drawing of the gates of the hospital may indicate that Josef could leave the hospital grounds, or at least show the importance he placed on being admitted to, and eventually leaving, the hospital.

Impact of the War on Psychiatric Patients

Patient records, such as those of Josef L., can illustrate how the war affected the mental health of the people in Straßburg. Patient files can also convey the feeling of uncertainty and persecution that was evident in those who

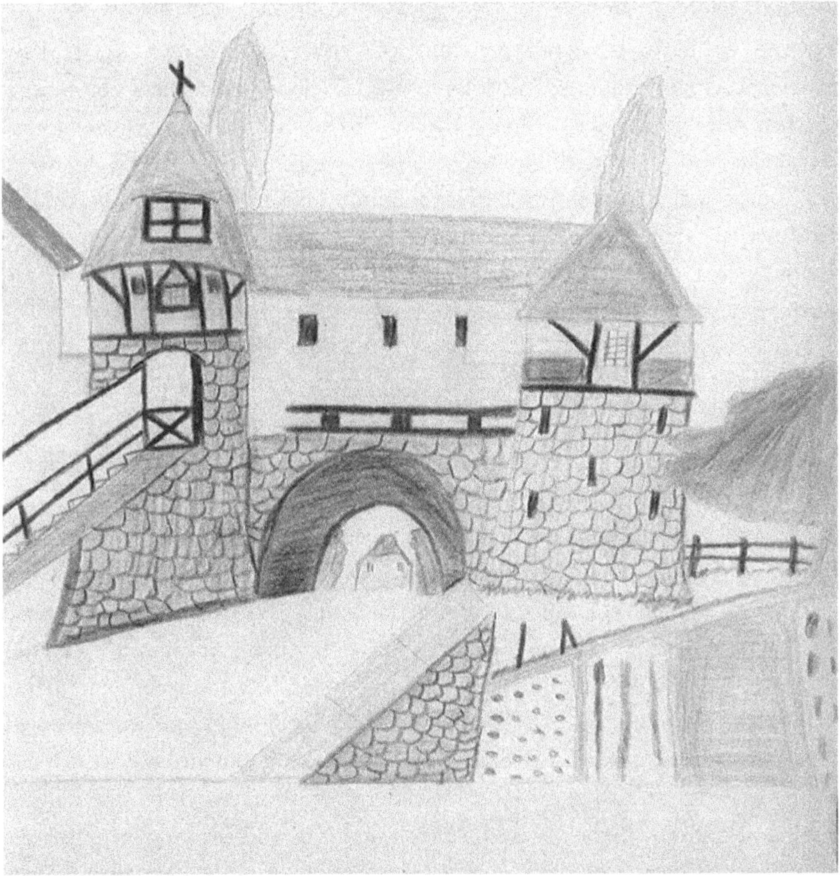

Fig. 4.3. Drawing of the Porte de l'Hôpital gates leading to the hospital by Josef L., 1942.[145]

were not considered a threat to the German system. This is particularly evident in the case of Johann H., an Alsatian patient, who was diagnosed with schizoid psychopathy and admitted to the psychiatric clinic on 20 September 1943.[146] Johann had no typical childhood illnesses and performed well in school. He became a locksmith's apprentice after school, which he enjoyed.[147] In his first instance of psychopathy, he became anxious when people spoke, and he would not speak or listen to music.[148] During Johann's second attack of psychopathy, he repeatedly said 'is someone down in the basement', highlighting his growing paranoia in a further example of the patient voice in a medical file. His third instance of psychopathy led to his hospitalization, following his belief that the Gestapo were following him and that he would be taken to the Schirmeck concentration camp.[149] This illustrates that the general population was aware and afraid of the concentration camps, albeit not the full extent of what occurred there.[150] Doctors note that this was a significant cause of anxiety and fear in the patient, leading them to diagnose 'Verfolgungsideen', or a persecution complex.[151] Johann was given electroshock therapy seven times, and Wassermann, Meinicke, and Kahn testing returned a negative result.[152] Dr Bostroem noted that outpatient treatment took place for four weeks, while he received electroshock therapy.[153] It appears that this electroshock therapy helped the ongoing fear and anxiety that Johann felt, as following his discharge and outpatient treatment he was not readmitted to the hospital.

Conclusion

The case study analysis demonstrates that there were multiple ways of treating patients in the clinic, which largely depended on the patient's illness, social status, and nationality, as well as the involvement of the parents. Nationality played a role in medical care, as those patients who were from Eastern Europe have much less information in their files. This also may be a result of language and the ability of the doctor and patients' families to communicate effectively, leading to barriers in understanding the treatments being provided. The influence of social class and wealth on the treatment of patients appears through the case of Susanna D., in which the doctor refers to the patient by a nickname, and corresponds extensively with the parents.[154] This issue of social class, wealth, discrimination, and occupation politics is explained in more detail in Chapter 3 on paediatric files, and should also be considered in psychiatric cases. Many parents signed consent forms illustrating consultation about their child's treatment, but to what extent they were informed about the risks, consequences, or alternatives to this treatment is unknown.[155] This is especially pertinent in the numerous cases of pneumoencephalography.[156]

In many cases, there was no apparent communication between the parents and the patients, particularly with patients that were not considered to be German. Some parents communicated directly with the clinic, requesting permission to visit their children, writing for information and updates on the welfare of their children, and also informing the clinic of patient histories and the condition of their child prior to admission.[157] The parents had some degree of agency in the treatment of their children, based on requests by parents for their child's transfer to another institution or to be cared for at home. It is also evident that not all transfers were the result of clinical intervention by doctors at the psychiatric clinic; the parents could be consulted and did have a say in the matter.

In the case of children admitted to the psychiatric clinic in Straßburg, they were not subject to euthanasia, or indeed to registration of disabilities or psychiatric illnesses as children were in Germany, despite being admitted with the same diagnoses. This was not the case for adult patients of the psychiatric clinic—as noted by Lea Münch—who were transferred to the killing centre at Hadamar.[158] It is unclear why this occurred with adults, but not with the child patients admitted to the same clinic. For paediatric patients, there was a financial benefit in retaining patients rather than referring them to other institutions, as Roelcke notes, in that the doctors depended on some long-term relationships with patients to ensure their practice continued.[159] Furthermore, the intention to assimilate the occupied population through provision of healthcare and surveillance of their mental condition may have been a reason for the lack of child transfers to killing institutions. The psychiatric clinic did provide innovative treatments such as electroshock therapy to the children who were admitted, which is indicative of a clinic focused on recent therapeutic standards and new treatments.

CHAPTER 5

Medical Research and Student Theses on Paediatrics

> The revised medical curriculum included newly designed lectures in racial hygiene, the science of heredity, population policy, military medicine, and the history of medicine. These subjects seemed particularly suitable for promoting Nazi ideology to medical students [...] lectures were intended to provide medical students with 'an understanding of both the written and unwritten laws of the medical profession and of doctors' ethics.' The revised curriculum [...] was intended to explicitly create a 'new type of physician' [...] This physician would be trained to internalize and then implement the Nazi biomedical vision of a homogeneous and powerful people (Volk) in his daily work. It involved shifting the focus of ethical concern and medical care away from the individual patient and toward the general welfare of society or the people.[1]

Elie Wiesel stated that 'it is impossible to study the history of German medicine during the Nazi period in isolation from German education in general'. This chapter will address the medical education provided in the Reichsuniversität Straßburg from 1941 to 1944.[2] It will shed further light on the students of the medical faculty, the research that was conducted at the children's clinic, and the use of children as research subjects. The treatment of patients by student doctors was of course heavily influenced by their education; how a student is taught to view a person is ultimately how they will treat a patient. The study of paediatrics, and of subjects pertaining to children and the use of the Kinderklinik in student research, will form the basis for this chapter. The theses completed by students will be examined to ascertain how Nazi ideology influenced their research and education. Many of these theses were conducted under the supervision of Dr Kurt Hofmeier in the paediatric

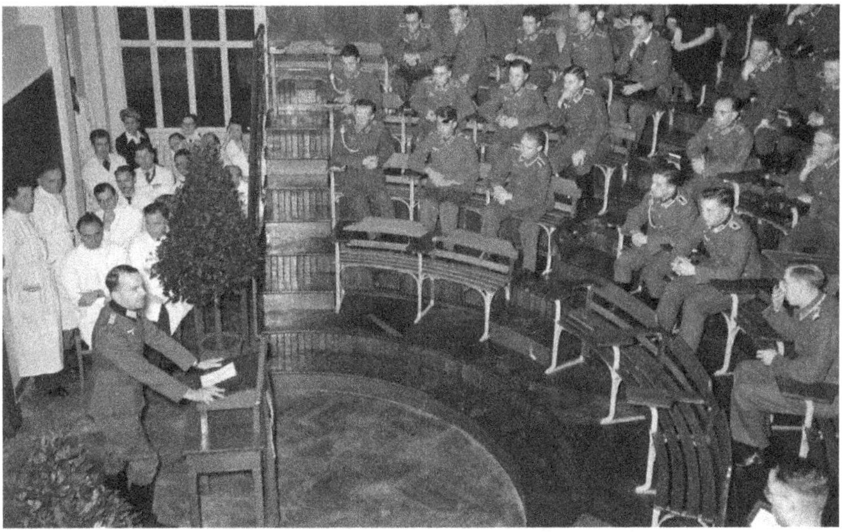

Fig. 5.1. Wehrmacht medical students at the inaugural lecture of Dr Johannes Stein in 1941 at the Reichsuniversität Straßburg medical faculty; behind him stand the directors of the medical faculty.[3]

clinic, but those that used children as subjects of study for their research, and those theses that were completed in conjunction with the paediatric department, will also be considered. The theses produced by the students in the Reichsuniversität Straßburg can help to understand the normal functioning of the clinics and the networks they had with one another, while also explaining how this version of 'everyday research' compared to other universities in Germany and internationally during this period.[4]

Ethics in Medical Research: Richtlinien

In order to examine medical research and the teaching of students during the era of National Socialism, it is helpful to first understand what ethical codes existed to regulate research. The Reichsrichtlinien, or *Richtlinien für neuartige Heilbehandlung und für die Vornahme wissenschaftlicher Versuche am Menschen* (Guidelines for Advanced Therapeutic Treatment and for the Conduct of Scientific Experiments on Human Beings) were a set of guidelines, established by the Reich health council and the minister of the interior in 1931.[5] These guidelines were drafted following the Lübeck tragedy of 1930, in which seventy-five children involved in a trial of a BCG (Bacille Calmette–Guerin) vaccine died as a result of contaminated vaccines.[6] However, the intention of the subsequent guidelines, and later the Nuremberg code, was not to forbid all research. It was imperative to situate the guidelines so that they were a workable compromise between the need to test modern medicine on humans, and the individual rights of the research subjects, in order to balance the risk for the individual taking part and the risk posed to society by not trialling a treatment or cure.[7]

The Guidelines for Advanced Therapeutic Treatment and for the Conduct of Scientific Experiments on Human Beings differentiated between therapeutic research and innovation, and scientific experimentation with no therapeutic benefit. For each of these, a different type of consent was required, and it also considered the different consent policies for minors. In the case of a new or innovative therapy, the patient had to be provided with all the information about the procedure in advance, and then give their consent. One caveat was that innovative therapy was allowed in the case of urgent care that could save the life of the patient, or prevent their suffering, where it was not possible to ask for consent beforehand. In the case of non-therapeutic experimentation, this was forbidden in all cases where informed consent had not been explicitly given. For patients under the age of eighteen, all experimentation was forbidden if it could constitute a risk to their health. Furthermore, animal experimentation had to be conducted before the same experiment was trialled in humans, to prove a baseline of safety and efficacy that justified the continuation of the experiment.[8]

If a doctor had signed the Richtlinien, they were obliged to follow it; however, the guidelines did not have the far-reaching power of a law to dictate what doctors should do.[9] Doctors were required to sign it at the beginning of their contract in public hospitals, but if their work was conducted outside public hospitals, then they did not have to sign the Richtlinien.[10] If a doctor had not signed these guidelines, they were not bound by these suggestions. The idea that these guidelines were not circulated widely appears to be false, as the main medical periodicals published the guidelines in 1931, including the most widely read medical journal at the time, the *Deutsche Medizinische Wochenschrift*.[11] Even during the Nazi era, it appears that the guidelines were disseminated, as they were present in medical textbooks, such as the introduction for medical students in *Der Ärzte-Knigge* by Carly Seyfarth.[12] However, as Volker Roelcke notes, just because they were widely circulated does not mean they were widely read, or taken seriously.[13] The issue of who exactly these guidelines applied to during the Nazi era is one of contention. In literature from the era in medical journals, in the case of research on human subjects, there appears to be very little discussion of the guidelines, or of a process of informed consent. This appears to be emulated in medical theses in the Reichsuniversität Straßburg and in the University of Gießen. In the case of human subject research, no reference is made to the process of informed consent, even in German subjects.[14] As established in the previous chapter, in the Reichsuniversität Straßburg, some first-class German patients have parent-signed consent forms for specific procedures, such as pneumoencephalography.[15] This is indicative that doctors were aware of the importance of patient consent, but not all patients were necessarily allowed to review their options and consciously consent to procedures. These consent forms did not explain to parents what procedures actually entailed, so this would not meet current standards of informed consent, as purely naming the procedure assumes knowledge on the part of the patient or their next of kin. Other consent forms in patient files just give consent for pneumoencephalography and 'associated procedures', illustrating that the standard of consent varied considerably from patient to patient. It is important to note this difference before examining case studies in Straßburg; German first-class patient files often have signed consent forms from their parents, but many other patient records contain no evidence of signed consent. This is not to say there was no consultation with parents; there may have been verbal consent, but the disparity between wealthy German families and other patients is evident. It must also be considered that with some patients, there may have been some logistical difficulties, particularly in wartime, to obtain consent, to call parents, have them visit, or sign forms with enough time to perform procedures in patients. That being said, telegrams and phone calls were always available with the local general practitioner—who may have admitted the child in the first place—who could often act as a proxy next of kin, affirming the diagnostic procedures of the doctors in the Reichsuniversität Straßburg.

Medical Education During National Socialism

Carola Sachse notes that German medical research and the German system of academic medicine was considered the world leader at the beginning of the twentieth century.[16] This is evidenced by considerable collaboration between Germany and prestigious research institutes such as the Rockefeller Foundation in the USA.[17] Indeed, many American and European scientific institutions were founded on the same principles as German medical schools. German scientists were integrated into international research, particularly when it comes to eugenics, which was a compulsory part of the German curriculum; however, it is important to note that eugenics was seen as a modern scientific theory in many countries in this era. As part of the prevalence of eugenics, the health of the national community was foregrounded, and took precedence over individual rights. André N. Sofair and Lauris C. Kaldjian describe this process of integration: 'This quasi-mystical image, later incorporated into Hitler's world view, portrayed society as an organism with its own health and identified human beings as functional or dysfunctional parts of a larger whole which became the focus of medical education.'[18]

Medical students were taught not only how care should be provided, but also to whom they should provide this care. Medical ethics during the Nazi era foregrounded the protection of the Aryan race and the German people, but conversely also aimed to 'eliminate' elements that could be seen as a threat to the 'Volk'. Lectures on ethics focused on the responsibility of the physician to the state, to their profession, and also to their patient. Due to the disruptive effect of the war on medical studies, many universities did not have ethics lectures in the final years of the conflict, or the third era of the Reichsuniversität Straßburg, as noted in the introduction. As Henry Sigerist noted, prior to Adolf Hitler's rise to power, the concept of individualism in healthcare in Germany was already fading in favour of the greater German Volk.[19] Ethical debates in German medicine pre-dated the Nazi regime, as figures such as Rudolf Ramm, Karl Binding, and Alfred Hoche focused on the good of the individual versus the good of the Volk.[20] There was extensive debate about the ethics of human research and the responsibility of the profession, but not so much about the day-to-day ethics of patient treatment.[21] Leonardo Conti wanted to install loyal Nazi party members to teach students, as most of them had joined the party before 1933 and were firmly in line with the ethics and ideology of the Nazi party. This led to the biased nature of ethics education for medical students from the outset, along with compulsory lectures on eugenics, racial biology, and other ideologically motivated areas of study.[22] Edmund D. Pellegrino states that 'ethical teaching has to be sustained by the ethical values of the larger community'.[23] Medical students were taught by people who actively advocated for the sterilization and extermination of the sick, with a strong basis in racial science and eugenics, so this was reflected in the syllabus, and, in turn, in the students' work.

As Reis, Wald, and Weindling state, the 'potential for abuse of power is inherent to medicine', and as a result, the teaching of medicine must recognize the decisive role that medical professionals had to play in the Holocaust.[24] Medical students are socialized to report to their superiors and do as they are told, in a very similar manner to soldiers.[25] Students during the Nazi era were called upon to do their 'duty' and were surrounded by social reinforcement of the ethics they were being taught. This is seen, as mentioned earlier, in the Alte Kämpfer appointed as clinic directors, such as Kurt Hofmeier, who encouraged the Nazi salute and wore his Wehrmacht uniform under his doctor's coat every day. In this way, it is conceivable that these students would carry out experiments based on what they saw on a daily basis as they emulated their professors and their peers.[26] It must also be noted, however, that clinical education is inherently necessary in any system of evidence-based medicine, and this vulnerability of patients potentially becoming research objects was no more likely in German medical education than in any other medical education.[27] Studying medicine, by its nature, is highly competitive; in an atmosphere of compliance with these ideals of duty and hierarchy, and state-sanctioned euthanasia, eugenics, and sterilization, it can be understood how medical students during the Nazi regime were indoctrinated. Sue Black notes that physicians, by their nature as trained professionals, are given permission to act in ways that would be criminal for the general public. She gives the example of dissecting a cadaver, which was once considered criminal but in the interest of furthering medical knowledge has become common practice.[28] Such medical exceptionalism in the view of advancing medical knowledge led to the perception of ethics and consent as secondary to the aim of increasing medical knowledge.[29]

Medical Education at the Reichsuniversität Straßburg

Those choosing to study medicine in the Reichsuniversität Straßburg were subject to a number of regulations. In applying for a place, the student had to attach a certificate to confirm their 'Aryan' identity that would be submitted to the dean of the university and the ministry for education (*Reichsministerium für Wissenschaft, Erziehung und Volksbildung*).[30] They also had to provide a letter of good character from the police—this naturally excluded those who were openly critical of the Nazi regime. This also applied to students in the Wehrmacht, as they had to supply this documentation when they joined. This political loyalty was often sworn under duress in occupied regions, as was the case of Alsatian students in the Reichsuniversität Straßburg. Of all medical theses in the Reichsuniversität Straßburg medical faculty, 9.6% were submitted by Alsatian students, who wrote their theses in German.[31] Of these twenty-eight Alsatian students, twenty of them remained after the war, but in order to regain their doctorate, they were required to repeat their medical thesis in French. Regarding the total number of students, the highest number in the Reichsuniversität Straßburg was in the 1942/1943 winter semester, when 620 students studied medicine. In the 1943 summer semester, 39% of all medical students were members of the Wehrmacht, while the highest number of medical students in total was recorded in summer 1944, with 1,683 enrolled medical students. Strasbourg seemed to have fewer female students than other universities, with only 7.8% of medical theses submitted by women, while the average for Germany was 29.8%.[32] In total, 292 medical theses were submitted to the Reichsuniversität Straßburg, of which thirty-three were conducted under the supervision of Dr Hofmeier in the children's clinic, almost twice the number previously identified by Patrick Wechsler in 1991. This is a significant finding as it confirms that producing research was the aim in founding the Reichsuniversität Straßburg, as it ranks seventh in terms of the most theses produced during the war out of twenty-four medical faculties in Germany at the time. In contrast, the Reichsuniversität Posen only produced two medical theses, while the Reichsuniversität Prag recorded sixty-seven medical theses.[33] This places the Reichsuniversität Straßburg firmly as the most productive medical faculty of the annexed territories, which had considerable ideological importance, and eighth of all universities in Greater Germany at the time.

As was standard, a number of students had external experts sit on their doctorate panel for supervision. Many students also travelled from other universities to complete their studies in Strasbourg, indicating that the Reichsuniversität Straßburg was well integrated into the German university system, with cooperation between departments and universities.[34] After the war in 1946, the medical, dental, and veterinary education of the universities of Leipzig, Halle, Jena, and Erlangen were examined by Colonel Robert M. Zollinger, Colonel Francois H.K. Reynolds, Lieutenant-Colonel George F. Jeffcot, and Captain Hans Schlumberger, and a report was then published by the US Department of War and the Navy, which had commissioned this work.[35] While this report did not directly concern the Reichsuniversität Straßburg, it shed some light on the manner of medical teaching in similar institutions during the Nazi regime. Issues such as consistent air-raid sirens requiring complete evacuation to air-raid shelters meant a loss of several hours of lectures, and these classes were not usually rescheduled. In 1944 in Strasbourg, the electricity network, water pipes, and the psychiatric clinic building had to be reconstructed due to bomb damage; this lack of basic facilities had a considerable impact on teaching practices.[36] Zollinger also noted that the number of enrolled students was difficult to decipher, given the transience of the students. In the Straßburg medical faculty, students who were members of the Wehrmacht were given preference on entry to medical studies; the number of medical students increased from 1,212 in 1943/1944 to 1,683 in the 1944 summer semester. However, with medical units of the Wehrmacht being moved across the Rhine in 1944, students moved to other faculties in the German Reich.[37]

The number of students at the Reichsuniversität Straßburg increased year on year despite these interruptions; the 1941/1942 winter semester had 896 enrolled students, while 1943/1944 boasted 2,270 students.[38] Based

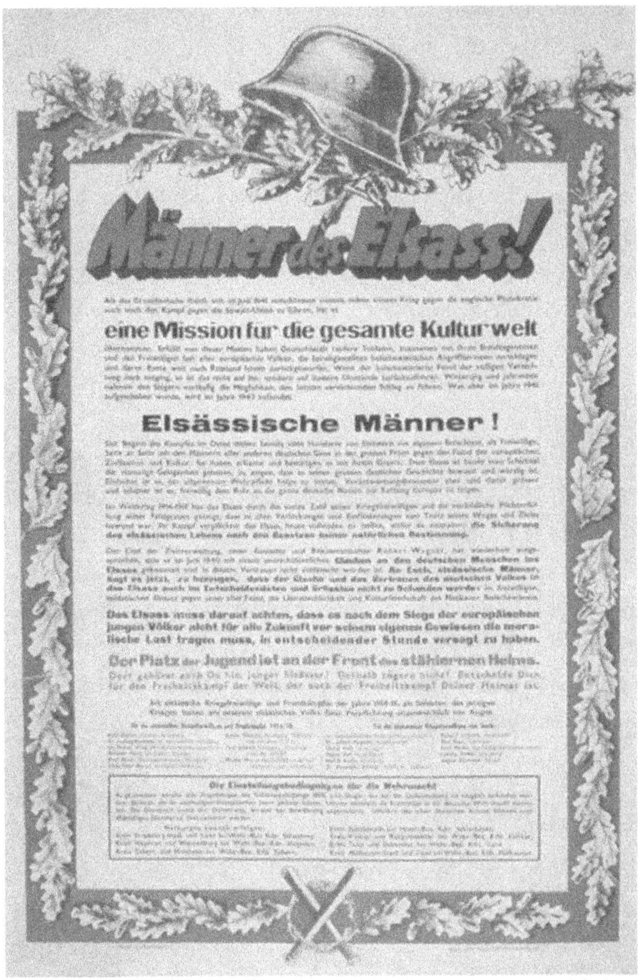
Männer des Elsass!
eine Mission für die gesamte Kulturwelt
Elsässische Männer!
Der Platz der Jugend ist an der Front des stählernen Helms.

Fig. 5.2. Propaganda poster from 1941 urging young Alsatian men to enlist in the Wehrmacht. Message states: 'Men of Alsace, a mission for the entire cultural world. Alsatian men, the place of the youth is at the front of the steel helmets.'[39]

on the 'Lebenslauf', or resumé and biography, of students provided at the back of their theses, many students took breaks in their studies to fight at the front.

Young men in Alsace were urged to enlist and join the war; however, this group formerly made up the majority of medical students. This had a considerable impact on the demographics of the student body, given that obligatory conscription was introduced in 1942. However, one advantage of students enlisting in the Wehrmacht that was not mentioned in the graphic above was that their tuition would be paid by the state. The report by Zollinger on medical education in Germany also remarked on the demographics of medical students in this era and how students comprised three categories. Fit young men who were in the army had their tuition paid by the state for their medical studies; those who were discharged from the army as a result of injury also had their tuition paid by the state; and those who were deemed unfit for military service had to pay their own tuition. This reflected, albeit to a lesser extent, the same hierarchical principles that were in practice for the patients at the Reichsuniversität Straßburg hospital; those who were considered of worth to the Volk were provided with the most, while those who were incapable of contributing to this collective, or were considered 'unworthy' to the German Volk, were not given such benefits. Therefore, adherence to the Reich was used as motivation, initially through incentivization, and later by conscription. The marked increase in women studying medicine is noted in the report, although they had to pay their own tuition fees and fell outside of this proposed structure.[40] A few women progressed to train as specialists, and served in civilian hospitals following their studies, while fit and discharged men could serve in either civilian or military hospitals.[41] Due to a shortage of manpower incurred by the war, women were more highly represented than usual in postgraduate study as the war continued. As mentioned earlier, paediatrics—prior to the eviction of Jewish physicians because of the rise of National Socialism—was one of the medical fields with the most female representation.[42] Despite this increased representation of women in postgraduate study, as noted in the Zollinger report, women were still in the minority.

The duration of medical studies decreased dramatically, from six years initially to just four and a half years by the end of the war. A core reason for this appeared to be the consistent interruptions to study; most of the students had their studies postponed by their military service. Therefore, Zollinger concluded that the real time that students spent in university was about three and a half years.

Medical Theses Conducted Under the Supervision of Dr Hofmeier

In general, students followed the topics of their supervisor quite closely, so it is to be expected that the students in paediatrics addressed similar topics and themes as Dr Hofmeier. Crucially, as these theses were conducted on patients considered incapable of consenting themselves but given a special status of protection under the Richtlinien, the theses on children do not discuss parental consent. This indicates that, at least within the clinic, this was not considered of particular importance. The theses also vary between the standard procedure of anonymizing patients, and providing full biographical information and use of proper names rather than pseudonyms, indicating a lack of a cohesive ethics strategy.

Hans-Joachim Gawantka's thesis, entitled 'The Significance of Pathological Hereditary Factors and Hereditary Diseases in Adoptive Parents and Adopted Children', was completed under the supervision of Dr Hofmeier in 1943. This study focused on the influence of heredity in adoptive children. This thesis is the most ideologically charged of all those that were supervised in the paediatric clinic. In its introduction, Gawantka quotes *Mein Kampf*; this is unusual in a scientific paper, as he uses ideological works that have no scientific basis as the introduction for this work.[43] His quote illustrates how the 'Führer' considers those who make a sacrifice in taking in a poor child to be noble:

> In the Führer's own words as he writes in Mein Kampf 'That it is a sign of the highest nobility and admirable humanity when a blameless sick person renounces giving birth to their own sick child, and gives their love and tenderness to a young poor unknown descendant of his people.'[44]

Gawantka's use of the quote suggests that the adoption of children was considered appropriate, providing this was done within the boundaries of which people were considered hereditarily valuable. Gawantka noted that children were being adopted at an earlier age, which meant not all of their inherited traits were evident. In his thesis, he noted that maternal age was affecting levels of so-called degeneracy, while also going into depth about the importance of early marriages to reduce levels of 'degeneracy' in any prospective children.[45] His thesis also deals with contemporary issues of heritability and eugenics, noting that issues such as alcoholism, psychopathy, idiocy, and mental illnesses were largely heritable.[46] It is these issues that Gawantka cites as being a concern when adopting children, as he notes that heritable traits, such as those for mental illness, would only become evident later in childhood. As a result of this, he advocated the importance of medical examination and of trying to retrieve paperwork for the potential adoptive child before adopting them.[47] This makes it clearer how the link between the Lebensborn home and the paediatric clinic was a crucial one, through the medicalization of belonging to the Volk, as well as the central role of paediatricians in medical examination which determined social inclusion. Ultimately, this central idea was important for sorting the occupied population into two groups: those who were suitable for integration into the German Volk, and those who were deemed medically 'unfit' for assimilation, which was the central role of the children's clinic. Gawantka noted that it was important to adopt racially and hereditarily valuable children and provide them with good parents and homes. This concern with heredity and mental ill health is prominent in normal contemporary research, but the ideological influence on Gawantka's thesis is evident. This research in his thesis was considered to be 'very necessary' by Dr Hofmeier, as it addressed questions posed by the NS Volkswohlfahrt and the Reichsgesundheitsführung on the topic of adoption, as well as addressing the concerns of doctors regarding adoption.[48] For this work, he received a grade of 'good' from Dr Busse, Dr Lehmann, and Dr Hofmeier. While this research can be classified as non-invasive literature research, as it does not directly concern experimentation on patients, it can be considered highly ideological, as it directly references eugenic concerns about the hereditary health of the population and the worth of children.

Wolfgang Wendel's thesis, entitled 'Two Cases of Juvenile Poikiloderma in the Inbred Area of Rimlingen, Lorraine', addressed the diagnosis of poikiloderma, a hypopigmentation disorder of the skin, which can develop over time or can be congenital in nature.[49] There was a significant interest in researching this illness in children to determine a hereditary cause. This thesis was jointly supervised by Dr Hofmeier, Dr Hirt, and Dr Achelis from Heidelberg. This study began in Straßburg, under the supervision of Dr Hofmeier, with research subjects at the children's clinic. However, it was finished in 1945; therefore, the supervision and institutional affiliation changed from Straßburg to the Ruprecht Karl Universität in Heidelberg with Dr Achelis as the co-supervisor. This illustrates how research and study continued following the Straßburg evacuation, and indeed indicates how this thesis could then be adopted in Heidelberg due to the broad interest of the research topics. Wendel's thesis draws heavily on previous research, establishing that the condition was quite variable and usually present in middle age, but he focused on the congenital presentation of the illness from birth. He quoted the unique histological markers of the illness, which appears not to have been his own histological analysis, but rather established through pre-existing research. It appears that Wendel tried to draw links between illnesses, noting how previous cases examined by doctors concluded that there was a link between poikiloderma and syndactyly, as well as malformations of the ear, as established through analysis of research by Thomson, a researcher at King's College London.[50] This illustrates that although much student research at the time was focused on insular themes relating to the political ideology of National Socialism, it still engaged with the international scientific community and cannot be termed 'pseudoscience'.

Wendel noted that the current best practice for treatment was vitamin C and could possibly be due to abnormal endocrine function. This concern with hormone research and its influence in causing disease follows both Hofmeier's research into nutrition and hormones and also contemporary research which focused on underlying causes as well as treatment of illnesses. In the congenital form of poikiloderma, Wendel noted that Thomson had researched differences in bone development of children with the condition through X-ray analysis. Two cases of poikiloderma had been examined in the Reichsuniversität Straßburg children's clinic by Dr Hofmeier and Dr Wendel. The first case noted in his study was of a five-year-old girl named Henriette H., whose parents had brought her to the hospital on 17 July 1942, where she was diagnosed with poikiloderma.[51] Her parents detailed that the child's grandparents, in Lorraine, had a similar skin condition, illustrating a familial link in the development of the illness. It appears that a non-hereditary cause of the illness is also examined, as it was noted that the child's home environment was very clean and airy, with no contaminants present.[52] The child was admitted to hospital for observation, where her general condition was noted to be very healthy, meeting all of the normal developmental milestones. She was sent to the dermatological clinic to be seen by Professor Leipold, who confirmed the diagnosis, and excised a calcified section of skin.[53] He advised Henriette's parents that the best treatment would involve dietary considerations for improving endocrine function, as well as topical treatments with a salicylic solution. He also noted that there were no bone abnormalities yet, but continued check-ups were recommended to ensure her proper development. In discussion with Dr Hofmeier at the children's clinic, it was noted that a second case of a child from the same area was admitted to the clinic. Hofmeier noted the influence of environment on the development of illness, as '[t]he author therefore went on behalf of Prof Hofmeier to the place and ascertained that the location Rimlingen in Lorraine is an area of consanguinity of the greatest extent',[54] illustrating that the condition may be as a result of 'inbreeding' in the racial group, leading to an increased prevalence of this otherwise rare congenital illness.[55] The second case was that of Paulette H., who was admitted to the children's clinic and also appeared otherwise to be a healthy child.[56] A comparative analysis of the two children was done, with a note stating that it would be recommended to follow both girls to adolescence to determine if there would be any dysmenorrhoea or gynaecological problems associated with the condition at the onset of puberty.[57] The thesis followed the comparative analysis of the children, wherein a genetic history table of both of their families was constructed, noting that they had shared ancestors and had a considerable amount of consanguinity.[58] As such, Wendel's thesis came to the conclusion that there was a recessive gene for poikiloderma on the X chromosome and it therefore primarily affected females. Due to this hereditary link, Wendel noted that he could not confirm if the illness was due to a reduced endocrine function.[59] Wendel finished his thesis by thanking Hofmeier for his help and supervision, and noted that the inclusion of photographs was prevented due to conditions of the war.[60] This note of the effect of the war on the production of a student's thesis is notable, as this does not occur in other theses of the paediatric department. Wendel's thesis includes human research on young patients, without apparent informed consent. It is not evident that this treatment was invasive, as it does not appear that the student himself treated the patient, and the only treatment indicated is topical ointment. This research can be categorized as Nazi medical research, given that it is heavily focused on heredity, consanguinity, and the Sippentafel, as well as a contemporary focus on hormones. There is no record of the grade received for this research, nor any evidence of publication of this thesis, so there is no indication as to its reception following completion.

Not all of the theses conducted under the supervision of Dr Hofmeier in the children's clinic were particularly influenced by National Socialism, and one was even referenced into the postwar era. Rosemarie von der Decken completed her thesis, entitled 'Hand-Schüller-Christian Disease in Fraternal Twins', in 1942. This thesis examined one case of Hand-Schüller-Christian syndrome, a rare condition which causes skeletal defects, bone lesions, and diabetes insipidus. Her research examined the difference in illness between monozygotic twins, and discovered a previously unknown hereditary link, as both twins were affected by this syndrome.[61] The children involved in this case study were Daniel and Christine, aged fifteen months at the time of admission to the clinic.[62] They were both referred from the infants home in Straßburg, where they were temporarily staying while their mother was recuperating from polyarthritis and rheumatism, and as they were illegitimate children, there was no one else to take care of them.

Comparative X-rays were conducted on both twins to illustrate the difference in skeletal structure that is evident in this syndrome, and this showed that the disease had progressed slightly further in Daniel, although neither of them had yet developed diabetes insipidus as was expected with this condition. Moreover, extensive patient records on treatments and tests done on both children were listed, including prophylaxis measures against rickets. Von der Decken also referenced other works on this illness, noting that not much was known about the syndrome, but that it resulted in developmental delays and 'idiocy', based on the results of R. Wagner's study.[63] The enduring relevance of the subject material after the Nazi era highlights the exceptional nature of this thesis. Von der Decken published her edited thesis in *Archiv für Kinderheilkunde* in 1943, including the findings, X-rays, and comparative analysis of the patients.[64] This research was considered important at the time, as it was published in a well-renowned journal.

However, not only was it considered of importance in the era, but in 1960, this thesis was referenced by Hans Forssman and Brita Rudberg in an article entitled 'Study of Consanguinity in Twenty-one Cases of Hand-Schüller-Christian Disease (Systemic Reticuloendothelial Granuloma)', and was listed as one of the core studies on this syndrome.[65] Although this syndrome is rare, it is notable that von der Decken's research was still considered of a high calibre many years after its publication.[66] In a short evaluation of her thesis, Dr Hangarter (professor of internal medicine, hereditary pathology, and constitutional research at the Reichsuniversität Straßburg) noted that this thesis 'deals with the very rare and important hereditary biology disease of Hand Schuller Christian of dizygotic twins', while the grade given by Dr Hirt, Dr Bickenbach, and Dr Hofmeier was 'very good'.[67] This thesis appears to have been well received and was published as a result. While there does not appear to be any evidence of informed consent, the nature of the experimentation involved in this thesis lends itself to the classification of 'normal research'. In the absence of concrete knowledge on how this syndrome developed, the use of twins in this instance was integral to understanding the genetic and environmental factors affecting the presentation of this illness. Therefore, while the children who were research subjects did not appear to benefit from the study, it also could not be classified as invasive or as damaging. While this study did involve research on twins, it could not be classified as Nazi research, as it did not further the war effort. It appears that a concern with heritability, 'illegitimacy', and disease progression was the motivating factor in choosing this topic for a thesis. Von der Decken notes that the prognosis is unclear, but the simultaneous occurrence of the disease in a pair of twins was noteworthy, given the possible familial occurrence of the disease. This focus on heritability and 'illegitimacy' as factors in illness were also concerns of Hofmeier in his work, and this is reflected in his students' theses.

Medical Theses Involving Paediatric Patients

Several students developed their research and thesis topic under a different supervisor, but carried out research on children. Therefore, while Dr Hofmeier was not necessarily involved in the supervision of these theses, they included research concerning paediatric care. Some of this was conducted within the children's clinic in Straßburg, while others focused on the children of Straßburg and the surrounding area. Edith Schneider's 1944 thesis, entitled 'Fingerprint Examinations for Straßburg Schoolchildren', was supervised by Professor Lehmann of the racial biology institute, but conducted research on Straßburg schoolchildren.[68] This thesis is notable as it included the local population, but also compared Alsatian children and those of German descent through fingerprint analysis. The main argument of the thesis was that fingerprint analysis could be used to determine inherent criminality based on the unique whorl patterns.[69] Despite the unique nature of fingerprints, Schneider groups fingerprints in her thesis by racial characteristics to determine if Alsatian children were more disposed to criminal actions than German children. Three hundred and eight six- to eight-year-olds in Straßburg schools were the basis for the study, which was a considerable number of the children in the city.[70] It is also notable that such collaboration existed between Straßburg schools and the racial biology institute to conduct a study on such a vast scale. Schneider also includes the research findings of previous researchers, encompassing a broad view of fingerprint patterns for different nationalities and social groups across the world, including Northern Europe, Eastern Europe, smaller regions within Germany, the USA, as well as general groups entitled 'Gypsies, Romania' and 'Jews, America'.[71] Her findings are unclear, and do not provide a logical conclusion as to whether the researchers believed that Alsatians were more inclined to be criminals based on their fingerprints. She also never made it clear what specific patterns in the fingerprints were supposed evidence of criminality.

This research involved human research on underage research subjects with no apparent indication as to the informed consent of their parents. While this research was non-invasive, it was heavily ideologically charged, given that it focused on race, criminality, and biological determinism. A similar study was conducted by Dr Hans Fleischhacker for his habilitation, where he took the handprints of Jews in the Litzmannstadt ghetto to illustrate differences in racial biology.[72] This is clearly Nazi medical research, as it adheres to one of the core elements that classify this research, and that is a central eugenic component to the research. The thesis of Edith Schneider similarly belongs to the field of Nazi medical research, as it also contains a central eugenic component. The rationale of this thesis involved finding ways to establish a predictable biological measurement of criminality, and thus an indication for segregating who should be integrated into Germany and who should not in relation to the assimilation policies by Zivilverwaltung. It is not clear what use was made of this research, as it appears to have remained unpublished, and there is no record stating what grade was received.

Johanna Wehrung's thesis was completed in 1944, entitled 'Explanations of the Euthanasia Problem Based on a Query Among Women'.[73] It was supervised by Dr von Neureiter, and concerned the topic of euthanasia. However, the opinions expressed in this study are pertinent to the study of paediatric patients, as these patients were vulnerable and unable to give consent for medical procedures, therefore medical opinions about their right to life particularly affected children. Wehrung initially detailed that the issue of eugenics was a very commonly discussed one in medical ethics for that era, and quoted extensively from the monograph by Binding and Hoche, *The Release of the Destruction of Life Unworthy of Life.*[74] Wehrung explained that the issue of euthanasia was not simply that of medical ethics, but was closely tied to the religious affiliation of the person, as well their financial and social situation.[75] The final two reasons illustrate why the elimination of life deemed 'unworthy' was in part an ideological concept, but also it was framed by the issue of 'wasting' money on those who could not in turn contribute financially to society. Wehrung quoted from Binding and Hoche: 'Should permissible elimination of life be limited to suicide as it is in current law, or should it be legally extended to the killing of fellow humans, and to what degree?'[76]

Wehrung wrote about questionnaires distributed to those of Reichsdeutsche descent and those of Alsatian descent. The questionnaires included situations in which one would answer whether euthanasia should be permitted in such an instance. Two hundred and fifty questionnaires were handed out, of which 150 were answered and returned. Of those, 88% stated that euthanasia should be allowed in some circumstances,[77] and 62% stated that the 'lebensunwerten lebens' should be eliminated by euthanasia.[78] Wehrung noted that a similar survey was conducted by Karl Bacher, a fellow student at the Reichsuniversität Straßburg, involving seventy medical students.[79] It is notable that two students conducted a similar study, both clearly influenced by the Meltzer survey conducted on parents of institutionalized children in Saxony, in which they were asked if they would theoretically consent to a painless shortening of their children's lives.[80] As Hohendorf noted, the parents' positive response was largely framed around the perception that this would be an act of mercy, but it was also heavily influenced by the societal and financial view of being a 'burden'.[81] Therefore, while the children in Straßburg were not subject to the 'euthanasia' programme, the consideration within the medical sphere of lives that were deemed 'unworthy of living' is evident.

In the conclusion of Wehrung's thesis, it was noted that those of Alsatian descent were more likely to agree with euthanasia, with only 10% of respondents stating that it should never be permitted, in comparison to 13% of Reichsdeutsche stating that it should never be permitted.[82] There is no comparative study to examine what the general population thought about this, so this study cannot be considered a representative one. It is interesting to note that despite this support from medical practitioners in Straßburg, there is no evidence that child euthanasia occurred. These points are discussed in more detail earlier in the chapter, but it seems that while euthanasia was a discussion, and an important topic of study, as evidenced by this thesis, the Reichsuniversität Straßburg was primarily focused on assimilation, integration, and Germanization of the population. It must also be noted that this perception of a person's hereditary worth was not unique to Nazi ideology.[83] However, that this many people who self-identified as Alsatian agreed with euthanasia in certain circumstances illustrates just how prevalently the ideological concept of the 'worth' of a person had infiltrated Straßburg, and possibly the greater Alsace region.

Conclusion

Given that the Reichsuniversität Straßburg was founded to be an example of Nazi research, many of the theses conducted by its students do not differ greatly from other similar research at the time. This solidifies Sara Seiler Vigoriot's point that Nazi doctors, and by extension Nazi medical students, did not have an immediately recognizable distinction that could set them apart from other doctors and scientists of their era.[84] Eugenics was a key theme in their work, but this in and of itself is not enough to mark their theses as typically 'Nazi'. The research conducted in the Reichsuniversität Straßburg was not what is popularly termed 'pseudoscience'.[85] Research done in these institutions under Nazi leadership during the Second World War did seem to reflect international research interests and concerns of the time. Research done both by students and by professors during this era played an important role in science in the postwar era and some of it was quite well regarded long after the Nazi era. This was evidenced by Rosemarie von der Decken, as her research was one of the core studies on Hand-Schüller-Christian syndrome in the late 1960s and was cited in Forssman and Rudberg's study. Of course, there was some research that was of little to no scientific value, being too weighted by Nazi ideology to be considered of a high scientific and objective standard; an example is Gawantka's thesis on heredity in adopted children. However, this very strongly ideological scientific work is in the minority of theses.

Overall, the theses do not mention the Richtlinien, nor do they adhere to existing ethics policies of the era. They do not mention getting consent for procedures, particularly in the case of minors who could not consent themselves. While the students do in general anonymize their patients, there are a number of cases where photographs with identifying features are used, along with the publication of surnames and addresses. The theses produced by the Reichsuniversität Straßburg, while quite numerous, are typical for 'normal' medical research of this era within the framework of the National Socialist regime. This chapter has provided just a few examples of the range of theses produced by students at the Reichsuniversität Straßburg; they were not a monolithic group, with some students more clearly aligned with National Socialist ideology, while others produced theses that were well regarded.

Sabine Hildebrandt makes an important point in *The Anatomy of Murder* which illustrates how we must consider the theses of students in this era to be an important source. She notes that in the postwar era, the doctors who served the population had been trained during the Nazi era, often being taught in universities with the motive of indoctrinating students with Nazi ideals.[86] Their theses reflected not only their own research interests, but also the research interests of their supervisor and of the university they studied in; therefore, the legacy of their Nazi supervisors effectively lived on into research in the postwar era.

CHAPTER 6

Paediatric Patients at the Internal Medicine Clinic

> For forced labourers [...] diseases were common [...] For the regime, the treatment of sick forced labourers was not primarily a matter of restoring health, but the restoration of their capacity to work.[1]

The treatment of children in paediatric departments in the 1940s focused mostly on the prevention of epidemic disease, improvement of nutrition, reducing infant mortality rates, and promoting vaccination campaigns. As a result, specialist children's clinics largely focused on younger children, while minors were also often represented in other clinics in hospitals, for example internal medicine. Internal medicine, or *innere medizin*, began as a speciality in the nineteenth century, focusing on the internal causes of the symptoms the patient experienced, through incorporating laboratory work, bacteriology, and the bedside assessment of patients. Thomas Beddies notes that childhood in this era was primarily associated with race, nationality, politics, and the state, thereby inherently affording some children the protections of the state, while others were not given such protections.[2] We have seen this discussed in previous chapters, through the issue of consent, nationality, and patient care. We know how race, nationality, income, and purported 'worth' to the regime impacted medical care, and this is seen in action with the presence of forced labourers in the internal medicine clinic. The impact of the war can be seen through the changing approach to forced labourers' medical care.

In the internal medicine clinic, some children with more complex needs such as heart problems requiring extensive monitoring are evident, but there are also forced labourers who were brought through the hospital in the third era of the Reichsuniversität Straßburg, in an attempt to return them to work as soon as possible. This treatment of very disparate patient groups in the same hospital, the same clinic, and often the same ward is emblematic of the third era of the Reichsuniversität Straßburg, when the former hierarchies began to break down, while the ideology behind it became more outwardly hostile, and can be seen through the lens of the change in the course of the war towards Allied victory. The clinics also played a fundamental role in maintaining the health of forced labourers and, above all, their 'worth' as a labour force for the benefit of the Reich economy. This chapter will examine the young patients in the internal medicine clinic, how their treatment changed as the war ground on, and ultimately how the war brought an end to the Reichsuniversität Straßburg itself.

Background of Internal Medicine and Structure of the Clinic

As described above, internal medicine focused on the internal causes of a patient's symptoms as a whole, not on individual sections of the body, and basing diagnostics on laboratory analysis and technology, rather than exclusively using the traditional physical examination. This distinction was much more evident in the nineteenth century, where laboratory assessment was not standard for coming to a differential diagnosis, and this combination of clinical assessment of patients with laboratory investigation was popular in Germany. Internal medicine, as evident in the following patient files, often deals with patients that have multiple comorbidities, or those with symptoms that cannot be easily and distinctly placed with one speciality. They also look more cohesively at the body as a whole, as symptoms in one area could lead to complications in another area. Chronic illnesses and infectious disease, as well as heart problems, are treated by internal medicine.

In examining the treatment of children in the Reichsuniversität Straßburg hospital, one has to address the presence of children at the internal medicine clinic. While the number of patients under eighteen was relatively low, approximately 10–15% of cases, they do reflect important facets of the Reichsuniversität Straßburg, how it functioned, and how it viewed minors, as well as their medical decision making.[3] Children were most often admitted in times of infectious disease epidemics, particularly for diphtheria, scarlet fever, and meningitis. This is reflected in the increased capacity of the internal medical clinic isolation ward, where more children could be accommodated with these illnesses. While infectious diseases were also present in the children's clinic, these records indicate that the children's clinic isolation ward was not as well equipped for seasonal increases in admissions for diphtheria, meningitis, and scarlet fever.[4] Priority was given to younger children in the children's clinic, while teenagers were more often accommodated in the internal medicine isolation ward.

The National Socialist administration restructured the French clinical services and combined all internal medicine departments of the Reichsuniversität Straßburg into a single medical clinic (Medizinische Klinik), headed by Dr Johannes Stein, the dean of the medical faculty and the director of internal medicine. The clinic was divided into three departments: Department I, which was located in the former Medizinische B, was directed by Johannes Stein and Hajo Wolbergs. Department II, located in the Medical A building, was managed by Gunnar Berg and later by Werner Hangarter, an Alsatian doctor. Department III, or the medical poliklinik, was managed by Professor Otto Bickenbach. In addition to these three departments, the medical clinic also contained a radiation treatment institute and a radiology department. It is clear that the main appeal in sending children to this clinic was the increased capacity for diagnostic testing, where the specific illness was not yet known, or it required specialist technology and equipment. Based on the Reichsuniversität Straßburg's central role in occupation in the west, along with its position as a centre for Nazi research, considerable sums of money were provided with the intention of accessing the latest in medical treatment.

Specialist Treatment and Referrals to the Internal Medicine Clinic

It also appears that the clinic had a specialist function to perform electrocardiograms (ECG) in more detail. Although there is some evidence that these were used in the children's clinic, for those that were admitted directly with heart concerns, particularly angina, it seems that they were accommodated directly at the internal medical clinic instead of the children's clinic, likely due to the increased availability of ECG machines. This is reflected in the patient files, where patients with angina are given routine ECGs, whereas in the children's clinic this was used less frequently. One such example of this treatment was provided in Chapter 3, in the case of Klaus D., who was monitored via a three-lead ECG.

Günther F., a German student, was born in 1928 and was admitted to the internal medicine clinic in 1943 with endocarditis.[5] His admission directly to the internal medicine clinic is indicative of the emergency nature of the case, which is marked as urgent. On 10 November 1943, the internal medicine clinic wrote to the patient's doctor, stating that Günther had unfortunately died of endocarditis, brought on by untreated rheumatoid arthritis. Günther's father wrote to the clinic, marked urgent, in late December. The clinic wrote to his father on 20 January, saying:

> your son was taken to hospital on 6.11.43 in a seriously ill and conscious condition, where he died within a few hours despite all the medical and nursing measures taken immediately. It was a general septic illness which probably started with an inflammation of the inner lining of the heart. We sympathize with you in the great loss you have suffered as a result of your son's death.[6]

That the clinic took the time to write directly to his father, not just to the referral general practitioner, and sympathized with his loss, emphasizes how this social hierarchy was embedded in medical care. Such sympathetic letters, or even any correspondence with the family, are of course not seen at the later stages of the war when forced labourers come to the Reichsuniversität Straßburg for medical care. The pathology institute conducted an autopsy to conclusively determine cause of death, which was sepsis, endocarditis, pleuritis and necrotizing pharyngitis, abscesses in the kidneys, and inflammation of the spleen and liver.[7] This is indicative of the importance of diagnostic pathological autopsies in internal medicine, to determine the cause of death in situations with multiple comorbidities.

Georgine S. was sixteen years old when she was moved from the Bürgerspital in Hagenau to the Reichsuniversität Straßburg internal medical clinic in January 1943.[8] She was originally from Lothringen, with no siblings, and as her father died in Lemberg, her mother was her only remaining family member. Georgine was admitted to the internal medicine clinic in January 1943 by her family doctor in Lemberg, Dr Backerange, for what he suspected to be aleukaemic lymphadenosis, which is swelling of the lymph tissue associated with leukaemia. The internal medicine clinic confirmed this diagnosis via X-ray, which showed multiple tumours, and thus the clinic proceeded to offer radiation treatment. While the swelling was reduced, the medial tumour could not be reduced, so further therapy with blood transfusions, solarson, and nuelsodorate were continued for fourteen days. The pathology department was central to diagnostics in the Reichsuniversität Straßburg, particularly in the case of cancer. Klinge analysed multiple tumours, that were hazelnut- and walnut-sized, of lymphatic tissue in the pathology institute and recommended further blood transfusions.[9]

During the course of her treatment, Georgine's weight dropped to 37kg, but as the treatment progressed, she did not regain much weight. The clinic

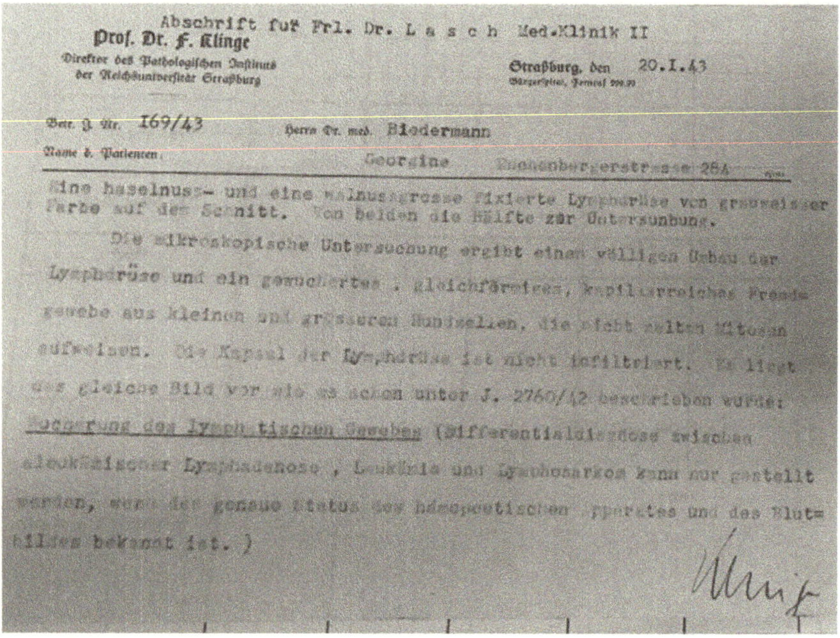

Abschrift für Frl. Dr. L a s c h Med.Klinik II

Prof. Dr. F. Klinge
Direktor des Pathologischen Instituts
der Reichsuniversität Straßburg

Straßburg, den 20.I.43

Betr. J. Nr. 169/43

Herrn Dr. med. Biedermann

Name d. Patienten: Georgine [illegible]

Eine haselnuss- und eine walnussgrosse fixierte Lymphdrüse von grauweisser Farbe auf dem Schnitt. Von beiden die Hälfte zur Untersuchung.

Die mikroskopische Untersuchung ergibt einen völligen Umbau der Lymphdrüse und ein gewuchertes, gleichförmiges, kapillarreiches Fremdgewebe aus kleinen und grösseren Bündeln, die nicht selten Mitosen aufweisen. Die Kapsel der Lymphdrüse ist nicht infiltriert. Es liegt das gleiche Bild vor wie es schon unter J. 2760/42 beschrieben wurde: Wucherung des lymphatischen Gewebes (Differentialdiagnose zwischen aleukämischer Lymphadenose, Leukämie und Lymphosarkom kann nur gestellt werden, wenn der genaue Status des hämopoetischen Apparates und des Blutbildes bekannt ist.)

Klinge

Fig. 6.1. Pathology analysis for Georgine S., 1943.[10]

request that she return in four weeks for a check-up, and rest until then. There is no documentation from the check-up, but on the fourth of March, her file notes only that they predict a poor outcome, and she is sent home the next day. In this sense, we see a degree of 'palliative care', wherein the clinic's treatments cannot be expected to improve the condition, and so the patient is released home for rest. This can be viewed in contrast to the forced labourers, who were discharged to work without recommended treatments even running their course.

The impact of war is clear in Luise S.'s patient file, as increased wartime stress, particularly aerial bombing raids, impacted her health. She was admitted to the internal medicine clinic in March 1944 with meningitis epidemica.[11] She was a fifteen-year-old Alsatian patient, whose parents paid for her third-class care. As noted in Chapter 3, the class of medical care corresponded to the health insurance reimbursement, but also for the cost of care, and was affiliated to social class in that those with better-paying jobs had a higher level of care. Luise's family history is noted, as her father was quite ill and coughed up blood, so he was sent to a sanatorium. Despite this, her two brothers and her mother were free from tuberculosis and quite healthy. Luise got whooping cough, pneumonia, measles, and varicella as a child, but it does not appear to have impacted her long-term health. She began to feel very unwell in the air-raid shelter in February, which developed into a fever, and because they were ordered to stay there, she could not go to hospital.[12] By March 1944, when she was admitted to hospital, aerial bombing was almost constant, with British RAF planes bombing Germany at night while American USAAF planes bombed during the day.[13] When Luise's temperature reduced, she went back to school, although she still felt unwell, but a few days later had a headache that was so severe she missed school, along with a return of her fever. Her mother called the nurse, who gave her aspirin and tea, but she vomited these up. By 5pm that evening, she was no longer responsive at all, and the local doctor referred her to the internal medicine clinic with a suspected diagnosis of meningitis.

As Shields and Bryan note, the delay in receiving medical care due to air raids, not to mention the conditions in the air-raid shelters, had considerable health implications, which is clear in Luise's case.[14] We also see that in the third era of the Reichsuniversität Straßburg, the guise of a beneficent regime began to dissolve as even German and Alsatian children's health was impacted by the encroaching war front. On admission, Luise was unconscious and unresponsive to external stimuli, but her breathing and heart rate were calm. She was given camphor, cibazol, oxygen and fluids, and extensive blood tests to determine an exact diagnosis. Doctors performed a lumbar puncture three times, which confirmed meningitis. In her medical notes, Luise's response to the lumbar puncture is noted: 'today patient is responsive, recognizes her surroundings and family members. During the lumbar puncture, which was performed again, she cursed and screamed.[15] Cerebrospinal fluid is still turbid.' This quote shows that her family had been visiting her in the clinic, and also that her pain and discomfort at the test was notable. After three weeks in the clinic, she complained of severe pain and stinging in her chest, which led to a bronchoscopy, although nothing was found. She was released from the clinic after one month of treatment, completely cured and with no neurological deficits.

Dieter H. is the youngest known patient to have been admitted to the internal medicine clinic, at eight years old, in August 1944.[16] He was a German schoolboy, whose father was an Oberstabarzt, and his parents paid privately for his care. Oberstabarzt was one of the highest ranks in the German army medical corps, so his care was affected by this as a result of financial circumstances, but also due to social hierarchy, particularly in the military. It is also quite possible that his father had connections to some of the staff in the hospital, which was reflected in the semi-informal register

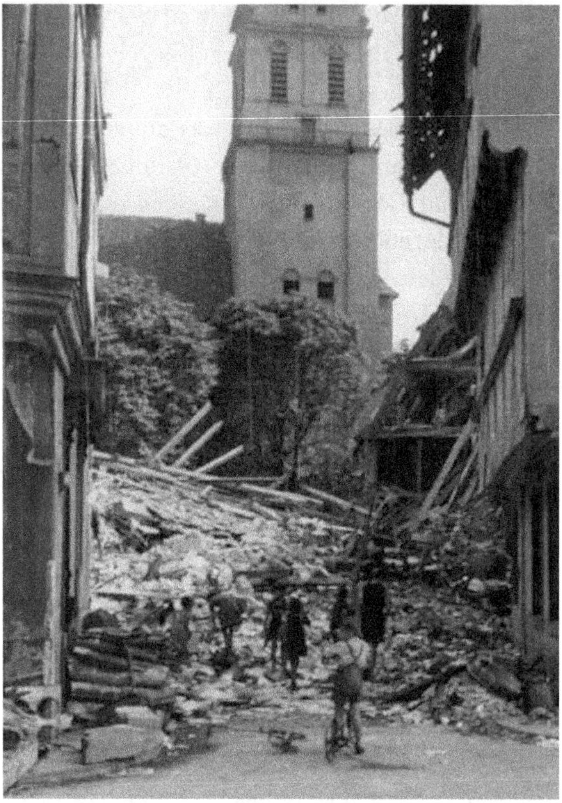

Fig. 6.2. Children playing in the rubble of buildings that were bombed on 11 August 1944 on Rue de Trois Gateaux in Straßburg.[17]

they had in exchanging letters about Dieter's medical care. It appears that even in the clinic, this was considered exceptional, as the staff referred to Dieter as 'bübchen', a term of endearment for a young boy, illustrating the higher status that he had due to his father's position in the army, his nationality, and his ability to pay for his medical care. This also marks the distinction between the treatment of children of a high-ranking figure in the German military in contrast to the forced labourers discussed later in the chapter. Dieter is referred to by informal but identifiable ways, while forced labourers are often not even directly named, or their names are misspelled and Germanized. The staff note that his parents and all three of his siblings were healthy, and although Dieter was in good general health, he had a slightly blue pallor, as well as a fever and swollen throat. He was admitted to the clinic in August with angina lacunaris. He was referred to the otolaryngology department, which recommended adenectomy, and possible later tonsillectomy depending on how much of an improvement was found. No further record for his admission was found, so it is believed that he did not require further surgery or hospital treatment, which is in part an indication of the quality of care that his parents could pay for privately. That treatment was dependent on the circumstances of the patient's improvement, with a clearly graduated system of increasingly serious therapies based on how the patient responded to each step, illustrating that patient treatment was possible in the clinic. That this then was not provided to forced labourers clearly indicates the differences in their treatment.

Treatment of Forced Labourers

Forced labourers were a central part of the National Socialist state, as civilian slave labourers. Originally they were primarily foreign labourers who joined on a voluntary basis—including Belgian, Dutch, and French workers from 1940 onwards—but this later expanded to coerced labour from Eastern Europe, and then forced labour. Within the forced labourers, however, there was a hierarchy, with Ostarbeitern (meaning Eastern workers) at the bottom, and their treatment was quite different according to this hierarchy.[18] They were captured as the Wehrmacht advanced, and then sent as forced labour wherever they were required, primarily in industrial work, agriculture, and domestic service.[19] This need for forced labour increased as the war progressed and more and more German civilians were drafted into the war effort, while the conflict simultaneously resulted in demand for more materials, leaving large gaps in the industrial workforce that was filled by forced labour. Those from the East received the worst rations, and were subject to harsher conditions than other forced labourers.[20] Ostarbeitern lived in guarded barracks, one of which was built on the grounds of the Reichsuniversität Straßburg.[21] As Eva Hallama notes, forced labourers' medical care was essentially determined by economics, with doctors informed that their medical insurance would extend so far as to return them to a functional work capacity, but no further.[22] This included children, as boys below the age of conscription were captured and used as forced labour, while young women were also taken for domestic service.[23]

The first forced labourers are found in the Reichsuniversität Straßburg patient records in October 1941 in the internal medicine clinic, and there are 228 foreign labourers from Eastern Europe; 8% of patients treated in the clinic, which would peak at 25% of patients treated in July 1943. The decree on 16 October 1942 'on workers in the East who are unfit for work' declared that the repatriation of foreign workers must be reduced, and this repatriation was based on a cost-benefit analysis to the employer in view of the increasing costs of train transport due to wartime shortages.[24] This ensured that workers from the East had to be provided with medical care so that they could remain fit for work for as long as possible. This medical care, as evidenced from their records, indicates a considerable emphasis on capacity to work, even returning patients who were not fully recovered, as long as their condition was stable enough to be of 'worth' to their employer again.[25] The October 1942 decree limited this care to 'a maximum of about eight weeks'.[26] The admission statistics to the internal medicine clinic II reflect this decree and the increased provision for medical care to ensure a workforce. While the issue of nationality and Eastern workers, or Ostarbeitern, is alluded to in the children's clinic, this becomes more apparent when addressing the internal medicine clinic records. Paediatrics in this era primarily focused on early childhood and infant nutrition, prevention of epidemic diseases, vaccination, and a focus on heritability of illnesses. Naturally, health issues that resulted from the workplace were not considered the remit of the children's clinic, and so forced labourers, including teenagers, were admitted to the internal medicine clinic for treatment.

Wojciech Kwieciński notes that

> Polish and Soviet forced labourers, who were considered 'subhumans' in the National Socialist ideology, were the most discriminated nationalities among the foreign workers in the war economy of the 'Third Reich'. Their entire living and working conditions were subordinated to racial ideology. Both the living conditions and the medical treatment reveal the main objectives of the Nazi state and its racist and dehumanised character.[27]

We can see this in the internal medicine clinic records, which can be contrasted with the treatment of Alsatians and Germans of a similar age: the focus remains for Ostarbeitern on their capacity to work, and not on relief of pain or adequate time to fully recuperate.

Michal G. was born in Ukraine in 1926.[28] It is not clear when he became a forced labourer at the trade association of Metz, who referred him to the internal medicine clinic in February 1944. He was referred to the otolaryngology clinic on arrival at the hospital, who conducted an examination which showed a fracture at the base of the skull leading to facial paralysis. As Graefe and Roelcke note, forced labourers were not diagnosed with less effort, but had a variety of diagnostic procedures provided, and were often transferred to other departments—like other patients—based on what was required, as evidenced in Michel's case. However, they note that 'the question of the correct diagnosis, and above all the prognosis, at least in very many cases, was not relevant from the perspective of the individual patient's wellbeing, but rather from the point of view of the question whether the patients, after a possible discharge, would be able to fulfil their function'.[29] In Michal's case, we see a clear process of referrals, careful diagnostics, and unusually, they request follow-up care, on weekdays at 7am and on Sundays at 11.30am.[30] It is unclear, though, if this follow-up care was ever provided, or if this was merely a suggestion in the event that his capacity for work was not considered sufficient after basic treatment, focused on Michal's ability to fulfil his functions after discharge. As Katarzyna Woniak explains, while doctors may have recommended certain treatments, referrals, or follow-up care, this was often not fulfilled because ultimately patients' health insurance would refuse to pay for treatments that were not essential to their capacity to work.[31] Michal was released back to the camp in March 1944, and there are no further records of his admission or attendance at the outpatient poliklinik. It is telling that he fractured the base of his skull but was only referred to the hospital after seven months, illustrating how it was not necessarily the injury in and of itself that led to hospitalization of forced labourers, but the impact this had on their capacity for work.

Iwan P. was born in 1928 in Russia, and was forced to work in Oberbrunn.[32] He was admitted to the internal medicine clinic in February 1944 for unspecified nervous heart problems and taboparesis. He was referred for diagnostic X-ray imaging, which confirmed serious peribronchitis of the right lung, but there was no recommendation for treatment. In March 1944, the internal medicine clinic wrote to Dr Dietz, who had referred Iwan for treatment, that the patient was 'discharged from the hospital as fit for work. The patient had a nervous heart condition. No pathological findings were found in the heart or lungs.'[33] However, as with other Ostarbeitern, there was no follow-up treatment plan provided. Extensive imaging was provided, along with blood tests, to confirm that Iwan's heart difficulties were not as a result of tuberculosis or other infectious diseases. Once this was confirmed, he was released back to the forced labour camp. This case shows how it was not the medical care of the individual that was the primary concern, but to prevent the spread of epidemic diseases, and also to ensure the minimum capacity to work.

Wassily D. was born in Ukraine and was seventeen years old when he was admitted to the internal medicine clinic in May 1943.[34] His name was Germanized on his admission file to 'Basil', while his other documents refer to him as Wassily. He was a forced labourer at Königshofffen, and was admitted to the clinic after a truck ran over his foot, crushing it. This reflects the systemic health disparities evident in the National Socialist healthcare system; while the healthcare benefits afforded to the German population did improve, this came at the expense of foreign labourers, who existed on the margins of society, being forced to work more difficult jobs. Although they too were given healthcare, many existed on meagre rations and suffered life-changing injuries that were not adequately treated, leading to lifelong difficulties, particularly those who worked in construction and manufacturing industries.[35] The Ostarbeiter lager in Königshofffen wrote a letter to the clinic, informing them 'here is an Eastern worker. He does not speak German. We ask for information and when we should fetch him again.'[36]

This letter is indicative of the general treatment of Eastern workers, as he was not named in the letter, and the main concern was not with the accident or Wassily's welfare, but with when he would be capable of working

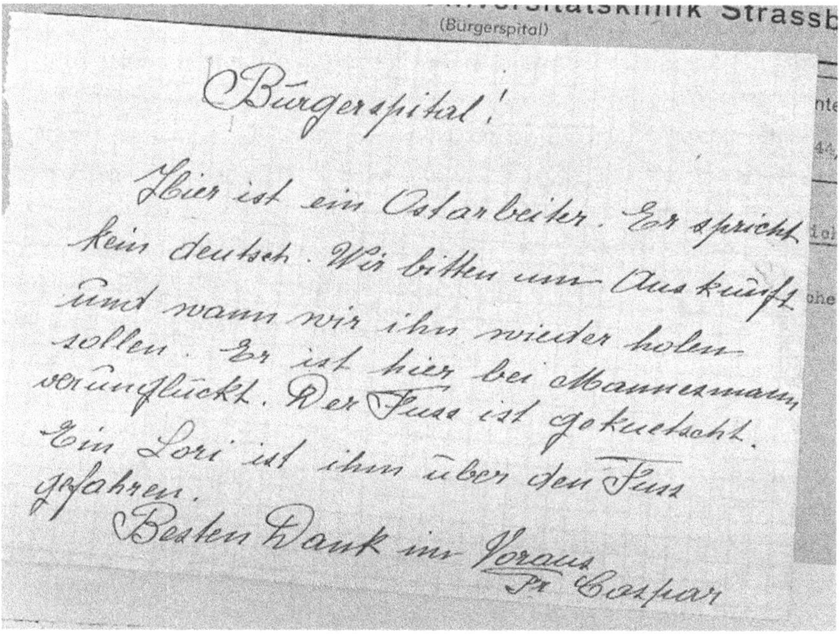
(Bürgerspital)

Bürgerspital!

Hier ist ein Ostarbeiter. Er spricht kein deutsch. Wir bitten um Auskunft und wann wir ihn wieder holen sollen. Er ist hier bei Mannesmann verunglückt. Der Fuss ist gekuetscht. Ein Lori ist ihm über den Fuss gefahren.

Besten Dank im Voraus

Fr Caspar

Fig. 6.3. Letter from forced labour camp to the Reichsuniversität Straßburg internal medicine clinic concerning Wassily, 1943.[37]

again. This is reflected in the letter from the medical clinic on 30 May in which he was declared fit for work, noting that there was significant distortion of the right ankle and right foot, but with no detectable fracture. The healing process was considered smooth, but notably, there was no recommendation for follow-up care, unlike in referrals for German or Alsatian patients.

Katherine S. was born in Ukraine, in Woroschilowgrad, in 1926.[38] It is unclear when she was forced to work at the Hausbergen train depot, but she was sent from there to the internal medicine clinic when she was seventeen years old in May 1943.[39] It is unclear why exactly she was admitted, but she was given a referral to the gynaecology clinic due to unexplained secondary amenorrhea. The gynaecology clinic wrote to the internal medicine clinic on 24 May that they recommended intensive hormone therapy to resolve the secondary amenorrhea. The internal medicine clinic then wrote to the Reichsbahn Betriebskrankenkasse Karlsruhe, who paid for her medical care, that 'we released the eastern worker Katerina S. into the camp ready for work. No significant pathological findings were found.'[40] The internal medicine clinic also specified that the secondary amenorrhea was likely due to a 'change in climate', and while hormone therapy was considered, it was not conducted. A similar case was mentioned by Woniak in her article, wherein a sixteen-year-old girl suffered menstrual disturbances which should have been medically treated, but the forced labour camp leader refused to give permission for this treatment, dismissing her as a 'dawdler'.[41] While in the clinic, she was not given hormone therapy, and was provided only with a light diet. This illustrates how fertility was not considered important for Ostarbeitern, as this was not integral to their capacity to work. It also indicates the extreme working conditions for Ostarbeitern, as stress and a lack of food are causes of secondary amenorrhea.[42] This can be contrasted to the treatment of Watzlaff in Chapter 4, who was Germanized and considered Aryan despite being born in Eastern Europe. We can gather then that as Katherine was not considered Germanizeable, preserving her fertility was not a concern, so she was given the bare minimum of medical treatment in order to regain her capacity to work. This case shows how although forced labourers were given medical care in the Reichsuniversität Straßburg, it was not patient-centric care, but care intended to make them fit to work.

By 1944, forced labourers came to be treated at the internal medicine clinic in the third era of the Reichsuniversität Straßburg, this belies how the impact of the war led to the façade of benevolence disappearing by 1944. Increased war work led the staff to abandon planned projects, staff members and students alike were being drafted into the Wehrmacht and serving at

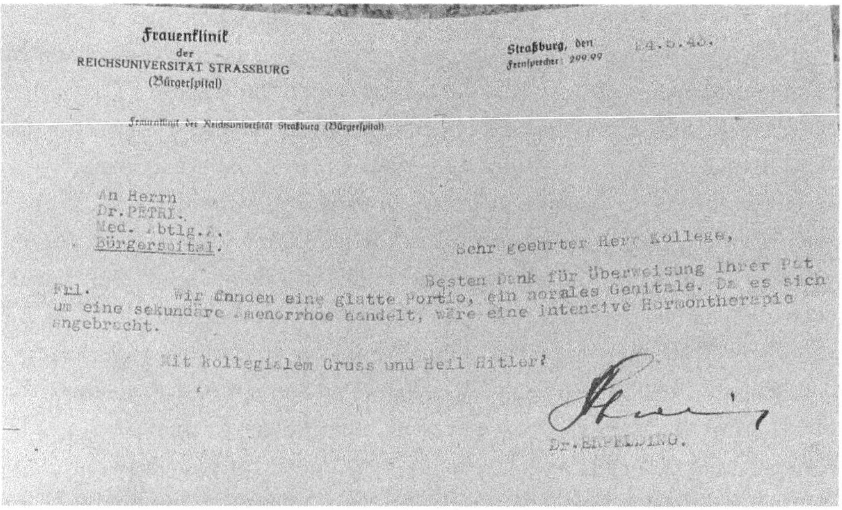

Frauenklinik
der
REICHSUNIVERSITÄT STRASSBURG
(Bürgerspital)

Straßburg, den 24.5.43.
Fernsprecher: 209.99

Frauenklinik der Reichsuniversität Straßburg (Bürgerspital)

An Herrn
Dr. PETRI.
Med. Abtlg. A.
Bürgerspital.

Sehr geehrter Herr Kollege,

Besten Dank für Überweisung Ihrer Pat Frl. Wir fanden eine glatte Portio, ein norales Genitale. Da es sich um eine sekundäre Amenorrhoe handelt, wäre eine intensive Hormontherapie angebracht.

Mit kollegialem Gruss und Heil Hitler!

Dr. [illegible]

Fig. 6.4. Letter from the gynaecology clinic to the internal medicine clinic recommending hormone therapy for Katherine in 1943.[43]

the front, and the remaining staff were left to care for an increased number of patients. It became harder for the staff to justify the beneficial treatment of the Alsatian population that had built up to that point, and so Germanization measures became more strict. The clinics and the hospital played a fundamental role in maintaining the health of the Volk, but also the health of the forced labourers, above all keeping the labour force going as the regime crumbled. This corresponds directly to the material shortages, the air raids, and the fall of the city and the hospital to Allied forces in November 1944. While breast milk banks, mothers' consultation hours, and extensive outpatient care initially may have satiated the population, using healthcare to win people over and make the regime seem benevolent in the first era, by the third era of the Reichsuniversität Straßburg, the mask had slipped. Foreign children were being used as forced labour, medical students were under threat, staff began to flee the encroaching war, and patients felt the impact; children spoke of fearing the Gestapo would come for them,[44] while such concerns were dismissed as paranoia. Buildings were being destroyed, and eventually, some patients were evacuated.

Final Days of the Reichsuniversität Straßburg

Accounts of the final days of the Reichsuniversität Straßburg were mostly written after the evacuation had happened, so it is difficult to analyse these sources, as they are particularly biased. One such source is that from the Police Judiciaries in 1945 in Strasbourg, who opened a case concerning Hofmeier denouncing students to the Gestapo for 'anti-German sentiment'.[45] Georgette Sittler accused Hofmeier of contacting the Gestapo about her, due to her keeping French books in her student dorm, which had been searched. All French published material had been banned in 1940, but quiet resistance was often tolerated unless French publications were read in public or disseminated. Georgette testified to the police that Hofmeier called her into his office one day in 1943 and reproached her for distributing French propaganda, which she claimed was false. He supposedly threatened to send her to Schirmeck, a forced labour camp.[46] When she heard this, she left the nursing school without any notice, and fled to Paris.[47] Despite her leaving the hospital and the city, her family were repeatedly called in for questioning by the Gestapo after her departure, and Hofmeier supposedly attempted to make her an example for the other students. While this case did not progress any further, testimonials indicated that he was particularly adamant that protocol was followed, such as giving the Nazi salute every morning and forcing the nurses to do likewise, along with policing their attendance at party meetings.[48]

The Police Judiciaries note that they were investigating

> actual information; Hofmeier and Weski denounced students to the SS and one of them was even sentenced to death after the attack on Hitler on 20 July 1943 [sic], for expressing regret at the failure of the attack. Other students were sent to the front in the safe companies (bewahrungskompanien), [nurse] Fischer was used by Hofmeier and Weski as an informant.[49]

Despite this convincing investigation and an interrogation of multiple former staff members, it is not clear who had supposedly been sentenced to death, or indeed where they got this information in the first place. All of the testimonies provided in 1945 are remarkably sparse, partly due to the nurses being reluctant to incriminate themselves. One such example is the testimony of Gabriele Krebs, a twenty-eight-year-old paediatric nurse who formerly worked under Hofmeier, who gave testimony in December 1945. She stated:

> He was a member of the party, I always saw him wearing the insignia. But outside of that I ignored his political activities [...] Personally I don't have to complain about him, but I do know

> that he made the student nurses give the Hitler salute and attend party meetings [...] I do not know if Hofmeier reported anyone. At the liberation of Strasbourg, he was in Germany. He hasn't reappeared here since.[50]

This adds another element to Hofmeier's adherence to the regime, as previous accounts mention only the Wehrmacht uniform, but he apparently also wore the party armband. Another example is the testimony of a paediatric nurse, Emilie Richert, who stated:

> During occupation I worked under Hofmeier who arrived there in September 1941 as the director of the children's clinic. I ignored his political activity. He must have been a member of the party because I saw him several times in uniform and wearing a badge. He had the function of Stabarzt, that is, he had a company of students under his command. I don't know if there were any incidents between him and them.[51]

The Police Judiciaries note that all those who were asked about the incident claimed ignorance, and not only this, they barely admitted to being aware of any political activity in the clinic. From their testimonies, it is evident that none of them were willing to incriminate themselves and possibly impact their own careers by association with such a politically motivated clinic, where many of them trained or developed their practice. The Police Judiciaries also do not record the questions that were asked during the course of the investigation, just the answers given by those being interviewed, but from these one can see that they answered carefully to indicate, not that these denunciations did not happen, but that they personally were unaffected by denunciations. None of them declare that intimidation of students and staff on political grounds never occurred, nor do they defend Hofmeier and say he would not have done this, but they state that they were unaware of the incident in question. As a result of this, the investigation was dropped. From this investigation, we can gather that in the third era of the Reichsuniversität Straßburg, the benevolent façade was abandoned, with forced labourers no longer at a distance so civilians could ignore them, where the threat of the Gestapo was very real for the students, and individual patients were more and more affected by air raids. This is evident in the case of Johann, the locksmith's apprentice who was treated in the psychiatric clinic, and whose fear of the Gestapo was dismissed as a persecution complex.

Evacuation of Patients and Staff

One of the central documents available to help understand the evacuation of the Reichsuniversität Straßburg hospital was written by Dr Kurt Hofmeier, partially in his position as director of paediatrics, but also in his former role in the military. He wrote this account for the Reich Ministry of Science, Education, and National Education on 1 December 1944 to provide an explanation of what exactly had happened to their strategically significant university and hospital.[52]

On 20 November 1944, Dr Kurt Hofmeier and Dr Johannes Stein, the dean of the medical faculty, discussed how they should be prepared in case of Allied invasion, and the decision was made to not evacuate the hospital, the patients, or the staff. The University, and by extension the hospital, were regarded as particularly significant and politically important, partially due to the optics of having a Nazi stronghold in France, which symbolized that they had not yet lost the war, despite the obvious impending defeat.[53] Stein noted that evacuation was not an immediate concern and scheduled a faculty meeting for the next day. Hofmeier seemed insistent that life should continue as normal and that civilians should stay in the city to continue working. This measure would prevent panic from resulting in a civilian retreat that might block roads and thus impede the military.[54] Such was their optimism that nursing student exams were scheduled up to 1946.[55] Hofmeier was particularly insistent that paediatric lectures should continue, scheduling one on the morning of the arrival of the Allied forces.

On the morning of 20 November, Hofmeier spoke to General Franz Vaterrodt, the commandant of Straßburg, who told him the city was not well equipped for defence, but still he did not get the impression that there was serious concern about a threat to the city.[56] Later that afternoon, he went to Dr Stein, the dean of the medical faculty and head of the internal medicine clinic, and spoke about the meeting with General Vaterrodt. Hofmeier's liaison between the general and the dean implies he held a key role in civilian administration and that he was trusted with sensitive information concerning the war. It is also clear that by this point the war had degraded former hierarchies to such an extent that a meeting between Hofmeier, a lieutenant of the former imperial German army and a chief medical officer for the Sanitätercorps, and Major General Vaterrodt, the commandant of Straßburg, could occur.[57] Hofmeier and Stein discussed the fact that 'the keeping open of the University can be regarded as particularly significant and politically important'.[58] Hofmeier's refusal to accept the reality of the situation belies his experience in the First World War and the false notion that the German army had not been defeated militarily. This mindset was shared among members of the Nazi party and German military command throughout other infamous German engagements, such as the Battle of Stalingrad in 1941, Kursk in 1943, and the Battle of Britain in 1940, where tactical withdrawals and rest were denied to active forces by indoctrinated commanders, who believed that the German army could not be beaten in the field. The movement of seventeen research institutes to the interior of the Reich was labelled as 'defeatist' by the chief of civil administration in Straßburg. Only eighteen civilian medical students remained in Straßburg following the order for all medical student companies of the Wehrmacht to be relocated to the interior of the Reich.[59] This illustrates how militaristic the medical faculty was, but also how few people were left in the hospital by the time the Battle of Straßburg began. The students had been militarized, as noted in Chapter 5, while Hofmeier styled himself as a soldier even in the clinic, highlighting how militarization of the medical faculty was an essential part of occupation. The Battle for Straßburg reflected German military ideals, wherein retreat was seen as completely unacceptable, regardless of how obvious their eventual defeat was. Moreover, this façade of military might extended to the civilian population too, where people were dissuaded from evacuating the city and the illusion of 'business as usual' was maintained. Antony Beevor noted that despite this policy of fighting until the last round, discipline broke down and soldiers began to throw away their ammunition and surrender. This helps to highlight the central position of Straßburg in an idealistic sense; once it was captured, although the war would last into 1945, the optimism of regaining occupied territories and incorporating it into a greater German Reich was seen as a distant dream and no longer logistically possible.[60] This is reflected in the final winter semester of medical studies in the Reichsuniversität Straßburg; although exams and courses were planned, it only lasted three days.[61] It is probable that the students were aware of the encroaching battle to some degree, as only ten of them attended Hofmeier's lecture on 21 November, in part because so many were members of the Wehrmacht and so were drafted into the war, but also because, as mentioned above, this ideological optimism had begun to fade.

Hofmeier noted that by the end of the meeting, there was no clear instruction from either the dean or the rector as to who should stay in Straßburg, and they continued to highlight the symbolic importance of retaining the university. The medical, surgical, and gynaecological clinics had been moving patients to Stephansfeld Heil-und Pflegeanstalt, a psychiatric institution in Alsace, for an indeterminate amount of time. Hofmeier noted that about 100 paediatric patients had been placed in Stephansfeld in a makeshift children's clinic.[62] General Vaterrodt confirmed that the roads to Stephansfeld were clear for transport if it became necessary to move more patients.

On 22 November, it is clear that the staff were made aware of the Allied position, as Hofmeier began to hand out certificates to the nurses, doctors, and technical assistants for them to leave. He also gathered the staff of the children's clinic and told them to leave Straßburg for a week. If it was not possible to return to Straßburg in a week, they were ordered to report to the clinic in Tübingen. Following bombing raids on Straßburg, which led to the destruction of the hygiene institute in October 1944, Adalbert Erler, Ernst Ahnrich, and Richard Dehm of the Reichsuniversität Straßburg were sent to the University of Tübingen to find suitable premises for the relocation of the university. By 20 November, agreement had been reached between the Reichsuniversität Straßburg, the University of Tübingen, and the Reich Ministry of Education to move teaching for the last three clinical semesters of medical studies to the new site.[63] This suggests the evacuation to Tübingen was well understood and planned among the staff, but was ultimately intended to be a short-term solution. The patients of the children's clinic also appear to have been well prepared, as Hofmeier mentioned only twenty patients remained at the clinic in Straßburg, under the supervision of a new Lithuanian medical assistant, Dr Elena Alexandraviciene.[64] It is assumed that these twenty patients were not evacuated due to their medical conditions, although why they were not moved and what specific illnesses they had is not mentioned. Some patients were released in anticipation of the Allied arrival. The record does not specify how many patients were released under such conditions, nor is there an explanation as to how this triage system was organized, or who made the final decision as to those who would leave and those who would stay.

Hofmeier went to see the Wehrmacht Lieutenant-Colonel Kaiser on 23 November, having heard gunfire and shells exploding outside his house. On his arrival, Kaiser told him that the Battle of Straßburg had just begun.[65] Hofmeier went to Dr Johannes Stein, the dean of the medical faculty and director of the internal medical clinic, who was having coffee with his daughter at the hospital, and informed him of the advance of the Allied troops. There were no further German staff members from the clinic in Straßburg by that morning, but Hofmeier suggested that Alsatian staff remain in the hospital. Hofmeier believed that if he stayed in the hospital, he would be imprisoned when the Allies arrived, so he planned his escape. He went to his office at the children's clinic, gathered his papers and files, and packed up his car. He noted that 'We drove very slowly, as the car was heavily overloaded' over the bridge to Kehl, where they arrived by about 10.30am.[66] It is unknown exactly what material and files Hofmeier took with him on his escape from Straßburg, and it is clear from his account that by 10am, the Allies had advanced almost to the gates of the hospital. Due to Hofmeier's insistence on remaining in Straßburg until the last available moment, the hospital was left in considerable disarray, but luckily, this also included leaving a large portion of paediatric patient files behind.[67] These remaining patient records serve as a poignant reminder of the impact of trauma on healthcare, especially in the case of the most vulnerable members of the population. These records show the practical implications of the institutional narrative of power, and theoretical framework of trauma, on the patient experience.

Conclusion

Despite its efforts to dethrone the Sorbonne, the Reichsuniversität Straßburg lasted only three years. While it may seem obvious to state that the war affected the Reichsuniversität Straßburg, it truly changed how the clinic's doctors and nurses saw and treated their patients. The war also profoundly impacted the patient demographic, from 1941, when the patients were largely local, to 1944, when patients were increasingly German, from further afield, with often more serious illnesses, and of course the presence of forced labourers in the clinics as patients. Patients were also subject to increased Germanization, as their place of birth or personal feelings of national identity were discarded to prioritize increasing the population of the German Volk. The internal medicine clinic became more integral to the functioning of the Reichsuniversität Straßburg hospital as the war progressed, as modern war created new difficulties that were harder to diagnose, with multiple comorbidities that needed to be distinguished from one another. This required an investment in new technologies and equipment that could be accommodated at the internal medicine clinic, but as the war progressed, there was less capacity to provide care as expected. The illusion of Alsatian autonomy, and of a benevolent regime, slowly gave way to euphoria, with multiple innovative treatments that were lauded and provided to the population. This, in turn, in the third era, crumbled, to reveal a considerable number of forced labourers that kept the regime going. It also revealed how the staff of the Reichsuniversität Straßburg, as well as the broader political system, viewed them as entirely dispensable; while children who could pay privately for their care were being offered trips to sanatoria for their health, teenaged forced labourers with barely healed skull fractures were sent back to work without any follow-up care to eke out the remaining labour from them. When the front finally reached Straßburg, despite their idealism, many staff at the Reichsuniversität Straßburg had already abandoned their posts. This chapter also illustrates how although paediatrics, and children in general, were viewed in a utopian way, this did not include all children—just those who could be envisioned as future soldiers to fight for the National Socialist state, who would be hereditarily healthy, and never in need of welfare provisions. This extends too to girls, for whom fertility was a concern only if they could be the mothers to future Aryan Germans, not those who were forced labourers from the East. As this chapter, and this book as a whole, has shown, the healthcare system, and particularly the Reichsuniversität Straßburg, was not only central to providing for this vision, but also integral to propagating and continuing this idealistic vision of childhood in service of an authoritarian state. When the state itself began to crack around them, this idealistic vision embedded in the Reichsuniversität Straßburg visibly diminished.

CHAPTER 7

Final Days of the Reichsuniversität Straßburg and the Immediate Postwar Consequences

> We know that the genetic make-up of a human being is basically decisive for the shaping of his or her path through life [...] Nevertheless, the environment has a decisive shaping influence on this hereditary material, especially in the childhood years [...] This is achieved by developing the favourable and suppressing the unfavourable dispositions [...] But the idea of the racial and hereditary biology of the German people should always precede everything else.[1]

The Reichsuniversität Straßburg was founded to be a centre for Nazi research and a stronghold of Nazi ideology in the occupied territory of Alsace. How this ideology came to influence paediatric patient care in the city of Straßburg has been the focus of this book. The place of the children's clinic in the Reichsuniversität Straßburg was not just to treat patients, but also to enforce assimilation of the population. The hospital, and by extension the children's clinic, became crucial to connecting the civilian administration and the de facto annexed population. The university clinics' medical services represent the political administration and attempts to secure the Alsatian population's obedience to occupying Nazi ideology which favoured certain elements of the population above others. This can be exemplified by the above quote from Dr Kurt Hofmeier detailing that although adoption of children orphaned by the war, particularly in Alsace, was intended, the primacy of the 'German Volk' was considered to be the most important element. This research has illustrated how paediatric healthcare was integral to the politics and processes of occupation in Alsace.

This book has questioned what factors influenced patient care; Nazi ideology certainly impacted treatment, and it seems that the clinics were primarily motivated by financial factors. Patient class, indicating their ability to pay privately for their care, was one of the most important differentiating factors between patients. Those who could pay more in turn received more correspondence with their parents, were accommodated in better rooms, were provided with more follow-up care as outpatients, and had more treatment options available to them. This patient class, and financial ability to pay, reflects not only monetary advantage, but also societal inclusion in occupied Alsace. In order to have the financial means to pay for care, one had, to some degree, to integrate into the Nazi system. Therefore, patient class not only indicates healthcare benefits, but also social benefits, which in turn were rewarded as part of the Reichsuniversität Straßburg hospital system. Questions about membership of the Hitler Youth and Bande Deutsche Mädel, as well as marriage loans and Sippentafeln, while on the surface may appear to be just administrative box-ticking exercises, played an important role; after all, membership of an organization normally should not impact healthcare outcomes, but between 1941 and 1944 in Straßburg, this was the central determinant of healthcare, particularly for children.

It appears that the children were somewhat prepared for the Allied arrival and the encroaching front lines, even though the students and civilians may not have been. The patients of the children's clinic also appear to have been well prepared, as Hofmeier mentioned that only twenty patients remained at the clinic in Straßburg, under the supervision of a Lithuanian medical assistant, Dr Elena Alexandraviciene.[2] It is assumed that these twenty patients were not evacuated due to their medical conditions, although what illnesses they had are not mentioned. Hofmeier's decision implies that some patients were released in anticipation of the Allied arrival. The record does not specify how many patients were released under such conditions, nor is there an explanation as to how this triage system was organized.

The End of the Reichsuniversität Straßburg

The Allies took three days to liberate Strasbourg, starting on the morning of 23 November 1944. In the immediate aftermath of the battle, surgical clinic I was used by the American and French troops as a field hospital, and Dr Ludwig Zukschwerdt, the former director of surgery at the Reichsuniversität Straßburg, continued to operate in surgical clinic II.[3] The hospital doctors who did not flee stayed in the private clinic of Dr Johannes Stein for two weeks. On 7 December, the remaining 250 staff members were placed on a train from Strasbourg to a prisoner of war camp between Marseilles and

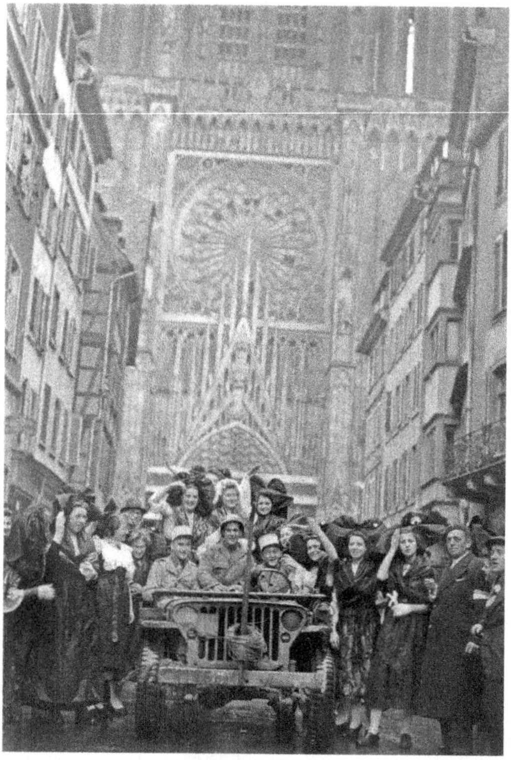

Fig. 7.1. Liberation de l'Alsace; Allied troops with Alsatian women at Strasbourg Cathedral, 1944.[4]

Aix-en-Provence, where they worked in a new hospital camp built to accommodate 1,500 patients.[5] The female Reichsuniversität hospital staff members were brought to a prisoner of war camp near Chartres, although it is not known if this group included Alsatian staff members. Despite being in a prisoner of war camp, they had considerable freedoms, and their capture did not diminish their intent to produce publications or anticipation that they would have a career after the war. Dr Fritz Klinge, the chair of pathology, is one such example; he took time in the Marseille camp to write a book, published in 1948, detailing his methods of teaching pathology in Strasbourg.[6]

It does not appear that there was any cohesive plan for the forced labourers who were present at the hospital when the Allies arrived; they were not taken to prisoner of war camps but left to make their way back home. There were multiple displaced persons camps (also known as DP camps) across Europe in the immediate aftermath of war, usually managed by the UNRRA (United Nations Relief and Rehabilitation Administration). Despite this, the UNRRA and the IRO did not have well-established protocols on how to deal with these displaced children; as Verena Busser states, their policy was to 'learn as they go', given the diversity of people's experiences both during and immediately after the war.[7] Many children had been orphaned as a result of air raids, others were forced labourers, some were mentally or developmentally delayed, which impacted their resettlement, along with, of course, the children who had survived the Holocaust either in hiding or in concentration camps.[8] As a result of this range of possible circumstances, and the fact that the UNRRA did not anticipate this unprecedented amount of child displacement, many children remained undocumented.[9] This return home was easier said than done, as they had to navigate limited transport options to get back to the East following the destruction from the war, and of course, their home countries were ransacked, with often very few family members left to return to. Unfortunately, their exact fate is unknown.[10]

Following their time as prisoners of war, the former staff of the Reichsuniversität Straßburg underwent a process of denazification, which varied slightly depending on the occupied region of Germany that they settled in, and largely kept their licences to practise medicine. Being a member of the Nazi party alone was not sufficient to have their licence revoked, simply because medicine was structured so that most doctors had to swear an oath, even if they did not personally believe it, in order to continue practising medicine. Therefore, several levels of participation were established, and realistically, unless they had committed grievous crimes, they evaded any prosecution. There was of course a considerable dearth of doctors in the aftermath of the war to tend to the extensive injuries of both civilians and the military, so many continued to practise in the postwar era, including Hofmeier, who began a private practice in Stuttgart. They were not brought to trial, with the exceptions of Hirt, Haagen, and Bickenbach. In their correspondence reflecting on their time in the Reichsuniversität Straßburg, Dean Georg Niemeier and Altrektor Schmidt mention that 'it was nice' and that the abrupt evacuation was a 'sad end' to the university.[11]

The university buildings had sustained considerable damage after the battle, but despite this, the overall layout and structure remains the same today, albeit considerably modernized. The French children's clinic had been evacuated to the Hôpital Parrot in Périgueux in 1940, and returned to Strasbourg at the end of August 1945.[12] The rest of the hospital was reinstated by the French in June 1945, but the buildings of the children's clinic retained their function as a military health facility until August.[13] In 1989, the children's clinic buildings were demolished and the clinic moved to the Hôpital Hautepierre, with the site of the former children's clinic later used for the construction of the Nouvel Hôpital Civil in 2008.[14]

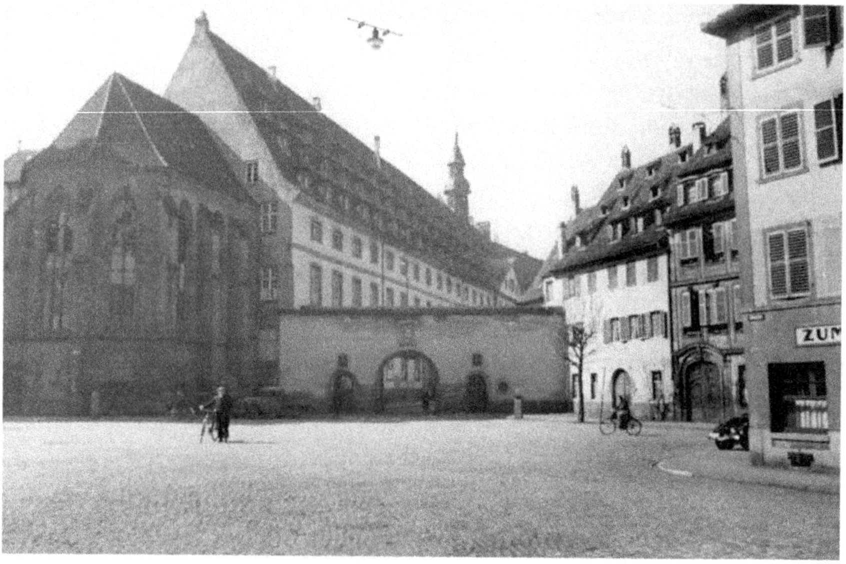

Fig. 7.2. Gates to the Reichsuniversität Straßburg hospital, 1941.[15]

Postwar Reception of the Former Children's Clinic Director, Dr Hofmeier

Hofmeier was one of hundreds of thousands who had to complete a denazification document, both under the French occupation forces and then again when he tried to get a job in Germany.[16] While many former directors of clinics were successful in getting another academic post, Hofmeier was not. He applied to the University of Mainz in the postwar era, but was unsuccessful for unknown reasons; his application is included in the dossier of rejected applications for the position.[17] In his 1949 denazification, the file includes a chronology of his military service, his publications, research positions, and personal information. We do not learn anything from this document about his involvement in the Lebensborn home, as he never received any financial compensation from the SS Lebensborn organization for his time there—he did this work voluntarily—and so the denazification officials remained unaware of this work. He was allowed to choose testimonies himself, from his banker, co-workers, and friends, which detail that he was a skilled and dedicated paediatrician, with no political affiliation. They had the effect of legitimizing his career, and his political position as one solely of joining the Nazi party to progress in career, rather than any actual belief in the ideology. As a result, Hofmeier was classified as a Mitläufer, and his medical

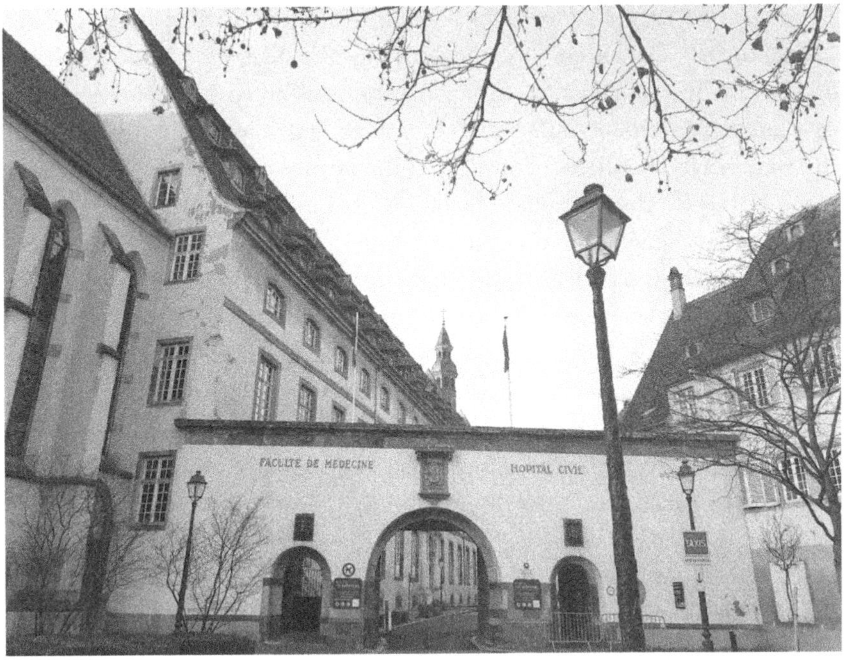

Fig. 7.3. Gates to the Faculté de Médicine at Hôpital Civile de l'Université de Strasbourg, 2020.

licence was reinstated as they considered him 'medically indispensable in paediatrics'. He returned to medical practice, albeit never in a research or academic role again.[18]

Despite the multiple denazifications, and his directorship of one of the most ideologically Nazified universities, Hofmeier's reputation as a paediatrician won out. His medical opinion appears to have been valued in the immediate postwar era, as he contributed in 1949 to the Fragekasten section in the *Deutsche Medizinische Wochenschrift*, one of the most popular medical journals at the time, so it is clear the editors thought his perspective was valuable.[19] His main research concerns—including the impact of environment on childhood development, constitution, infection control, and nutrition—remained pertinent after the war, as evidenced in his publications such as *Deutsche Nachkriegskinder* in 1954 and *10 Jahre Nachkriegskinder* in 1962.[20] These addressed issues such as intelligence testing, the impact of physical environment and social environment, childhood development, nutrition, infection control, and details on the question of childhood constitution and the impact on health; these were all subjects he had published on during the war. Hofmeier published many books in the postwar era, most popular of which was *Alles Uber Dein Kind*, originally published in 1971, which went through five editions.[21] On his seventy-fifth birthday, the *Stuttgarter Zeitung* published a piece on his contribution to paediatrics, and noted how Hofmeier had campaigned to reduce infant mortality rates and improve nutrition during the war, briefly mentioned that he was the former director of the children's clinic in the Reichsuniversität Straßburg, and focused on his establishment of a successful paediatric practice in Stuttgart in 1948.[22]

He privately saw patients at his Stuttgart practice, and while his reputation was clearly not impacted by his involvement with the Reichsuniversität Straßburg, he never held an academic position again. He did support SOS Kinderdorf, a non-profit organization of villages providing social, educational, and medical facilities to impoverished children, particularly in the postwar era, which was possibly reflective of his experience during wartime, where he saw so many orphaned and homeless children as a result of the Allied bombing.[23] It cannot be denied, though, that he saw these children in racialized terms; those who would be worth something to the Volk and those who would not. Indeed, this is reflected in his unpublished memoirs, 'Mein Zeit so es ist', in which he dedicates an entire chapter to 'Zur Judenfage' and denies any knowledge of differences between different social groups in Germany prior to the war. His memoirs finish with this quote on the topic of the 'Jewish question':

> What differentiated the Jews from us was their religion, but they were never presented to us as a foreign race. They were also like Prussian citizens and that they had any rights deprived was not known to me, and was not the case [...] With these few words I want to conclude what I remember from the Jewish problem from that time. One can perhaps say the following, that the Jews were not loved, that one did not seek a community or initiate contact, but there was no talk of hatred toward Jews, or even worse, racial hatred.

This quote is typical of the refusal to engage with this 'open secret' of exclusion and persecution during the Nazi era among those who had not openly committed war crimes. It was thought that being cleared by denazification documentation was sufficient, to the extent that in the postwar era, these were called Persilscheine, a pun on the popular laundry detergent Persil, which claimed to eliminate all stains and wash things completely white.[24] It is telling that he chose the final chapter of his memoirs to focus exclusively on Jews while simultaneously not mentioning his actions during the Second

World War, his early membership of the Nazi party, or indeed his position in the Reichsuniversität Straßburg, which was predicated on the expulsion of Jews from Straßburg. This is an example of—as Sheila Faith Weiss calls it—political whitewashing in the postwar era, by seeming to address the issue at hand while simultaneously glossing over the wartime realities.[25] This quote refers specifically to Prussia and the period of his childhood, and not Nazism; however, Hofmeier's claim of being entirely unaware of the deprivation of rights to Jewish people is untrue. Considering he published work discussing how some children were more hereditarily valuable than others, and that those who were considered lesser should be 'suppressed', this is a clear reflection and adherence to National Socialist ideas, at which the core was the suppression of the Jewish people.[26] Hofmeier was appointed as director of the Kaiserin Auguste Viktoria Haus in 1938 as a direct consequence of the expulsion of its former director, Werner Gottstein, on the grounds that he was Jewish.[27] He also appears to be fully aware of the exclusion of Jewish doctors, and was actively participating in it through his comment that 'it is inconceivable to us that it was considered right to appoint a Jewish doctor as the successor'.[28] His involvement with the Deutsche Gesellschaft für Kinderheilkunde was as a result of the 'voluntary' resignation of Jewish members, who were then replaced by members of the NSDAP, including Hofmeier and Gruninger.[29] Given his close relationship with the commandant of Strasbourg from 1941, and his involvement in the Nazi party, Hofmeier must also have been aware that Straßburg was declared 'Judenrein' by 1940. During the war, he was a zealous adherent of National Socialism, and had joined the party early enough to be considered an Alte Kämpfer.

While he did not mention the Reichsuniversität Straßburg in his memoirs, despite this being his last academic position, he clearly held his time in Straßburg close to his heart. This is evidenced by his attendance at the Rektor Schmidt's seventieth birthday party in Tübingen in 1970, where the former staff members of the Reichsuniversität Straßburg gathered and reminisced about what they considered the highlights of their careers, which they remembered fondly.[30] This would be the last known meeting of the staff of the Reichsuniversität Straßburg.

Reflection on Patient Records

This book is primarily based in archival analysis of patient files which have not been previously examined. It has been a privilege to have access to these files, to recover them, and to read them to understand how the Reichsuniversität

Straßburg functioned in terms of clinical practice rather than institutional research. That being said, these patient files were created by National Socialist doctors and nurses, whose intention was to deny treatment and care to those they did not consider 'worthy' of it. With this in mind, this book has presented these case files as they are, and has read them against the grain, to illustrate the inherently unequal, racist, and ableist treatment that these doctors promoted and practised in the name of Nazism.

From this reading of the patient files, we can see how this hospital functioned on top of a pre-existing financial status hierarchy, as seen in Günther F. and Francine L.'s cases. Günther F.'s father was contacted personally by the hospital, whereas Watzlaff Z. was discharged from hospital after only three days with minimal treatment based on financial status. This can also be viewed as a reason for the lack of referral to other hospitals, despite the presence of serious illnesses, as if the patient stayed in the Reichsuniversität Straßburg, the hospital could continue to financially benefit from them.

Through the records of Susanna D. and Wida K., it is evident that attitudes to nationality and Germanization became more strict as the occupation progressed through the three eras. Those with German nationality, such as Susanna D., were provided with consent forms before treatment, in contrast to Wida K. Furthermore, the administrative designation of Reichsdeutscher, and the increasing prevalence of this designation, can be seen to correspond with the progression of Germanization, and indeed the progressing racial profiling of the population as those who would benefit the German Volk and those who would not.

In examining the case records of Johann B. and Renatus T., we can see how ideology shaped the diagnoses that were given, as Johann H. was diagnosed with a persecution complex based on being aware of the Gestapo at a young age. We can also see this in the intelligence tests that were part of Renatus T.'s file, with questions based around Nazi beliefs, so that if the child was not integrated into the Nazi system, their intelligence would be considered lower than that of their peers.

We also see the impact of the war as it progressed through patient files, as Luise S.'s health declines while she is in an air-raid shelter, and children are admitted with injuries as a result of bombing raids. Children are orphaned because of the conflict, some with fathers fighting on the front lines as in the case of Irmgard D., Dieter H., and Georgine S. The impact of the war can be most clearly seen with the forced labourers, of course, as their very presence in the clinic indicates that the war is being lost, with no more capacity to repatriate them, and the bare minimum of medical treatment being provided to maintain their 'human capital', as in the case of Katherine S. and Wassily D.

Final Thoughts and Summary of Results

The result of this work is primarily that the records from the Reichsuniversität Straßburg have been detailed and described in relation to an important demographic group. It has also examined the staff, students, and directors who treated these individuals, and how this treatment was informed by the political system in which they operated. This book has mentioned the unique political situation of the city of Strasbourg during National Socialism, and how the three-era structure of the hospital reflects that. This book has detailed the individual cases and stories of patients who were treated at the hospital, and in doing so it shifts the focus from individual doctor-centric histories to looking at the population more broadly and the institutional narrative that dictated and impacted daily treatment in a clinic based on inherently exclusionist ideas. Cathy Caruth's concept of 'let the archives speak' is particularly poignant in the case of this research; one can understand how this trauma of wartime occupation and Nazi ideology manifested and impacted children's care in the Reichsuniversität Straßburg through examining the archives.[31] In analysing these patient files, it can be seen how trauma developed under this institutional power; both the larger institution of the Nazi-occupied zones, but also the smaller institution of the hospital. Another practical implication of this research is to flip the narrative from the more traditional history of clinic directors, to a more broad study of the practical impact this had on a vulnerable population. The recommendation from this research is to further understand how medicine operated under such ideological conditions, by not only looking at victims of criminal research, but also by examining the everyday research of such a regime. The Nazi regime was, for millions of people, an everyday occurrence. Their day-to-day lives were encapsulated in this regime that touched every part of their existence. This is clear from the patient records; they show that patients' parents married and had children with the help of marriage loans, their parents were forced into conscription with the Wehrmacht, they became objects of interest due to the fact they were twins, they were emotionally impacted by the evacuation of the city, and they were indoctrinated through the schools. As part of everyday life, these patients got sick and were sent to hospital. They were treated, and returned home, as was the case in most of those admitted to the Reichsuniversität Straßburg. Despite this seemingly mundane 'ordinary everyday' research, it highlights the practical impact of an ideology on the regular medical care of the population.

Therefore, the question of whether the research conducted on children at the Reichsuniversität Straßburg was adherent to the Nazi ideology that was central to the foundation of the university can be answered with both yes and no. The children's clinic did not appear to conduct any criminal research, but it did reinforce the ideology that some children, by virtue of their place of birth, their parents, or their hereditary illnesses, were more 'useful' to the German Volk than others. In this sense, then, although the Reichsuniversität Straßburg children's clinic did not contribute to experiments conducted in the name of National Socialism, the department was central to fulfilling the aim to integrate the population into a new Germany. Furthermore, Kurt Hofmeier's eager involvement with the Lebensborn programme illustrates that he took these ideas particularly seriously and was content to support the Nazi system. The research in the children's clinic, and indeed research on paediatric patients, concerned the areas of nutrition, heredity, twin research, prevention of infectious disease through vaccination and other preventative measures, childhood development, social concerns such as adoption and children born out of wedlock, and a focus on the environment and how this impacted childhood. While many of these areas were affiliated with Nazi research, such as the concern with social issues and illegitimacy, twin research and heredity, and the control of the environment, these were not solely the concern of Nazi medicine. These concerns were prevalent at the time and much of the research done in the children's clinic at the Reichsuniversität Straßburg was very much in line with international research of that era. Indeed, the ideas of the impact of race and social mixing being harmful to childhood development, while indicative of Nazi ideology, were not unique to the 'Third Reich'.

The Reichsuniversität Straßburg was established in 1941 with the intention to 'dethrone the Sorbonne', as a central part of the new 1,000-year German empire. Despite these lofty ambitions, the university lasted only three years. Although the university, and thus the hospital contained within it, lasted a short period of time, the intentions behind it were evident as it progressed through its three key eras. The first, during which the Alsatian population seemed to have some degree of autonomy while the university was being organized, gave way to the second phase in just one year. In the second era, the university was formally inaugurated, and with it came the Alte Kämpfer to firmly solidify the place of National Socialist ideas in the next generation of students, in their medical practice, in the local population, and in research.

The university was—symbolically—not a new one, unlike other Reichsuniversitäten, as they believed that Alsace was a historic part of Germany, and that its people were native Germans. This can be seen in the patient statistics provided in this book, as the clinics provided a central place wherein the population could be both monitored and administratively converted to German nationality. In this manner, the university was central not only to medical research, but also to the practical daily task of 'Germanization' which characterized the second era of the Reichsuniversität Straßburg. In this sense, while this book mentions 'normality', it must be noted that this normality changed dramatically as the eras progressed. In the third era, the more extreme criminal research of August Hirt, Eugen Haagen, and Otto Bickenbach takes place, which can only be facilitated in such an extremist university, founded on the intention of racist medical research. While this was happening, hints of the degradation of the structures of the Reichsuniversität Straßburg can be seen in patient files, as children and their families are being impacted by bombing raids, and their long waits in air-raid shelters begin to impact their health. We see this idealistic separation of those 'worthy' of medical care start to disintegrate as forced labourers and their children begin to be seen in the hospital wards, where this separation can't remain a secret to the local population. We see this in patient files, where children fear the Gestapo, along with medical students, and their adherence to this social system becomes both medicalized and pathologized.

This book has sought to make the issue of paediatrics under National Socialism more salient, and indeed, more tangible. While, of course, there were horrific human experiments conducted in the name of National Socialism, it is my central thesis that one can only fully comprehend the extent of the ethical divergence by first understanding what 'normal' was during this time. This study goes beyond the political and the rhetorical to the experiential, asking how exactly the patients experienced this 'normality', and asks how difficult normality was under such an ideological system for the children who never chose to be part of that system.

Appendices

1. Map of Reichsuniversität Straßburg Hospital with Key Indicating Buildings. ADHVS

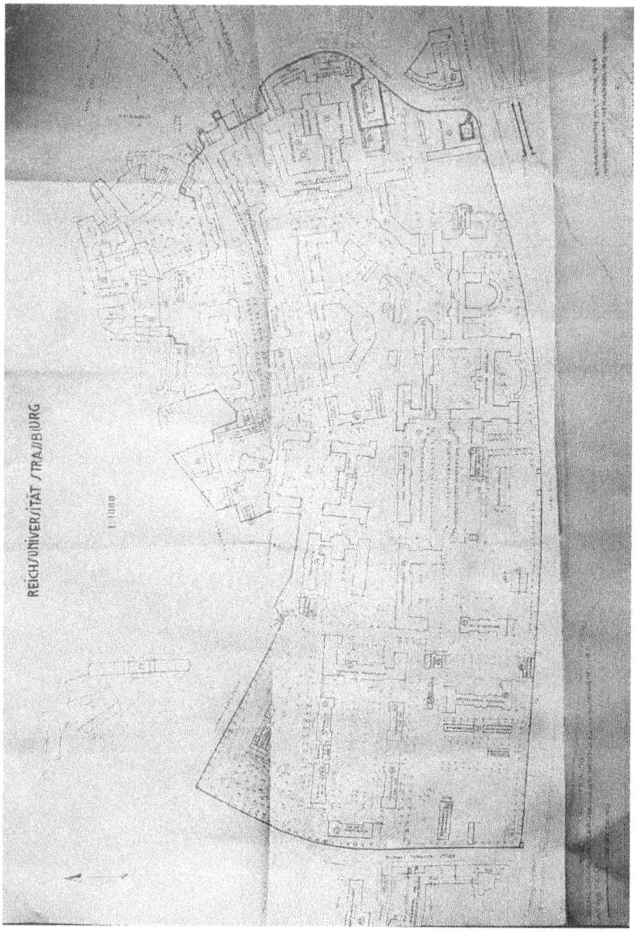

2. Full List of Paediatric Clinic Staff

Surname	First Name	Nationality	Position	Title	Entry	Exit
Schneegans	Ernest	Alsatian	Assistenzarzt	Dr. med.	Nov. 1940	Summer 1941
Hofmeier	Kurt	German	Director	Prof. Dr. med.	1940	1944
Mehl	René	Alsatian	Assistenzarzt	Dr. med.	Nov. 1940	March 1942
Melle-Dietz	Élisabeth	Alsatian	Volontärassistentin, Assistenzärztin	Dr. med.	Nov. 1940	Oct. 1944
Gachot-Heyl	Almuth	German	Volontärassistentin	Dr. med.	June 1941	Nov. 1944
Von Bentheim	Hermine	German	Assistenzärztin	Dr. med.	June 1941	Nov. 1944
Steinmaurer	Hansjörg	German	Oberarzt	Doz. Dr. med. habil.	Nov. 1941	Nov. 1944
Willer	Charles	Alsatian	Assistenzarzt	Dr. med.	Nov. 1941	Nov. 1944
Wenner	Ernst	Luxembourger	Volontärassistent, Assistenzarzt	Dr. med.	Nov. 1941	Nov. 1944
Von der Decken	Rosemarie	German	Pflichtassistentin, Volontärassistentin, Assistenzärztin	Dr. med.	Nov. 1941	Nov. 1944
Link-Amos	Marlène	Alsatian	Pflichtassistentin, Assistenzärztin		Nov. 1941	Nov. 1944

Surname	First Name	Nationality	Position	Title	Entry	Exit
Ulrich-Heil	Marguerite	Alsatian	Volontärassistentin	Dr. med.	Spring 1941	Summer 1941
Siebert-Hohagen	Margarete	Unknown	Volontärassistentin		Nov. 1941	Feb. 1943
Strohm	Hugo	German	Assistenzarzt	Dr. med.	Jan. 1942	Nov. 1944
Pappert-Trier	Grete	Unknown	Assistenzärztin	Dr. med.	March 1942	Sept. 1944
Wilhelm	Ludwig	Unknown	Assistenzarzt	Dr. med.	March 1942	Nov. 1944
Kiehl	Wolfgang	German	Assistenzarzt, kommissarischer Oberarzt	Dr. med. habil.	June 1942	Nov. 1944
Geissler	Liese	Unknown	Assistenzarzt	Dr. med.	June 1942	Sept. 1942
Strohe	Ingeborg	German	Volontärassistentin, Assistenzärztin	Dr. med.	Nov. 1942	Nov. 1944
Von der Decken	Christel	German	Wissenschaftliche Hilfskraft	Dr. med.	Feb. 1943	April 1943
Nägele	Hans	Unknown	Assistenzarzt	Dr. med.	July 1943	Nov. 1944
Bader-Sartorious	Emma	German	Assistenzärztin	Dr. med.	Feb. 1943	Nov. 1944
Bouma-Teyé	Johan	Dutch	Assistenzarzt	Dr. med.	Dec. 1943	Nov. 1944

Suhr	Larissa	Unknown	Volontärassistentin		Feb. 1943	Nov. 1944
Unshelm	Egon	German	Oberarzt	Prof. Dr. med.	1943	1944
Woringer	Pierre	Alsatian	kommissarischer Chefarzt	Dr. med.	Nov. 1940	Autumn 1941
Wörth	Lina	Unknown	Leitende Ärztin (Waisenhaus 'Karl-Roos-Haus')	Dr. med.	Nov. 1940	Autumn 1941
Wollesen	Ingeborg	Unknown	Wissenschaftliche Hilfskraft		Aug. 1942	Oct. 1942
Gerard-Haukohl	Rosemarie	German	Pflichtassistentin		Aug. 1944	Aug. 1944
Schubert-Menne	Elli	German	Pflichtassistentin		Aug. 1944	Nov. 1944
Alexandraviciene	Elena	Lithuanian	Ass.Arzt	Dr. med.	Sept. 1944	Nov. 1944
Apffel	Charles	Alsatian	kommissarischer Chefarzt 'Säuglingsheim'	Dr. med.	Aug. 1940	Nov. 1941

3. Sample of Admission Diagnostic Questions from the Paediatric Clinic

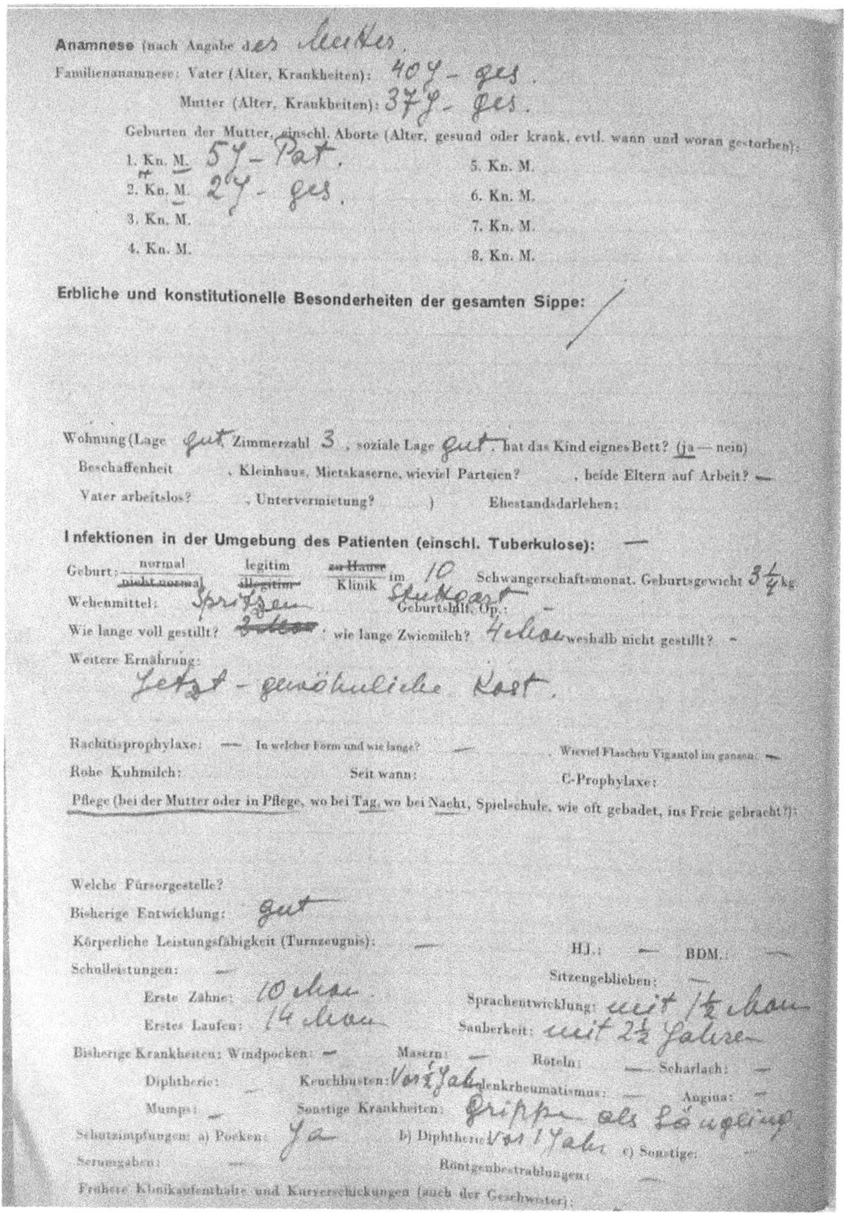

Anamnese (nach Angabe der Mutter.

Familienanamnese: Vater (Alter, Krankheiten): 40 J. – ges.

Mutter (Alter, Krankheiten): 37 J. – ges.

Geburten der Mutter, einschl. Aborte (Alter, gesund oder krank, evtl. wann und woran gestorben):

1. Kn. M. 5 J. – Pat.
2. Kn. M. 2 J. – ges.
3. Kn. M.
4. Kn. M.
5. Kn. M.
6. Kn. M.
7. Kn. M.
8. Kn. M.

Erbliche und konstitutionelle Besonderheiten der gesamten Sippe: /

Wohnung (Lage gut, Zimmerzahl 3, soziale Lage gut, hat das Kind eignes Bett? (ja — nein)
Beschaffenheit , Kleinhaus, Mietskaserne, wieviel Parteien? , beide Eltern auf Arbeit? —
Vater arbeitslos? , Untervermietung?) Ehestandsdarlehen:

Infektionen in der Umgebung des Patienten (einschl. Tuberkulose): —

Geburt: normal / ~~nicht normal~~ legitim / ~~illegitim~~ ~~zu Hause~~ / Klinik im 10 Schwangerschaftsmonat. Geburtsgewicht 3¼ kg
Wehenmittel: Spritzen Stuttgart Geburtshilfl. Op.: —
Wie lange voll gestillt? ~~3 Mon~~ wie lange Zwiemilch? 4 Mon weshalb nicht gestillt? –
Weitere Ernährung:
Jetzt – gewöhnliche Kost.

Rachitisprophylaxe: — In welcher Form und wie lange? — Wieviel Flaschen Vigantol im ganzen: —
Rohe Kuhmilch: Seit wann: C-Prophylaxe:
Pflege (bei der Mutter oder in Pflege, wo bei Tag, wo bei Nacht, Spielschule, wie oft gebadet, ins Freie gebracht?):

Welche Fürsorgestelle?
Bisherige Entwicklung: gut
Körperliche Leistungsfähigkeit (Turnzeugnis): — HJ.: — BDM.: —
Schulleistungen: — Sitzengeblieben:
Erste Zähne: 10 Mon. Sprachentwicklung: mit 1½ Mon
Erstes Laufen: 14 Mon Sauberkeit: mit 2½ Jahren
Bisherige Krankheiten: Windpocken: — Masern: — Röteln: — Scharlach: —
Diphtherie: — Keuchhusten: Vor ½ Jahr Gelenkrheumatismus: — Angina: —
Mumps: — Sonstige Krankheiten: Grippe als Säugling
Schutzimpfungen: a) Pocken: Ja b) Diphtherie: Vor 1 Jahr c) Sonstige: —
Serumgaben: — Röntgenbestrahlungen: —
Frühere Klinikaufenthalte und Kurverschickungen (auch der Geschwister):

4. Racial Hygiene Twin Examination from Otto Dahm's Thesis

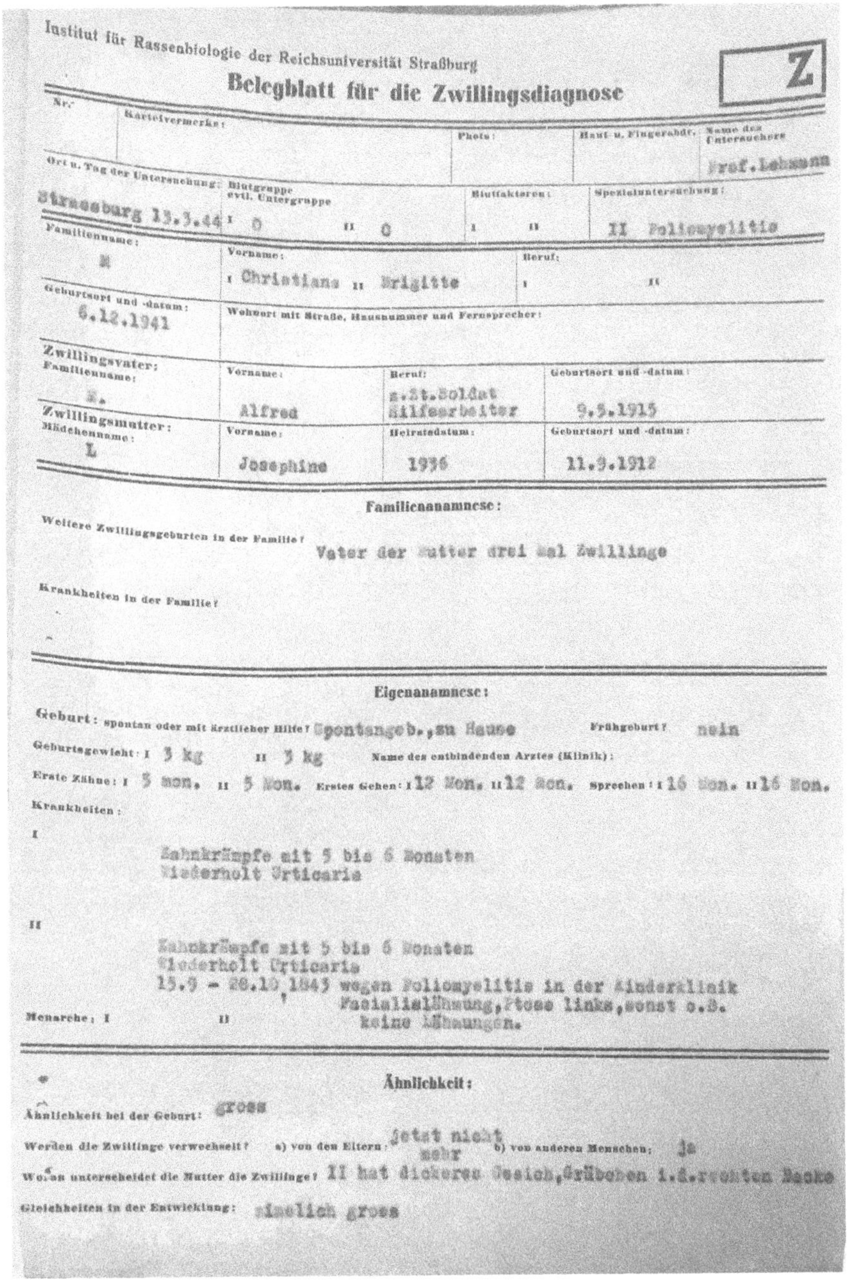

Institut für Rassenbiologie der Reichsuniversität Straßburg

Belegblatt für die Zwillingsdiagnose Z

Nr.: | Karteivermerke: | Photo: | Haut- u. Fingerabdr.: | Name des Untersuchers: Prof. Lehmann

Ort u. Tag der Untersuchung: Strassburg 13.3.44
Blutgruppe evtl. Untergruppe: I 0 II 0
Blutfaktoren: I II
Spezialuntersuchung: II Poliomyelitis

Familienname: M
Vorname: I Christiane II Brigitte
Beruf: I II

Geburtsort und -datum: 6.12.1941
Wohnort mit Straße, Hausnummer und Fernsprecher:

Zwillingsvater: Familienname: M.
Vorname: Alfred
Beruf: z.Zt. Soldat Hilfsarbeiter
Geburtsort und -datum: 9.5.1915

Zwillingsmutter: Mädchenname: L
Vorname: Josephine
Heiratsdatum: 1936
Geburtsort und -datum: 11.9.1912

Familienanamnese:

Weitere Zwillingsgeburten in der Familie? Vater der Mutter drei mal Zwillinge

Krankheiten in der Familie?

Eigenanamnese:

Geburt: spontan oder mit ärztlicher Hilfe? Spontangeb., zu Hause Frühgeburt? nein

Geburtsgewicht: I 3 kg II 3 kg Name des entbindenden Arztes (Klinik):

Erste Zähne: I 5 Mon. II 5 Mon. Erstes Gehen: I 12 Mon. II 12 Mon. Sprechen: I 16 Mon. II 16 Mon.

Krankheiten:

I

Zahnkrämpfe mit 5 bis 6 Monaten
Wiederholt Urticaria

II

Zahnkrämpfe mit 5 bis 6 Monaten
Wiederholt Urticaria
15.9 - 28.10.1943 wegen Poliomyelitis in der Kinderklinik
Fazialislähmung, Ptose links, sonst o.B.
keine Lähmungen.

Menarche: I II

Ähnlichkeit:

Ähnlichkeit bei der Geburt: gross

Werden die Zwillinge verwechselt? a) von den Eltern: jetzt nicht mehr b) von anderen Menschen: ja

Woran unterscheidet die Mutter die Zwillinge? II hat dickeres Gesicht, Grübchen i.d. rechten Backe

Gleichheiten in der Entwicklung: ziemlich gross

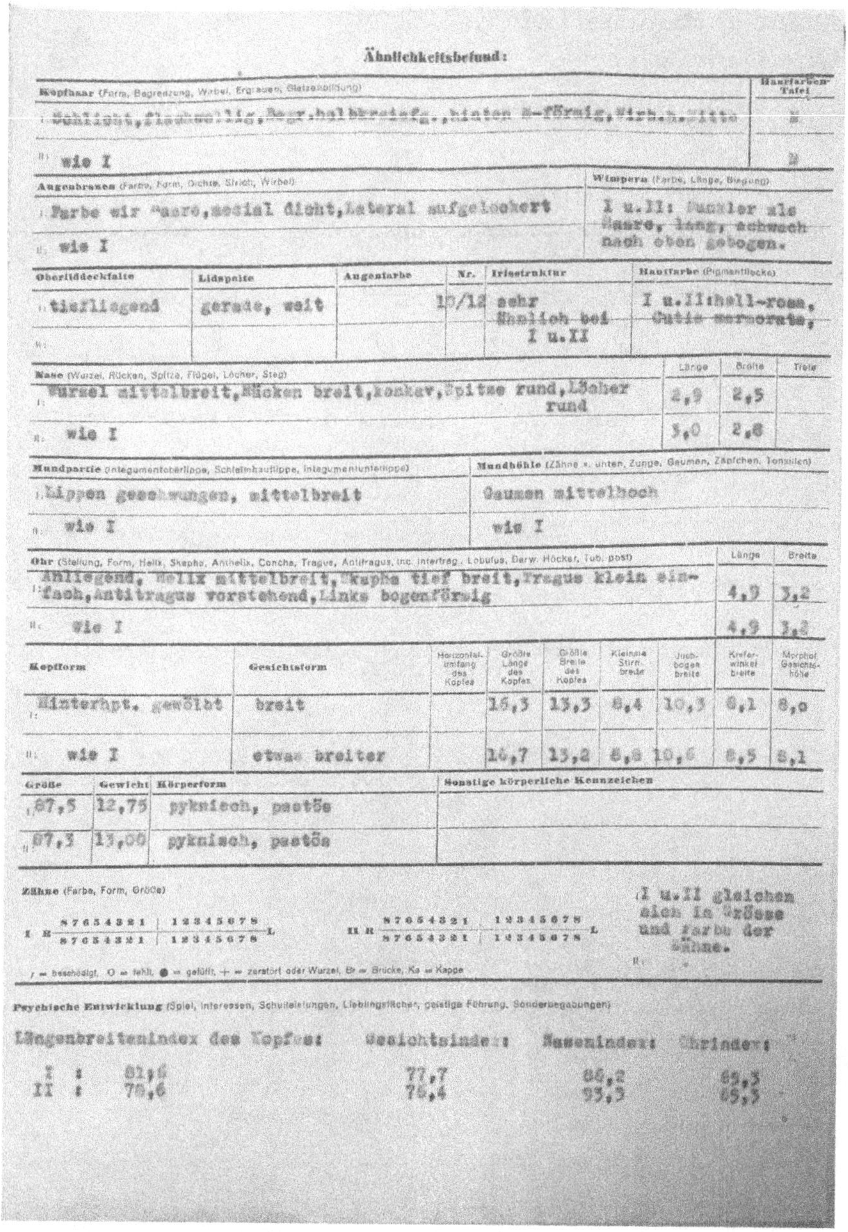

Ähnlichkeitsbefund:

Kopfhaar (Form, Begrenzung, Wirbel, Ergrauen, Glatzenbildung) — Haarfarben-Tafel

I: Schlicht, flachwellig, Begr. halbkreisfg., hinten M-förmig, Wirb. [illegible] Mitte — [illegible]

II: wie I — [illegible]

Augenbrauen (Farbe, Form, Dichte, Strich, Wirbel)

I: Farbe wie Haare, medial dicht, lateral aufgelockert

II: wie I

Wimpern (Farbe, Länge, Biegung)

I u. II: Dunkler als Haare, lang, schwach nach oben gebogen.

	Oberliddeckfalte	Lidspalte	Augenfarbe	Nr.	Irisstruktur	Hautfarbe (Pigmentflecke)
I:	tiefliegend	gerade, weit		10/12	sehr ähnlich bei I u. II	I u. II: hell-rosa, Cutis marmorata,
II:						

	Nase (Wurzel, Rücken, Spitze, Flügel, Löcher, Steg)	Länge	Breite	Tiefe
I:	Wurzel mittelbreit, Rücken breit, konkav, Spitze rund, Löcher rund	2,9	2,5	
II:	wie I	3,0	2,8	

	Mundpartie (Integumentoberlippe, Schleimhautlippe, Integumentunterlippe)	Mundhöhle (Zähne o. unten, Zunge, Gaumen, Zäpfchen, Tonsillen)
I:	Lippen geschwungen, mittelbreit	Gaumen mittelhoch
II:	wie I	wie I

	Ohr (Stellung, Form, Helix, Skapha, Anthelix, Concha, Tragus, Antitragus, Inc. intertrag., Lobulus, Darw. Höcker, Tub. post)	Länge	Breite
I:	Anliegend, Helix mittelbreit, Skapha tief breit, Tragus klein einfach, Antitragus vorstehend, Links bogenförmig	4,9	3,2
II:	Wie I	4,9	3,2

	Kopfform	Gesichtsform	Horizontalumfang des Kopfes	Größte Länge des Kopfes	Größte Breite des Kopfes	Kleinste Stirnbreite	Jochbogenbreite	Kieferwinkelbreite	Morphol. Gesichtshöhe
I:	Hinterhpt. gewölbt	breit		16,3	13,3	8,4	10,3	8,1	8,0
II:	wie I	etwas breiter		16,7	13,2	8,8	10,6	8,5	8,1

	Größe	Gewicht	Körperform	Sonstige körperliche Kennzeichen
I	87,5	12,75	pyknisch, pastös	
II	87,3	13,00	pyknisch, pastös	

Zähne (Farbe, Form, Größe)

I R 87654321 | 12345678 L / 87654321 | 12345678

II R 87654321 | 12345678 L / 87654321 | 12345678

I u. II gleichen sich in Grösse und Farbe der Zähne.

/ = beschädigt, O = fehlt, ● = gefüllt, + = zerstört oder Wurzel, Br = Brücke, Ka = Kappe

Psychische Entwicklung (Spiel, Interessen, Schulleistungen, Lieblingsfächer, geistige Führung, Sonderbegabungen)

	Längenbreitenindex des Kopfes:	Gesichtsindex:	Nasenindex:	Ohrindex:
I :	81,6	77,7	86,2	65,3
II :	78,6	76,4	93,3	65,3

- 15 -

Fall 2. (Diskordantes Auftreten der Poliomyelitis)

Christiane und Brigitte L. (52)

Proband: Brigitte.

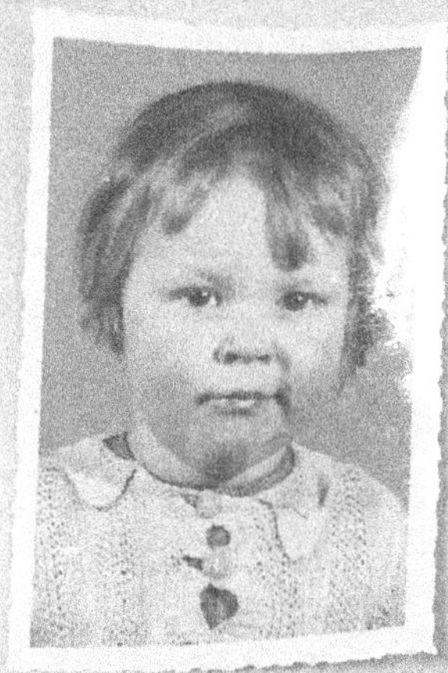

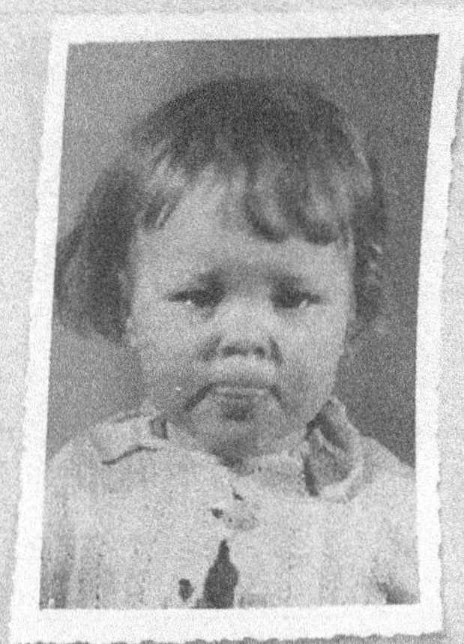

Christiane Brigitte (Proband)

Vorgeschichte :

Nach Angabe der Mutter war 6 Wochen vor der Aufnahme Brigittes ein kleiner Vetter von ihr auf einer Treppe gefallen. Der Junge konnte nach dem Fall zunächst gut laufen. 3 Wochen später konnte er jedoch, nach-dem er vorher einige Tage mit Fieber im Bett gelegen hatte, nicht mehr richtig gehen. Als der Junge fiebernd im Bett lag, hatte Proband ihn besucht. Rund zwei Wochen später hatten beide Zwillinge Fieber, das nicht gemessen wurde. Die Mutter nahm an, dass es vom Zahnen käme. Nach 3 Tagen waren beide Kinder entfiebert. Die Zwillinge fühlten sich wohl. Einen Tag nach der Entfieberung merkte die Mutter, dass Proband beim Lachen und Weinen

5. Statistical Analyses of Paediatric Patient Files in the Children's Clinic

Nationality	**Number of Patients**
Alsatian	555
Reichsdeutscher	127
German	90
Lothringen	27
Italian	7
French	6
Volksdeutscher	2
Polish	2
Ukranian	2
Luxembourger	2
Belgian	1
Yugoslavian	1
Swiss	1
Lithuanian	1
Unknown	34
illegible Nationality	11
Total	869

Prevalence of nationalities in the children's clinic

Diagnosis	**Number**	**Diagnosis**	**Number**
abscess	6	impetigo	4
anaemia	3	influenza	2
angina	34	laryngitis	2
appendicitis	6	mastoiditis	5
asthma	8	meningitis	31
atrophy	6	nephritis	9
brain swelling	2	neuropathy	3
bronchitis	32	osteomyelitis	2
burns	4	otitis media	39
cancer	2	paralysis	7
congenital heart defects	6	pneumonia	89
conjunctivitis	2	polyarthritis	7
debility	7	prematurity	41
diphtheria	50	purpura werlhof	2
disordered eating	9	rhinopharyngitis	4
dyspepsia	46	scabies	11
eczema	5	scarlet fever	80
encephalitis	16	seizures	13
endocarditis	6	sepsis	4
enteritis	8	stomatitis	8
fever	9	syphilis	5
hepatitis	5	TB	42
idiocy	3	tetanus	5
icterus gravis	5	toxicosis	13
typhus	14	tumour	2
unknown	12	vomiting	8

Diagnoses present in the children's clinic

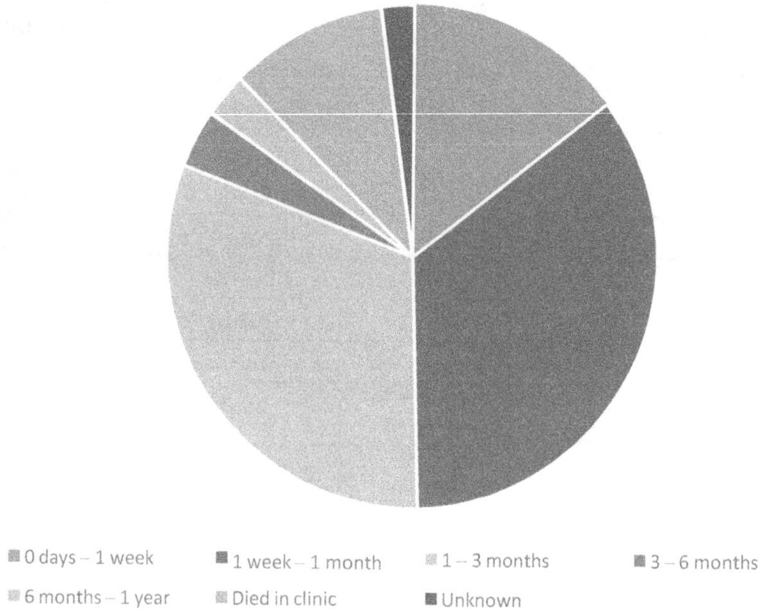

Age range of patients in the children's clinic

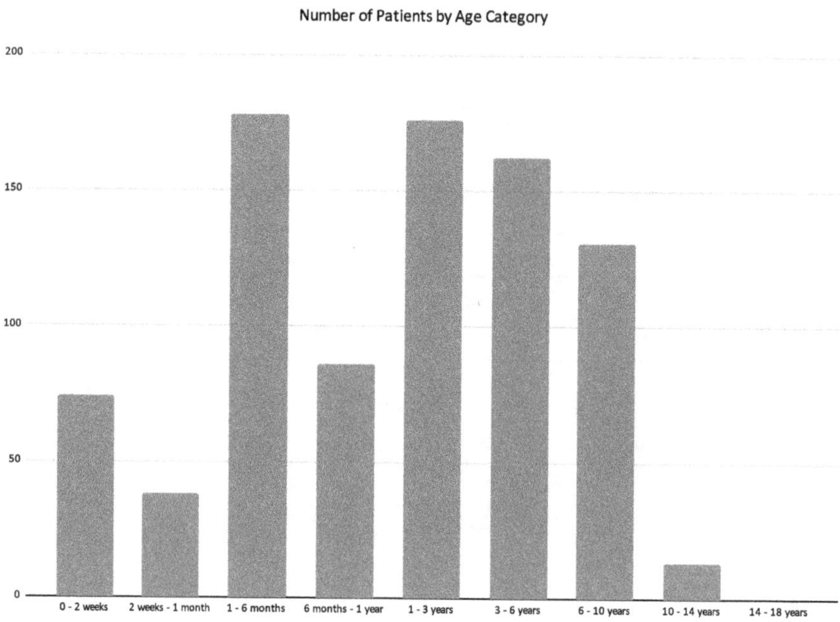

Duration of stay of paediatric patients in the children's clinic

6. Statistical Analyses of Paediatric Patient Files in the Psychiatric Clinic

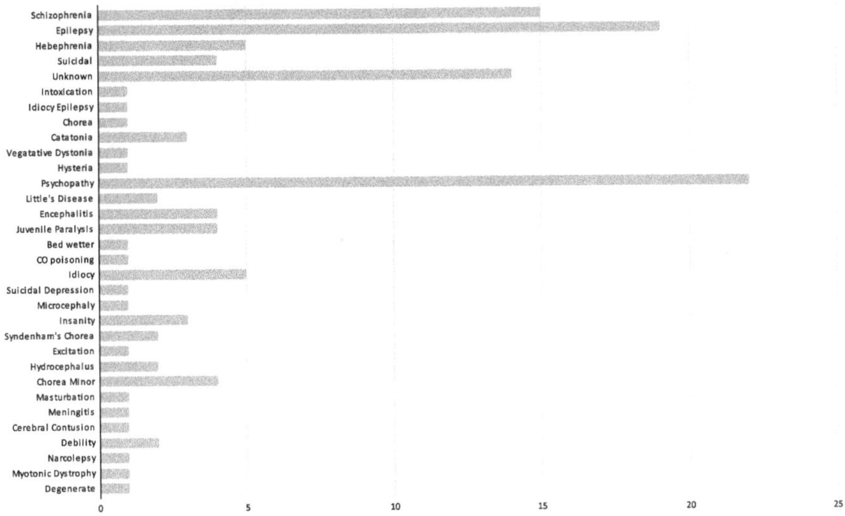

Primary diagnoses of paediatric patients admitted to the psychiatric clinic. ADHVS Psych.

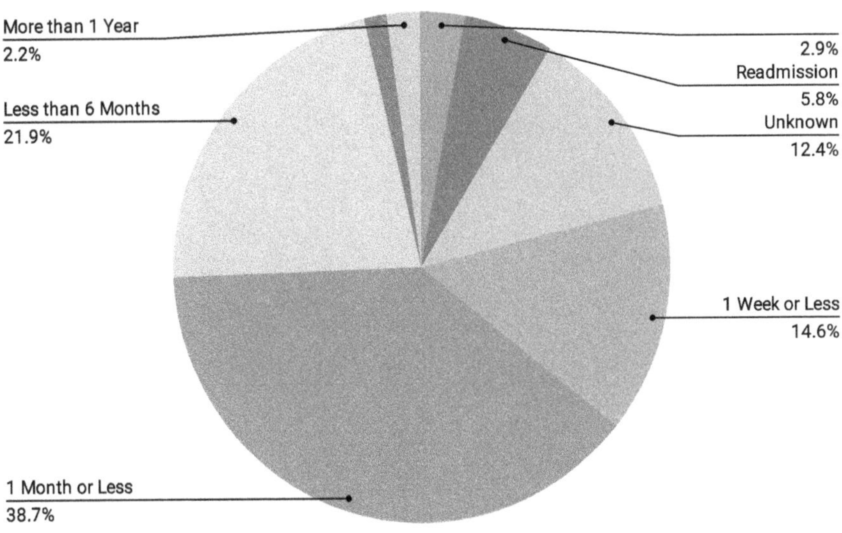

Duration of stay of paediatric patients admitted to the psychiatric clinic. ADHVS Psych.

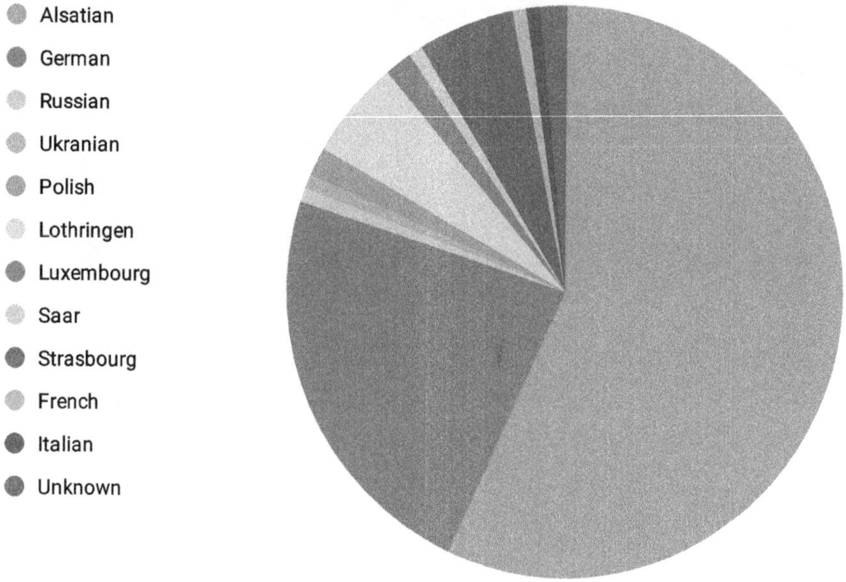

Nationality of paediatric patients admitted to the psychiatric clinic. ADHVS Psych.

7. Example of an Intelligence Test Used in the Psychiatric Clinic. ADHVS

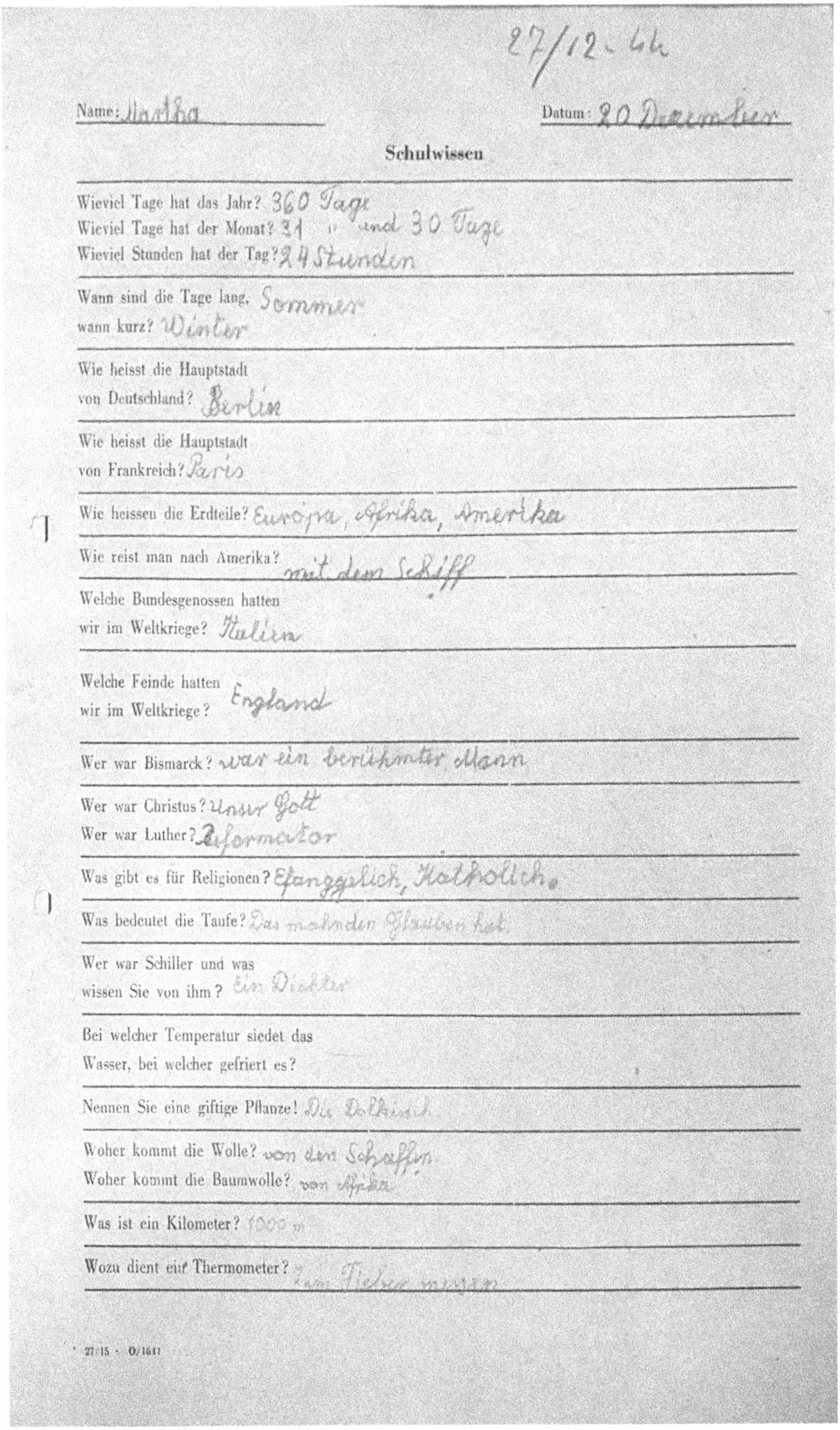

27/12-44

Name: Martha   Datum: 20 Dezember

Schulwissen

Wieviel Tage hat das Jahr? 360 Tage
Wieviel Tage hat der Monat? 31 " und 30 Tage
Wieviel Stunden hat der Tag? 24 Stunden

Wann sind die Tage lang. Sommer
wann kurz? Winter

Wie heisst die Hauptstadt
von Deutschland? Berlin

Wie heisst die Hauptstadt
von Frankreich? Paris

Wie heissen die Erdteile? Europa, Afrika, Amerika

Wie reist man nach Amerika? mit dem Schiff

Welche Bundesgenossen hatten
wir im Weltkriege? Italien

Welche Feinde hatten
wir im Weltkriege? England

Wer war Bismarck? war ein berühmter Mann

Wer war Christus? Unser Gott
Wer war Luther? Reformator

Was gibt es für Religionen? Efanggelich, Katholich.

Was bedeutet die Taufe? Das man den Glauben hat.

Wer war Schiller und was
wissen Sie von ihm? Ein Dichter

Bei welcher Temperatur siedet das
Wasser, bei welcher gefriert es?

Nennen Sie eine giftige Pflanze! Die Tolkirsch

Woher kommt die Wolle? von den Schaffen.
Woher kommt die Baumwolle? von Afrika

Was ist ein Kilometer? 1000 m

Wozu dient ein Thermometer? zum Fieber messen

27/15 · O/1611

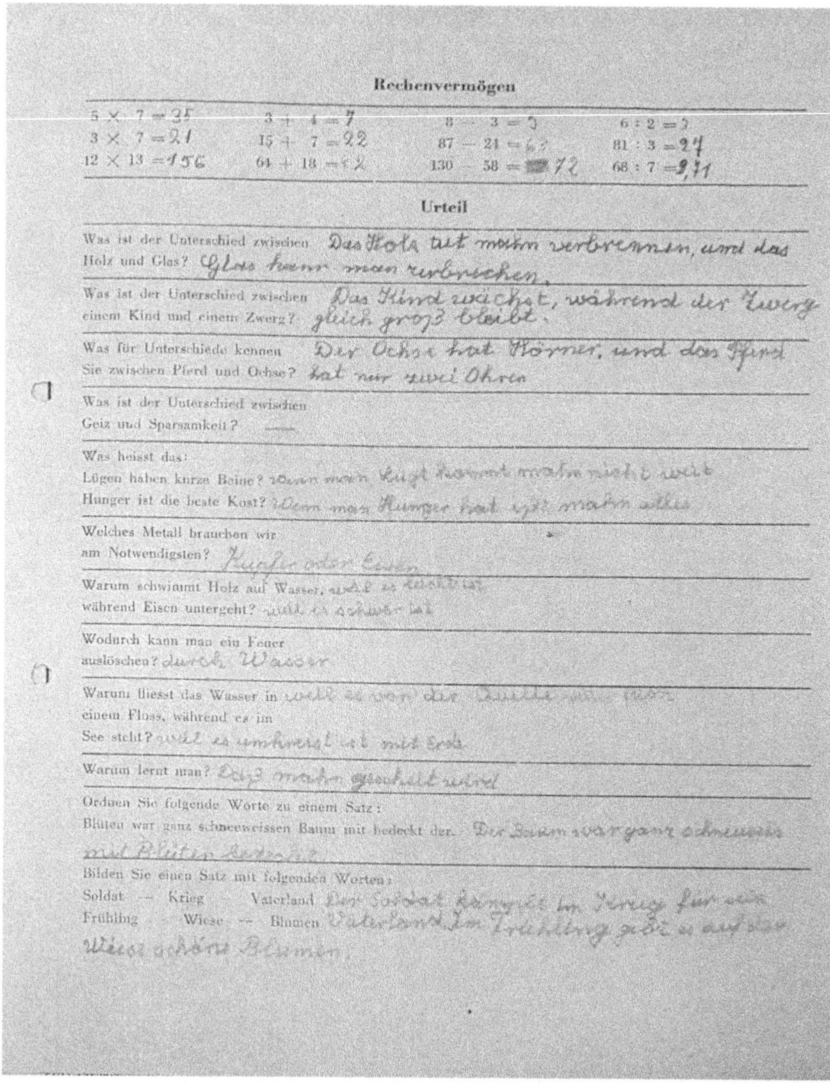

Rechenvermögen

5 × 7 = 35	3 + 4 = 7	8 − 3 = 5	6 : 2 = 3
3 × 7 = 21	15 + 7 = 22	87 − 24 = 63	81 : 3 = 27
12 × 13 = 156	64 + 18 = 82	130 − 58 = 72	68 : 7 = 9,71

Urteil

Was ist der Unterschied zwischen Holz und Glas? Das Holz tut mahn verbrennen, und das Glas kann man zerbrechen.

Was ist der Unterschied zwischen einem Kind und einem Zwerg? Das Kind wächst, während der Zwerg gleich groß bleibt.

Was für Unterschiede kennen Sie zwischen Pferd und Ochse? Der Ochse hat Hörner, und das Pferd hat nur zwei Ohren

Was ist der Unterschied zwischen Geiz und Sparsamkeit? ——

Was heisst das:
Lügen haben kurze Beine? wenn man lügt kommt mahn nicht weit
Hunger ist die beste Kost? Wenn man Hunger hat ißt mahn alles

Welches Metall brauchen wir am Notwendigsten? Kupfer oder Eisen

Warum schwimmt Holz auf Wasser, weil es leicht ist
während Eisen untergeht? weil es schwer ist

Wodurch kann man ein Feuer auslöschen? durch Wasser

Warum fliesst das Wasser in einem Floss, während es im See steht? weil es von der Quelle [illegible]
weil es umkreist ist mit Erde

Warum lernt man? Daß mahn gescheit wird

Ordnen Sie folgende Worte zu einem Satz:
Blüten war ganz schneeweissen Baum mit bedeckt der. Der Baum war ganz schneeweiß mit Blüten bedeckt.

Bilden Sie einen Satz mit folgenden Worten:
Soldat — Krieg — Vaterland Der Soldat kämpft im Krieg für sein Vaterland.
Frühling — Wiese — Blumen Im Frühling gibt es auf der Wiese schöne Blumen.

Ergänzen Sie sinngemäss die Lücken in dem Folgenden:

Gegen vier ____ kam Günther wieder an ____ Strand. Er war vom Gehen ____ geworden und ____ nieder. Wenige Schritte ____ ihm ent____ spielten ein____ Kinder im Sande. Plötzlich ____ er ein kläg____ Geheul. Die Kinder hatten ____ Hund ____ Wasser gew____. Das Tier versuchte ver____ den Boden wieder zu ____. Es konnte kaum noch ____. Günther ver____ den Hund mit ____ Stock herauszu____. Es ____ ihm nicht. Da ging er bis an die Hüften ins ____ und hob den ____ her____. Sowie er den Rücken hatte ergr____ der grösste Knabe ____ wieder, um ihn noch ____ ins ____ zu ____. Günther hielt den ____ fest und ____ ihm, dass das Tier er____ würde.

Setzen Sie aus folgenden Buchstaben Worte zusammen, und zwar bilden Sie mehrere Worte. Es dürfen aber keine weitere Buchstaben verwendet werden, und es müssen alle angeführten Buchstaben in den betreffenden Worten vorkommen!

c, e, g, i, r, s.

In dem Folgenden sind einige Sinnfehler enthalten.
Bezeichnen Sie diese!

Um vier Uhr an einem windstillen Morgen im Winter — die Sonne war eben aufgegangen — wurden die Einwohner des Fischerdorfes durch das Nebelhorn geweckt. Wegen der schneidenden Kälte dicht in Pelze gehüllt, eilten sie zum See hinunter, der ganz zugefroren war. Es konnte einer den anderen im dichten Nebel kaum auf zwei Schritte erkennen. Draussen auf dem Wasser, etwa 15 km entfernt, sahen sie ein grosses Schiff im Sinken. Man hörte deutlich die Hilferufe der Schiffbrüchigen. Auf den vom Sturm gepeitschten Wellen schwamm ein kleines Boot daher. Die Insassen ruderten mit aller Gewalt, konnten aber nicht ans Ufer kommen. Da warf ein von der Sommersonne gebräunter Junge seine dünnen Kleider ab und ging mutig ins Wasser. Obgleich er riesengross und kräftig war, gelang es ihm doch, das Boot ans Ufer zu ziehen und die Insassen zu retten.

8. Questionnaire on Eugenics Conducted at the Reichsuniversität Straßburg Hospital Provided in Johanna Wehrung's Thesis, 1944. AFMS

F r a g e b o g e n !

Alter : ....Konfession : ....

Beruf : ....Reichsd.oder Els.: ....

---

1. Ein Mensch liegt mit qualvollen Schmerzen im Sterben. Der Arzt stellt schon die Todesanzeichen fest.
Halten Sie es für richtig, wenn durch ein schmerzlinderndes Mittel dem Sterbenden seine letzten Stunden erleichtert werden dadurch aber vielleicht der Todeseintritt um ein geringes beschleunigt wird ?

Begründung :

2. Halten Sie es für richtig, dass ein Patient, der an einem mit keinem Mittel zu heilenden Leiden krankt, das nach ärztlichen Erfahrungen in absehbarer Zeit zum Tode führt, durch irgend ein Mittel von seinem Leiden erlöst wird ?
Sollte dies nur auf besonderes Verlangen geschehen ?

Begründung :

3. Stellen Sie sich vor, dass bei einem Menschen infolge angeborener Geistesschwäche oder einer später aufgetretenen Geisteskrankheit eine weitgehende Verblödung aufgetreten ist. Der betreffende ist dadurch für die Volksgemeinschaft völlig wertlos, ja sogar eine Last geworden.
Würden Sie befürworten, dass es erlaubt ist, solche Menschen auf schmerzlose Weise aus der Welt zu schaffen ?
Sollte dies mit oder ohne Einwilligung, ja sogar gegen den Willen der Angehörigen geschehen ?

Begründung :

4. Sollten die unter 1, 2 und 3 angeschnittenen Entscheidungen getroffen werden von
 a) dem behandelnden Arzt
 - würden Sie der Ärzteschaft das gleiche Vertrauen entgegenbringen, falls dem Arzt derartige Rechte eingeräumt werden -
 b) einem Ausschuss, der sich zusammensetzen würde aus dem behandelnden Arzt, einem Facharzt für die betreffende Krankheit und einem Juristen.

Begründung :

9. Statistical Analysis of Paediatric Cases in the Internal Medicine Clinic (Courtesy of Christian Bonah and Lea Münch)

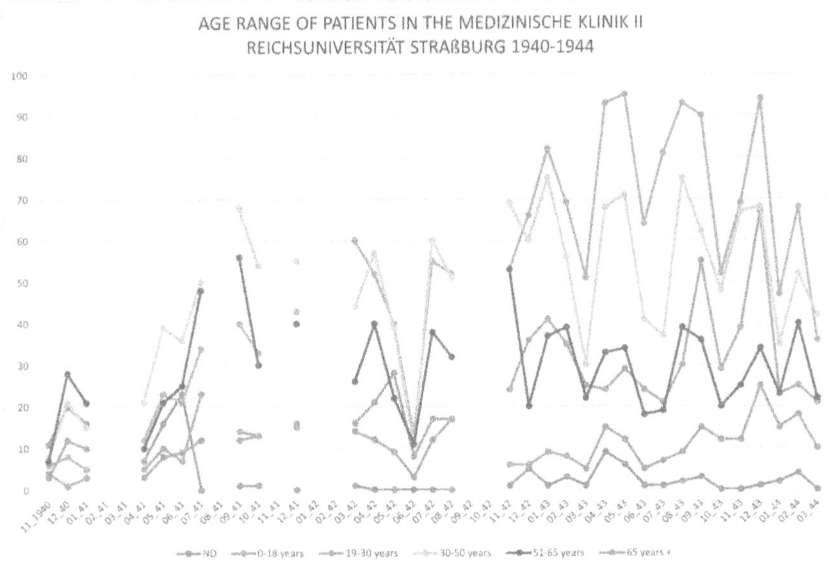

10. Full List of Dr Kurt Hofmeier's Publications

Year	Title	Journal/Publisher	Co-Author
1923	Untersuchungen über die Blutkonzentration. Verteilung der Erythrozyten in den verschiedenen Gefässegebieten und Wirkung des Adrenalins auf Erythrozytenzahl und Volumen	Zeitschrift für des gesamte experimentellen Medizin, 35, 191–202	
1923	Hautnekrose bei Scharlach	Zeitschrift für Kinderheilkunde, 36, 151–156	
1923	Individualismus bei pathogenen Bakterien	Verhandlungen der 36. Versammlung der Deutschen Gesellschaft für Kinderheilkunde, 254–258	
1927	Über die Rolle des Ekto-und Endoplasmas der Typhusbazillen bei Immunitätsreaktionen I. Komplementbindungs versuche	Zeitschrift Immunität Forschung, 50, 71–87	
1927	Über die Rolle des Ekto-und Endoplasmas der Typhusbazillen bei Immunitätsreaktionen II. Bakterizide und Phagozytose	Zeitschrift Immunität Forschung, 50, 509–524	

1927	Über den Verwendungsstoffwechsel der Diphtheriebazillen	Klinischen Wochenschrift 6 Jahrgang, 15	H. Braun
1928	Die kongenitale Übertragung der Infektionskrankheiten	Handbuch der Pathologen Mikroorganismen, Bd I. 523–564	H. Braun
1928	Unterscheidung der echten Paratyphus-B von den Breslau- Enteritis-Bakterien auf Ammonchlorid-Rhamnose-Agar	Klinischen Wochenschrift 7 Jahrgang, 1692	
1929	Die Vererbungsfrage in der Lehre von der Immunität gegen Infektionskrankheiten	Handbuch der Pathologen Mikroorganismen, Bd I. 1109–1146	H. Braun and G. Holzhausen
1929	Zur Ernährungsphysiologie der Diphtheriebazillen. II. Die Nahrungsbedürfnisse der Diphtheriebazillen in syntheischen Nährböden in quantitativer Hinsicht	Zentrallblatt für Bakteriologie. 113, 530–534	H. Braun and F. Mündel
1935	Zur Differentialdiagnose von Krämpfen im Kindesalter	Kinderärztlicher Praxis. 6 Jahrgang.	
1935	Fehlerziehung und Krankheit	Gesundheit und Erziehung, 48 Jahrgang, 10–14	
1936	Über Abhärtung, Ein Mittel der Einbeziehung	Kinderärztlicher Praxis. 7 Jahrgang, 222–227	

Year	Title	Journal/Publisher	Co-Author
1936	Naturgemäße Behandlung der Lungenentzündung bei Kindern	Hippokrates, 757–762	
1937	Erbanlagen und Erziehung	Monatsschrift für Kinderheilkunde, 68, 82–86	
1937	Vererbung und Immunität	Klinischen Wochenschrift, 16 Jahrgang, 329–333	
1937	Über spinale Kinderlähmung	Zeitschrift ärztliche Fortbildung, 34 Jahrgang	
1937	Prophylaxe und Behandlung der Erkältungskrankheiten beim Säugling und Kleinkind	Medizinische Welt, 8	
1937	Konstitution und Infektionskrankheiten	Kinderärztlicher Praxis. 9 Jahrgang	
1938	Die Bedeutung der Erbanlagen für die Kinderheilkunde	Ferdinand Enke Verlag Stuttgart, 200 pages	
1938	Grundsätze und Erfahrungen bei der Frühgeburtenaufzucht	Monatsschrift für Kinderheilkunde, 73, 397–405	Kürt König
1938	Über Wert und Grenzen der aktiven Immunisierung gegen Diphtherie	Zeitschrift Immunität Forschung, 93, 436–456	Anneliese Jansen
1938	Die Beurteilung der Wirksamkeit der aktiven Immunisierung gegen Diphtherie	Münchener medizinische Wochenschrift, 85 Jahrgang, 1035–1036	

1938	Poliomyelitis vom zerebralen Typ bei eineiigen Zwillingen	Zeitschrift für menschliche Vererbung und Konstitution Lehre, 22, 224–237	K. Dinckler
1938	Ist die sog. Säuglingsgymnastik zu empfehlen?	Zeitschrift ärztliche Fortbildung, 35 Jahrgang, 14	
1938	Biologische Medizin in der Kinderheilkunde (Übersicht über die Jahre 1935-1936)	Hippokrates, 772–776, 789–800, 817–824, 879–880	Kürt König
1938	Gefährdeten Säuglings und Kleinkinder und Ihre gesundheitsfürsorgerische Versorgung	Öffentliche Gesundheitsdienst E. Volksgesundheit, 4 Jahrgang, 11; 224–237	
1938	Über die erbliche Bedingtheit infektiöser Erkrankungen des Nervensystems	Monatsschrift für Kinderheilkunde, 75	
1939	Die Ernährung des Kleinkindes	Deutsche medizinische Wochenschrift, 665–668, 715–717	
1939	Die körperliche und geistige Erziehung der Kinder und Jugendlichen	Ferdinand Enke Verlag Stuttgart	
1940	Zur Frage der Rachitisverhütung	Archiv für Kinderheilkunde, 120, 49–59	
1940	Über die allgemeine Rachitisprophylaxe	Öffentliche Gesundheitsdienst E. Volksgesundheit, 6 Jahrgang, 117–124	

Year	**Title**	**Journal/Publisher**	**Co-Author**
1942	Erbwissenschaft und Adoption - Die Bedeutung von Krankheiten Erbanlagen und Erbkrankheiten bei Adoptiveltern und Adoptivkindern	Gesundheitsführung, 6, 160–168	
1943	Anleitung für Ernährung und Pflege der Kinder im ersten Lebensjahr	Strasbourg	
1944	Die englische Krankheit <Rachitis> : Wesen und Bekämpfung. Bearb. im Auftrag der Reichsarbeitsgemeinschaft für Mutter und Kind	Berlin; Reichsgesundheitsverlag	
1944	Lehrbuch für Säuglings- und Kinderschwestern	Stuttgart: Ferdinand Enke Verlag	Gerhard Joppich, KAVH, Reichsministerium des Innern
1949	Über eine wasserlösliche Vitamin-D2-Milcheiweißverbindung	Deutsche medizinische Wochenschrift, 74, 41, 1245–1246	

1949	Fragekasten	Deutsche medizinische Wochenschrift, 79 Jahrgang, 589–590	
1954	Das biologische Anrecht des Kindes. Ein ärztlicher Beitrag zum Erziehungsproblem	Friedrich-Karl Schattauer-Verlag	
1961	Alles Über dein Kind; Auskunft und Nachschlagewerk nach Altersstufen über die körperliche und seelische Entwicklung, Pflege und Erziehung des Kindes für alle Eltern, Lehrer und Erzieher	Gieseking Bielefeld	Werner Schwidder, Friedrich Müller
1982	Das Neugeborene - das Kleinkind körperl. u. seel. Pflege; Erkrankungen d. Säuglings	Reinbek bei Hamburg Rowohlt	Werner Schwidder, Friedrich Müller
1982	Das Schulkind - spätes Jugendalter kleine Krankheitslehre, Schutzimpfungen, Unfälle - Vergiftungen	Reinbek bei Hamburg Rowohlt	Werner Schwidder, Friedrich Müller

Bibliography

Primary Sources

Archival Unpublished Sources

Archiv der Universität Wien

AT-UAW/MED PA 502; Steinmaurer, Hans Jörg Medizinische Personalakten, Letter 5 April 1940.

Archives Départementales du Bas-Rhin, Strasbourg

126 AL 77 B Medizinalwesen Prüfung des Säuglings und Kleinkinderpflegerinnen.

126 AL 37, n°4.

126 AL 77 A. 14 September 1941 Verordnung zu Ordnung des Säuglings und Kinderpflegeberufs im Elsass.

126 AL 77 A. Strasbourg 18 June 1941; Chef der Zivilverwaltung im Elsass, Richtlinien für Säuglingsschwestern in der nachgehenden Säuglingsfürsorge (vorbeugende Familienhilfe), Ordnung des Säuglings- und Kinderpflege Berufs im Elsass.

126 AL 77 B. Medizinalwesen Prüfung des Säuglings und Kleinkinderpflegerinnen.

126 AL 77 E. Kinder und Saüglingspflegeschule Straßburg Medizinalwesen. Säuglings-und Kinderpflege' Eröffnung einer Schule an der Kinderklinik der Reichsuniversität Straßburg,

Strassburger Neueste Nachrichten, 22 November 1941.

126 AL 77 F. 11 April 1944, Letter from Uni Kinderklinik Oberin Reiter to Chef der Zivilverwaltung Dr Sprauer concerning the exam results of nursing students, Notdienstverpflichtung der Säuglings u Kinderschwestern Schülerinnen der Lehranstalt bei der Universität Kinderklinik in Straßburg.

142 AL 436. Unterricht und Erziehung Universität Heidelberg, NSDAP letter to Oberstadtskommissar Stadtichsgesundheitsamt, 1 December 1942.

1558 W 52167. René Mehl.

1558 W 77322. Antrag auf Einstellung eines Assistenten, 5 February 1942 Leiter der Dozentenschaft Prof. Anrich, 'In politischer und charakterlicher Beziehung keine Bedenken'.

1558 W 77322. Hans Jörg Steinmaurer Personalfragebogen, NSDAP number 1.611.493 joined 26 April 1933.

1558 W 7877757. Politische Beurteilung der Dr Karl Willer, 26 March 1942.

1558 W 52167. René Mehl.
1558 W 229 16473 Apffel, Charles.
1095 W 17 2391. Service Regional Police Judiciaire.

Archives de L'Etablissement Public de Santé Alsace Nord, Stephansfeld (Now Relocated to Archives Départementales Du Bas-Rhin)

AEPSANS. Case of Karl F. 355 1942, Admission file to Stephansfeld Heil-und Pflegeanstalt.
AHUS. Case of Dieter H., 194 (case number 9/1208).

Archives de la Faculté de Médecine, Université de Strasbourg, Strasbourg Thesis Archive

Otto Dahms, 'Poliomyelitis Bei Zwillingen', Diss. Med. (1944).
ADHVS, RUS Collection, Prüfungsunterlagen Dissertationen 1–242.
Hans-Joachim Gawantka, 'Die Bedeutung krankhafter Erbanlagen und Erbkrankheiten bei Adoptiveltern und Adoptivkindern', Diss. Med. (1943).
Hellmuth Will, 'Auftreten von Nervenerkrankungen Bei Kindern Im Zugangsgebiet Der Universitätskinderklinik Strassburg', Diss. Med. (1943).
Johanna Wehrung, 'Erläuterungen zum Euthanasie-Problem aufgrund einer Rückfrage bei Frauen' Diss. Med. (1944).
Karl Robert Bacher, 'Zum Euthanasieproblem', Diss. Med. (1943).
Referat über die Dissertationsarbeit Rosemarie von der Decken, 31 August 1943.
Rosemarie von der Decken, 'Hand-Schüller-Christian'sche Erkrankung bei zweieiigen Zwillingen', Diss. Med. (1942).
Rudolf Gross, 'Gedankništörungen bei der Schockbehandlung das manisch-depressiven Formenkreises', Diss. Med. (1944).
Werner Hesseling, 'Sterblichkeit und Todesursachen an der Straßburger Universitätskinderklinik vom 1.1.1941 bis 31.12.1942', Diss. Med. (1944).
Wolfgang Wendel, 'Zwei Fälle von jugendlicher Poikilodermie im lothringischen Inzuchtgebiet Rimlingen', Diss. Med. (1945).
Doktorprufung als Hans-Joachim Gawantka.
Edith Schneider, 'Fingerleistenuntersuchungen bei Straßburger Schulkindern', Diss. Med. (1944).

Archives du Département d'Histoire de la Vie et de la Santé, l'Ancien Bâtiment d'Anatomie, Hôpital Civile, Université de Strasbourg.

ADHVS, Collection René Burgun, Album de photographies 'Führerschule der deutschen Ärzteschaft Alt-Rehse', 1941, In Erinnerung an den Lehrgng 2/41 für Ärzte vom 13. März bis 5. April 1941 in Alt-Rehse. signé, Oberstarzt.

Pathology collection:

Case number 514/43
Case of Georgine S., 1943 (pathology case number 169/43).
Case of Günther F., 1943, Short Pathology Record (dissection number 613).

Paediatric collection: Amis des Hôpitaux Universitaires Association

Case of Helga T., 1943 (case number 2437/43).
Case of Monika T., 1943 (case number 2436/43).

Case of Ernst Z., 1942 (case number 1270/41).
Case of Francine L., 1943 (case number 1638/43).
Case of Karl Heinz B., 1943 (case number 725/43).
Case of Klaus D., 1943 (case number 659/43).
Case of Margarete O., 1944 (case number 865/44).
Case of Peter G., 1942 (case number 411/42).
Case of Ulof H., 1944 (case number 559/44).
Case of Wida K., 1942 (case number 336/42).
Case of Erich M., 1943 (case number 657/43).
Case of Hedwig H., 1942 (case number 341/42).
Case of Irene E., 1943 (case number 452/43).
Case of Johann B., 1941 (case number 590/41).
Case of Irmgard D., 1943 (case number 3100/43).

Psychiatric collection:
Case of Andreas N., 1942 (K27/520).
Case of Emilie G., 1942 (case number K27/481).
Case of Georg E., 1942 (case number K27/269).
Case of Johann H., 1943 (case number K27/508).
Case of Josef L., 1942 (case number K27/491).
Case of Karl F., 1942 (case number K27/519).
Case of Ludwig F., 1944 (case number unknown).
Case of Melitta S. 1944 (case number K27/873).
Case of Renatus T., 1944 (case number K26/260).
Case of Susanna D, 1943 (case number K27/170).
Case of Watzlaff Z., 1944 (case number K27/951).
Case of Johann H., 1943 (case number K27/508).
Case of Robert M., 1943 (case number K27/428).
Case of Herbert H., 1943 (case number K27/420).

Internal medicine collection:
Case of Georgine S., 1943 (case number 9/2130).
Case of Günther F., 1943 (case number 9/2201).
Case of Katherine S., 1943 (case number 9/483).
Case of Wassily D., 1943 (case number 9/418).
Case of Iwan P., 1944 (case number 9/3344).
Case of Michal G., 1944 (case number 9/3327).
Case of Luise S., 1944 (case number 9/3547).

Archives de la Ville et de l'Eurométropole, Strasbourg
1 FI 103 129. Ruelle des Trois-Gâteaux vers l'église Sainte-Madeleine après le bombardement aérien du 11 août 1944.
1 FI 132 40. Retour des réfugiés alsaciens en gare de Strasbourg. 1940. Photographed by Hellmuth Struckmeyer-Wolff.
1 FI 139 11. Inauguration de la 'Reichsuniversität Straßburg'. 23 Novembre 1941. Photographed by Charles Spehner.
1 FI 132 7. Retour des réfugiés alsaciens, convoi ferroviaire. 1940. Photographed by Struckmeyer-Wolff.

1 FI 135 24. Réception des jeunesses hitlériennes par le Gauleiter Robert Wagner, place Broglie en présence du Dr Robert Ernst.
1 FI 144 7. Place de l'Hôpital, entrée principale des hospices civiles. 1941.
7AH 358 inventory lists.
7AH120. DRK-Schwestern.
7AH47 *Direction Generale Krisenmaßnahmen Bergung und Rückführung aus den Bergungsgebieten.*
7AH486. Letter of Dr Hofmeier concerning breast milk bank in the Kinderklinik.
7AH90. Arztliche Betreuung. Dr Stein letter, 26 January 1944.

Bibliothèque Nationale et Universitaire de Strasbourg
NIM35806. Elsässer, sprecht Euere deutsche Muttersprache! 1940 Strasbourg.
NIM18718. Gesund gewarden durch Frauenmilch: Mutter gib deinen Milchüberfluss an die Frauenmilchsammelstelle der NSV. in der Kinderklinik der Reichsuniversität Strassburg.
NIM18815. Männer des Elsass, Eine Mission für die gesamte Kulturwelt. Elsässiche Männer, Der Platz der Jugend ist an der Front des stählernen Helms. Strasbourg, 1941.
NIM18747. Tradition bewahren, bei der Sparkasse sparen, Stadtsparkasse Strassburg, Thomasplatz 9, 1941. Bibliothèque nationale et universitaire de Strasbourg.
NIM18720. Diene Deinem Volk. Komm als Schwester in die NSV. Arbeit. Verantwortlich: NSDAP, Gauleitung Baden, Amt fuer Volkswohlfahrt, Abt. Propaganda.

Bridgeman Images Archive, Berlin
BIAB. SZT6310684, Opening of the Reichsuniversitaet Strasbourg, 1941 (28.11.1941), photographed by Scherl.
BIAB. SAI188962900022217 Liberation de l'Alsace 1944, René Saint Paul.

Archives Nationales de France, Pierrefitte-sur-Seine
BB30/1797 Procès de Germanisation VIII 1948.

Bundesarchiv Berlin
R 76 IV 27. Account of the evacuation of Strasbourg, Dr Kurt Hofmeier.
R76 IV 46. Concerning the reconstruction of the Psychiatric clinic Reichsuniversität Straßburg rebuilding costs 1944.
R9361-VIII Kartei / 3590565 NSDAP Zentralkartei, Bostroem, August.
R 76 IV/29. Otto Dahms, 'Poliomyelitis bei Zwillingen', Diss. Med. Bundesarchiv Berlin.

Humboldt Universität Archiv, Kaiserin Auguste Victoria Haus Bestand, Berlin
UAH. Lebenslauf Dr Hofmeier, Personalakten der Dozent Dr Kurt Hofmeier Medizinische Fakultät (Geschlossen 1938–1941).

International Tracing Service Digital Archive, Bad Arolsen
4.1.0/ 82452169. 100% breast feeding rate noted in letter from Dr Kiehl, 15 July 1943.

4.1.0/82449011. Fernschrieben über Reichsvereinigung der Juden in Deutschland—Heilanstalt der Rothschild'schen Stiftung in Nordrach/Baden.
4.1.0/82450597. Letter from Hofmeier to Ebner, 28 May 1943.
4.1.0/82452131. Letter from Ebner to Bissing, 1 June 1943.
4.1.0/82452169. Kiehl to Ebner, Kurzer Bericht, 15 July 1943.
4.1.0/82452190. Aktenvermerk Ebners, 13 November 1943.
4.1.0/82452192. Letter from Kiehl to Dr Ebner, 7 December 1943.
4.1.0/82466612. Speisezettel, menus of the Lebensborn home 'Schwarzwald'.
4.1.0 / 82451648. Correspondence and other documents concerning the birth of abnormal children.
4.1.0 / 82451649 Correspondence and other documents concerning the birth of abnormal children.

Landesarchiv Baden-Württemberg, Abt. Generallandesarchiv Karlsruhe

LA-BW. GLA. Holdings 235, no. 29990. Letter from the Directorate of the Institute for Experimental Cancer Research to the Ministry of Culture and Education from 26 April 1940.

Landesarchiv Baden-Württemberg, Abt. Hauptstaatsarchiv Stuttgart

J175 BU2006. Ein Bild Meiner Zeit; So War Es. Memoir. Dr Kurt Hofmeier.
J191. Obituary. Stuttgarter Zeitung no. 203, 4 September 1989.
Stuttgarter Nachrichten no. 214, 10 September 1971.
Stuttgarter Zeitung no. 208, 10 September 1971.

Landesarchiv Baden-Württemberg, Abt. Staatsarchiv Siegmaringen

Wü 13 T 2 Nr. 2133/014. Dr Kurt Hofmeier Entnazifizierung.

National Library of Medicine Bethesda MD; Historical Audiovisiuals Archive

9504906, Robertson, James. *A Two Year Old Goes to Hospital: A Scientific Film.* 1954.

Published Primary Sources

Baedeker, Karl, *Das Elsass, Strassburg und die Vogesen. Reisehandbuch* (Leipzig: Karl Baedeker, 1942).
Binding, Karl and Hoche, Alfred, *Die Freigabe der Vernichtung lebensunwerten Lebens, ihr Maß und ihre Form* (Leipzig: F. Meiner, 1920).
Coerper, Carl and Coerper, Anneliese, *Deutsche Nachkriegskinder: Methoden und erste Ergebnisse der deutschen Längsschnittuntersuchungen über die körperliche und seelische Entwicklung im Schulkindalter* (Stuttgart: G. Thieme, 1954).
Czerny, Adalbert, 'Straßburgs neue Kinderklinik', *JB Kinderheilkunde* 73 (1911): 1–8.
Deutsche Bücherei (dir.): *Jahresverzeichnis der deutschen Hochschulschriften 1943* (59. Jahrgang) (Leipzig: 1962), p. 431 (A. Hartmann, G. Möckel), and Hermann Voss: Die Medizinische Fakultät der Reichsuniversität Posen. *Deutsches Ärzteblatt* 72.31 (1942): 356–57.
Deutsche Medizinische Wochenschrift (1939), Kurt Hofmeier and F. Holz, 'Über die Wirkung von Fischleberöl Konzentrat (vitamin d3) auf die rachitis des Kindes', *Deutsche Medizinische Wochenschrift* (1941).

Dritte Anordnung zur Wiedereinführung der Muttersprache vom 18. August 1940, *Verordnungsblatt des Chefs der Zivilverwaltung im Elsaß 1940* 1.2 (24 August 1940).
Følling, Ivar Asbjørn, 'Über Ausscheidung von Phenylbrenztraubensäure in den Harn als Stoffwechselanomalie in Verbindung: mit Imbezillität', *Hoppe-Seyler's Zeitschrift für physiologische Chemie* 227.1–4 (1934): 169–81.
Hagen, Wilhelm, Thomae, Hans, and Ronge, Anna, *10 Jahre Nachkriegskinder* (München: J.A. Barth, 1962).
Hofmeier, Kurt and Dinckler, K., 'Poliomyelitis vom zerebralen Typ bei einiigen Zwillingen', *Zeitschrift für menschliche Vererbung und Konstitütions Lehre* 22 (1938): 224–37.
Hofmeier, Kurt, Schwidder, Werner, and Müller, Friedrich, *Alles über dein Kind: Auskunfts- und Nachschlagewerk nach Altersstufen über die körperliche und seelische Entwicklung, Pflege und Erziehung des Kindes für alle Eltern, Lehrer und Erzieher* (Bielefeld: Gieseking, 1970).
Hofmeier, Kurt, 'Erbwissenschaft und Adoption; Die Bedeutung von Krankhaften Erbanlagen und Erbkrankheiten bei Adoptiveltern und Adoptivkindern': 160–68.
Hofmeier, Kurt, 'Fragekasten', *Deutsche Medizinische Wochenschrift* 79 Jahrgang (1949): 589–90.
Hofmeier, Kurt, 'Über die erbliche Bedingtheit infektiöser Erkrankungen des Nervensystems', *Monatsschrift für Kinderheilkunde* 75 (1938): not paginated.
Hofmeier, Kurt, *Die Bedeutung der Erbanlage für die Kinderheilkunde* (Stuttgart: Ferdinand Enke Verlag, 1938).
Hofmeier, Kurt, *Körperliche und geistige Erziehung der Kinder und Jugendlichen* (Stuttgart: Ferdinand Enke Verlag, 1939).
Jensch, Nikolaus, *Untersuchungen an Entmannten Sittlichkeitsverbrechern. Sammlung psychiatrischer und neurologischer Einzeldarstellungen* (Leipzig: Thieme, 1944).
Klinge, Fritz, *Der Sektionskurs und was dazu gehört. Auch zur Zusammenarbeit des Pathologen mit dem Arzt* (Stuttgart: Georg Thieme Verlag, 1948).
Les Hospices Civils de Strasbourg, Les Grands Hospices Français, vol 1. EDARI, Strasbourg (1932).
Meltzer, Ewald, *Das Problem der Abkürzung 'lebensunwerten Lebens'* (C. Marhold, Halle a. Saale, 1925).
Otmar Freiherr von Verschuer, 'Twin Research from the Time of Francis Galton to the Present Day', *Proceedings of the Royal Society of London* (1939), 62–81.
Personal-und Vorlesungsverzeichnis der Reichsuniversität Straßburg. Sommer-Semester, 1943 (Henitz Verlag: Straßburg, 1943).
Personal-und Vorlesungsverzeichnis der Reichsuniversität Straßburg. Winter-Semester, 1943–1944 (Henitz Verlag: Straßburg, 1943).
Personal-und Vorlesungsverzichnis der Reichsuniversität Straßburg, Winter-Semester, 1941–1942 (Henitz Verlag: Straßburg, 1941).
Personal-und Vorlesungsverzichnis der Reichsuniversität Straßburg, Sommer-Semester, 1942 (Henitz Verlag: Straßburg, 1942).
Ramm, Rudolf, *Ärztliche Rechts- und Standeskunde. Der Arzt als Gesundheitserzieher* (De Gruyter: Berlin, 1942).
Schweizerische Gesellschaft für Psychiatrie (1937) Bericht über die wissenschaftlichen Verhandlungen auf der 89 Versammlung der Schweizerischen Gesellschaft für Psychiatrie in Münsingen b. Bern am 29–31 Mai 1937. *Schweizer Archiv für Neurologie und Psychiatrie* 39 (suppl.): 1–240.
Rohmer, Paul, *La Clinique Infantile et l'Enseignant de la Pédiatrie à Strasbourg* (Strasbourg: Les Editions Universitaires, 1931).

Seyfarth, Carly, *Der Ärzte-Knigge: über den Umgang mit Kranken und über Pflichten, Kunst und Dienst der Krankenhausärzte* (Leipzig: Georg Thieme, 1938).
Sigerist, Henry E., *Einführung in die Medizin* (Leipzig: G. Thieme, 1931).
Steinmaurer, Hans Jörg, 'Nachweis von Freiem Diphtherietoxin im Patientenblut', *Medizinische Klinik* 41 (1939).
Sydney Thomson, M., 'Poikiloderma Congenitale', *British Journal of Dermatology* 48 (1936): 221–34.
Tredgold, A.F., *Mental Deficiency (Amentia)* (New York: William Wood and Company, 1920).
Wood, C., 'A Training of Nurses for Sick Children', *Nursing Record* 1.36 (1888): 507–10.
Wyllie, A.M., 'Treatment of Mental Disorders by Cardiazol', *Glasgow Medical Journal* 129 (1938): 269–79.
von der Decken, Rosemarie, 'Hand-Schüller-Christian'sche Erkrankung bei zweieiigen Zwillingen', *Archiv für Kinderheilkunde (*1943).
Zollinger, Robert M., Reynolds, Francois H.K., Jeffcot, George F., and Schlumberger, Hans, *Medical, Dental and Veterinary Education and Practice in Germany as Reflected by the Universities of Leipzig, Jena, Halle and Erlangen* (Washington, DC, 1945), http://hdl.handle.net/2027/umn.31951d03595646d
'Richtlinien für neuartige Heilbehandlung und für die Vornahme wissenschaftlicher Versuche am Menschen', *Deutsche Medizinische Wochenschrift* 57.12 (1931): 509.
'Gesetz über das Deutsche Rote Kreuz', 9 Dezember 1937.

Secondary Sources

'Histoire / Général Franz Vaterrodt / Condamné à Mort Pour La Reddition de Strasbourg—Les DNA Archives', accessed 5 September 2019.
'KL-Natzweiler and the Faculty of Medicine of the Reichsuniversität Straßburg: interconnecting stories', exhibition at Centre européen du résistant déporté Natzweiler-Struthof, May 2022–February 2023, 'The Faculty of Medicine of the Reichsuniversität'.
'Strasbourg: un "Nouvel Hôpital Civil"', *Le Figaro*, 31 March 2008.
'Victims of Biomedical Research under NS. Collaborative Database of Medical Victims', Research Centre Leopoldina, German National Academy of Sciences, Halle, Germany.
Abraham, Thomas, *Polio: The Odyssey of Eradication* (London: Hurst & Co., 2018).
Andersen, Margaret, 'Kinderreicher Familien or familles nombreuses? French pronatalism in Alsace', *French History* 34, 2020. https://doi.org/10.1093/fh/crz069
Bacopoulos-Viau, Alexandra and Fauvel, Aude, 'The Patients Turn: Roy Porter and Psychiatry's Tales Thirty Years On', *Medical History* 60 (2016): 1–18. https://doi.org/10.1017/mdh.2015.65
Barnes, Pam, 'Thirty Years of Play in Hospital', *International Journal of Early Childhood* 27.1 (1 March 1995): 48. https://doi.org/10.1007/BF03178105
Beddies, Thomas, *'Du hast die Pflicht, gesund zu sein!': der Gesundheitsdienst der Hitler-Jugend 1933–1945* (Berlin: BeBra Verlag, 2010).
Beddies, Thomas, *Die Patienten der Wittenauer Heilstätten in Berlin 1919–1960* (Husum: Matthiesen, 1999).

Beevor, Antony, *Ardennes 1944: Hitler's Last Gamble* (London: Viking, 2015).
Benz, Ute and Benz, Wolfgang, *Sozialisation und Traumatisierung: Kinder in der Zeit des Nationalsozialismus* (Frankfurt: Fischer Verlag, 1992).
Black, Sue, *All that Remains: A Life in Death* (London: Penguin, 2019).
Boake, Corwin, 'From the Binet Simon to the Wechsler Bellevue: Tracing the History of Intelligence Testing', *Journal of Clinical and Experimental Neuropsychology* 24.3 (2002): 383–405. https://doi.org/10.1076/jcen.24.3.383.981
Bonah, Christian, Beddies, Thomas, Michl, Susanne, and Jung, Frank, *Zwangsversetzt—Vom Elsass an Die Berliner Charite: Die Aufzeichnungen Des Chirurgen Adolphe Jung, 1940–1945* (Berlin: Schwabe Verlag, 2019).
Bonah, Christian, Lepicard, Étienne, and Roelcke, Volker, *La médecine expérimentale au tribunal: implications éthiques de quelques procès médicaux du XXe siècle européen* (Paris: Éd. des Archives contemporaines, 2003).
Bonah, Christian and Münch, Lea, 'La Medizinische Klinik II (Médicale A): vie quotidienne et patients', in *La faculté de médecine de la Reichsuniversität Straßburg et l'hôpital civil sous l'annexation de fait nationale-socialiste 1940–1945: Vie des cliniques au quotidien, experimentations humaines criminelles, collections medico-scientifiques, biographies des victims et du personnel de la faculté de médecine et préconations concernant les politiques mémorielles*, eds. Christian Bonah, Florian Schmaltz, and Paul Weindling (Strasbourg: Presses universitaires de Strasbourg, 2022): 81–115.
Bonah, Christian and Schmaltz, Florian, 'The Reception of the Nuremberg Code and its Impact on Medical Ethics in France: 1947–1954', *Wiener Klinische Wochenschrift* 130 (2018): 199–202.
Bonah, Christian, '"The Strophantin question": Early Scientific Marketing of Cardiac Drugs in Two National Markets (France and Germany, 1900–1930)', *History and Technology* 26 (2013): 135–52. https://doi.org/10.1080/07341512.2013.833039
Bonah, Christian, 'Le drame de Lübeck: la vaccination BCG, le "procès Calmette" et les Richtlinen de 1931', in *La médecine expérimentale au tribunal: implications éthiques de quelques procès médicaux du XXe siècle européen*, eds. Christian Bonah, Volker Roelcke, and Étienne Lepicard (Pantin: Archives Contemporaine, 2003): 65–94.
Bonah, Christian and Schmaltz, Florian, 'From Nuremberg to Helsinki: The Preparation of the Declaration of Helsinki in the Light of the Prosecution of Medical War Crimes at the Struthof Medical Trials, France 1952–1954', in *Human Research Ethics and the Helsinki Declaration*, eds. Ulf Schmidt and Andreas Frewer (Oxford: Oxford University Press, 2019): 293–315.
Bonah, Christian and Schmaltz, Florian, 'From Witness to Indictee: Eugen Haagen and his Court Hearings from the Nuremberg Medical Trial (1946–47) to the Struthof Medical Trials (1952–54)', in *From Clinic to Concentration Camp: Reassessing Nazi Medical and Racial Research, 1933–1945*, ed. Paul Weindling (London: Routledge, 2017): 293–315. https://doi.org/10.4324/9781315583310-14
Bruns, Florian and Chelouche, Tessa, 'Lectures on Inhumanity: Teaching Medical Ethics in German Medical Schools Under Nazism', *Annals of Internal Medicine* 166.8 (18 April 2017): 591. https://doi.org/10.7326/M16-2758
Bryant, Michael S., *Confronting the 'Good Death': Nazi Euthanasia on Trial, 1945–1953* (Boulder, CO: University Press of Colorado, 2005). https://doi.org/10.26530/OAPEN_625241

Buddrus, Michael, '"HJ im Kampf um ein gesundes Volk". Die "Gesundheitsführung der deutschen Jugend" und die HJ-Medizinalorganisation', in *Totale Erziehung für den totalen Krieg: Hitlerjugend und nationalsozialistische Jugendpolitik*, ed. Michael Buddrus (Berlin: De Gruyter, 2003). https://doi.org/10.1515/9783110967951

Buddrus, Michael, *Totale Erziehung für den totalen Krieg: Hitlerjugend und nationalsozialistische Jugendpolitik* (Berlin/Boston: De Gruyter, 2003). https://doi.org/10.1515/9783110967951

Bundesarztkammer, Träger der Paracelsus-Medaille, available at www.bundesaerztekammer.de/page.asp?his=0.2.1825.1830

Buser, Verena, 'Child Survivors and Displaced Children in the Aftermath Studies. An Overview', in *Freilegungen: Rebuilding Lives—Child Survivors and DP Children in the Aftermath of the Holocaust and Forced Labor* (Göttingen: Wallstein, Bad Arolsen International Tracing Service, 2017): 27–40.

Caruth, Cathy, 'The Body's Testimony: Dramatic Witness in the Eichmann Trial', *Paragraph* 40.3 (2017): 259–78. https://doi.org/10.3366/para.2017.0234

Cohen, Boaz, 'Research on Child Holocaust Survivors and Displaced Persons: Goals and Challenges', *Freilegungen: Rebuilding Lives—Child Survivors and DP children in the Aftermath of the Holocaust and Forced Labor* (Göttingen: Wallstein, Bad Arolsen International Tracing Service, 2017): 265-275.

Cohen, Boaz and Horvath, Rita, 'Young Witnesses in the DP Camps: Children's Holocaust Testimony in Context', *Journal of Modern Jewish Studies* 11:1 (2012): 103–25. https://doi.org/10.1080/14725886.2012.646704

Colaianni, Alessandra, 'A Long Shadow: Nazi Doctors, Moral Vulnerability and Contemporary Medical Culture', *Journal of Medical Ethics* 38.7 (1 July 2012): 435–38. https://doi.org/10.1136/medethics-2011-100372

Craig, John Eldon, *A Mission for German Learning: The University of Strasbourg and Alsatian Society 1870–1918*, PhD thesis (Ann Arbor, 1977).

Crew, David F., 'Alltagsgeschichte: A New Social History "From below"?' *Central European History* 22 (1989): 394–407. https://doi.org/10.1017/S0008938900020550

Czech, Herwig, 'Hans Asperger, National Socialism, and "Race Hygiene" in Nazi-Era Vienna', *Molecular Autism* 9 (19 April 2018): 29. https://doi.org/10.1186/s13229-018-0208-6

Czech, Herwig, 'Von der "Aktion T4" zur "dezentralen Euthanasie" Die niederösterreichischen Heil- und Pflegeanstalten Gugging, Mauer-Öhling und Ybbs', in *Fanatiker, Pflichterfüller, Widerständige*, ed. Dokumentationsarchiv des österreichischen Widerstandes (Wien, 2016): 219–266. www.doew.at

Davis Biddle, Tami, 'British and American Approaches to Strategic Bombing: Their Origins and Implementation in the World War II Combined Bomber Offensive', *Journal of Strategic Studies* 18 (1995): 91–144. https://doi.org/10.1080/01402399508437581

Defrance, Corine and Hüther, Frank, 'Un nouveau personel pour une nouvel université? Les défis du recrutement des enseignants à Mayence, 1945–1949', in *La France et la denazification de l'Allemagne après 1945*, eds. Sébastien Cahuffour, Corine Defrance, Stefan Martens, and Marie-Bénédicte Vincent (Brussels: Peter Lang, 2019): 45–64.

Deutsche Gesellschaft für Kinder-und Jugendmedizin e.V. Die Stiftung für internationale Kindergesundheit der DGKJ (vormals 'Hermann-Mai-Stiftung'), available at www.dgkj.de/unsere-arbeit/projekte-fuer-die-kindergesundheit/stiftung-fuer-internationale-kindergesundheit/die-stiftung-fuer-internationale-kindergesundheit-der-dgkj

Dickinson, Edward Ross, *The Politics of German Child Welfare from the Empire to the Federal Republic* (Cambridge, MA: Harvard University Press, 1996).

Docking, Kate, 'Medical Misconduct: The Nurses of Ravensbrück Concentration Camp, 1939–1945', *UK Association for the History of Nursing* 8.1 (2020).

Durand De Bousingen, Denis, 'La Clinique Infantile de l'Hôpital Civil (1910–1989). Une Réalisation Modèle Au Service Des Enfants Malades', *Histoire & Patrimoine Hospitalier: Mémoire de La Médecine à Strasbourg* 23 (2010): 4–11.

Eghigian, Greg, 'A Drifting Concept for an Unruly Menace: A History of Psychopathy in Germany', *Isis* 106.2 (2015): 283–309. https://doi.org/10.1086/681994

Ehret, Sophie, 'Entre rupture et entente avec la ville: la congrégation des Soeurs de la Charité de Strasbourg de 1914 à 1945', MA. Diss. (Université de Strasbourg, 2003): 194–97.

Elias, Tania, 'La Cérémonie Inaugurale De La Reichsuniversität De Strasbourg (1941)', *Revue d'Allemagne et Des Pays de Langue Allemande* 43.3 (July 2011): 341–61.

Eulner, Hans-Heinz, 'Kinderheilkunde', in *Die Entwicklung der medizinischen Spezialfächer an den Universitäten des deutschen Sprachgebietes*, ed. Hans-Heinz Eulner (Stuttgart: Ferdinand Enke Verlag, 1970): 202–22.

Eulner, Hans-Heinz, *Die Entwicklung der medizinischen Spezialfächer an den Universitäten des deutschen Sprachgebietes* (Stuttgart: Ferdinand Enke Verlag, 1970).

Faulstich, Heinz, *Hungersterben in der Psychiatrie 1914–1949 mit einer Topographie der NS-Psychiatrie* (Freiburg im Breisgau: Lambertus, 1998).

Fiebrandt, Maria, *Auslese für die Siedlergesellschaft Die Einbeziehung Volksdeutscher in die NS-Erbgesundheitspolitik im Kontext der Umsiedlungen 1939–1945* (Göttingen: Vandenhoeck & Ruprecht Verlag, 2014). https://doi.org/10.13109/9783666369674

Figiel, Dominik, 'The Experience of the Hitler Youth: Boys in National-Socialism', *The Journal of Education, Culture, and Society* 5.2 (2014): 112–25. https://doi.org/10.15503/jecs20142.112.125

Forcade, Olivier, Dubois, Mathieu, and Grossmann, Johannes, *Exils intérieurs: les évacuations à la frontière franco-allemande (1939–1940)* (Paris: Presse universitaires Paris Sorbonne, 2017).

Forssman, Hans and Rudberg, Brita, 'Study of Consanguinity in Twenty-one Cases of Hand-Schüller-Christian Disease (Systemic Reticuloendothelial Granuloma)', *Acta Medica Scandinavica* 168.5–6 (12 January 1960): 427–29, https://doi.org/10.1111/j.0954-6820.1960.tb06673.x

Fuchs, Julien, 'Youth Movements in Alsace and the Issue of National Identity, 1918–1970', in *Borderland Studies Meets Child Studies: A European Encounter*, ed. Machteld Venken (New York/Frankfurt: Peter Lang, 2017): 85–114.

Gelinada, Grinchenko, 'Forced Labour in Nazi Germany in the Interviews of Former Child Ostarbeiters', in *Reclaiming the Personal: Oral History in Post-Socialist Europe*, eds. Natalia Khanenko-Friesen and Gelinada Grinchenko (Toronto: University of Toronto Press, 2017): 176–204. https://doi.org/10.3138/9781442625235-010

Graefe, Flora and Roelcke, Volker, 'Zwangsarbeiter in der Medizin—Zivile "Fremdarbeiter" als Arbeitskräfte und Patienten am Universitätsklinikum Gießen im Zweiten Weltkrieg', in *Die Medizinische Fakultät der Universität Gießen 1607 bis 2007.*

Band I IDie Medizinische Fakultät der Universität Gießen im Nationalsozialismus und in der Nachkriegszeit: Personen und Institutionen, Umbrüche und Kontinuitäten, ed. Sigrid Oehler-Klein (Giessen: Franz Steiner Verlag, 2007): 381.

Graefe, Flora, *Arbeitskraft, Patient, Objekt; Zwangsarbeiter in der Gießener Universitätsmedizin zwischen 1939 und 1945* (Frankfurt/New York: Campus Verlag, 2011).

Grandhomme, Jean-Nöel, 'La "mise Au Pas" (Gleichschaltung) de l'Alsace-Moselle En 1940–1942', *Revue d'Allemagne et Des Pays de Langue Allemande* 46.2 (July 2014): 443–65. https://doi.org/10.4000/allemagne.1844

Greenhalgh, I. and Butler, A.R., 'Sanatoria Revisited: Sunlight and Health', *The Journal of the Royal College of Physicians of Edinburgh* 47.3 (1 September 2017): 276–80. https://doi.org/10.4997/jrcpe.2017.314

Grinchenko, Gelinada and Olynyk, Marta D., 'The Ostarbeiter of Nazi Germany in Soviet and Post-Soviet Ukrainian Historical Memory', *Canadian Slavonic Papers* (2012). https://doi.org/10.1080/00085006.2012.11092715

Hallama, Eva, 'Between the Projection of Danger, Objectification, and Exploitation: Medical Examination of Polish Civilian Forced Labourers Before their Deportation into the German Reich', *Acta Universitatis Lodziensis. Folia Philosophica. Ethica—Aesthetica—Practica* 37 (2020): 35–50. https://doi.org/10.18778/0208-6107.37.04

Haüpl, Waltraud, *Die ermordeten Kinder vom Spiegelgrund: Gedenkdokumentation für die Opfer der NS-Kindereuthanasie in Wien* (Vienna: Bohlau Verlag, 2006). https://doi.org/10.7767/boehlau.9783205116240

Heinemann, Isabel, *'Rasse, Siedlung, deutsches Blut': Das Rasse- und Siedlungshauptamt der SS und die rassenpolitische Neuordnung Europas* (Göttingen: Wallstein, 2003).

Héran, Jacques, *Histoire de la médecine à Strasbourg* (Strasbourg: La Nuée Bleue, 1997).

Hildebrandt, Sabine, 'The Women on Stieve's List: Victims of National Socialism Whose Bodies Were Used for Anatomical Research', *Clinical Anatomy* 26.1 (2013): 3–21. https://doi.org/10.1002/ca.22195

Hildebrandt, Sabine, *The Anatomy of Murder: Ethical Transgressions and Anatomical Science During the Third Reich* (New York/Oxford: Berghahn Books, 2016). https://doi.org/10.2307/j.ctvgs09f3

Historique, www.diaconesses.fr/qui-sommes-nous/historique

Hoffbeck, Valentine, 'De l'arriéré Au Malade Héréditaire: Histoire de La Prise En Charge et Des Représentations Du Handicap Mental En France et Allemagne (1890–1934)', PhD thesis (University of Strasbourg, 2016).

Hohendorf, Gerrit, '"Death as a Release from Suffering": The History and Ethics of Assisted Dying in Germany Since the End of the 19th Century', *Neurology, Psychiatry, and Brain Research* 22.2 (2016): 56–62. https://doi.org/10.1016/j.npbr.2016.01.003

Hohendorf, Gerrit, Beschränkter Zugang, 'Die Selektion der Opfer zwischen rassenhygienischer "Ausmerze", ökonomischer Brauchbarkeit und medizinischem Erlösungsideal', in *Die Nationalsozialistische Euthanasie-Aktion T4 Und Ihre Opfer: Geschichte Und Ethische Konsequenzen Für Die Gegenwart*, eds. Petra Fuchs, Wolfgang U. Eckart, Christoph Mundt, Maike Rotzoll, Paul Richter, and Gerrit Hohendorf (Paderborn: Ferdinand Schoningh, 2010): 310–24. https://doi.org/10.30965/9783657765430_038

Histoire, Général Franz Vaterrodt, 'Condamné à mort pour la reddition de Strasbourg', *Dernièrès Nouvelles d'Alsace*, 23 March 2010, http://sitemap.dna.fr/articles/201003/13/condamne-mort-pour-la-reddition-de-strasbourg,strasbourg,000006351.php (accessed 23 June 2022).

Hopfer, Ines, *Geraubte Identität Die gewaltsame 'Eindeutschung' von polnischen Kindern in der NS-Zeit* (Vienna: Bohlau Verlag, 2010). https://doi.org/10.26530/OAPEN_437141

Humann, Detlev, '"Alte Kämpfer" in der neuen Zeit. Die sonderbare Arbeitsvermittlung für NS-Parteigänger nach 1933', *Vierteljahrschrift für Sozial- und Wirtschaftsgeschichte* 98.2 (2011): 173–94.

Humbert, Geneviève, 'Capter la Jeunesse', in *Alsace 1939–1945. La grande encyclopedie des années de guerre*, eds. Bernard Reumaux and Alfred Wahl (Strasbourg: La Nuée Bleue, 2009): 577–91.

Information on the history of the German Red Cross available at www.drk.de/das-drk/geschichte/das-drk- von-den-anfaengen-bis-heute/1930/1937

Ishaque, Mariam, Wallace, David J., and Grandhi, Ramesh, 'Pneumoencephalography in the Workup of Neuropsychiatric Illnesses: A Historical Perspective', *Neurosurgical Focus* 43 (2017). https://doi.org/10.3171/2017.6.FOCUS17238

Jolley, Michael Jeremy, 'A Social History of Paediatric Nursing 1920–1970', PhD thesis (University of Hull, 2003).

Kaelber, Lutz, 'Child Murder in Nazi Germany: The Memory of Nazi Medical Crimes and Commemoration of "Children's Euthanasia" Victims at Two Facilities (Eichberg, Kalmenhof)', *Societies* (2012): 157–94. https://doi.org/10.3390/soc2030157

Kalman, Julie, 'Presence and Absence of the Shoah in Strasbourg: A Regional Narrative', *Journal of Contemporary History* 52.2 (2017): 229–49. https://doi.org/10.1177/0022009416664019

Kevles, Daniel J., *In the Name of Eugenics: Genetics and the Uses of Human Heredity* (Cambridge, MA: Harvard University Press, 2004).

King, C.R., 'The Historiography of Medical History: From Great Men to Archaeology', *Bulletin of the New York Academy of Medicine* 67 (1991): 407–28.

Kipfelsperger, Tanja Maria, *Die Associationsanstalt Schönbrunn und der Nationalsozialismus die Konfrontation einer katholischen Pflegeanstalt mit Zwangssterilisierung, NS-'Euthanasie'-Maßnahmen und 'Klostersturm'* (Munich: Utz Verlag, 2021).

Klee, Ernst, *Das Personenlexikon zum Third Reich* (Frankfurt: Fischer, 2007).

Kolata, Jens et al., *In Fleischhackers Händen: Wissenschaft, Politik und das 20. Jahrhundert* (Tübingen: Museum der Universität Tübingen, 2015).

Konrad, Ota, 'Die Geisteswissenschaften an der Prager Universitat (1938/9–1945)', in *Universitäten und Hochschulen im Nationalsozialismus und in der frühen Nachkriegszeit. Gefälligkeitsübersetzung*, eds. Karen Bayer, Frank Sparing, and Wolfgang Woelk (Stuttgart: Steiner, 2004): 219–49.

Kravetz, Melissa, *Women Doctors in Weimar and Nazi Germany: Maternalism, Eugenics, and Professional Identity* (Toronto: University of Toronto Press, 2019). https://doi.org/10.3138/9781442629653

Kwieciński, Wojciech, 'Medizinische Versorgung polnischer Zwangsarbeiter in der Region Bielefeld', *Acta Universitatis Lodziensis. Folia Philosophica. Ethica—Aesthetica—Practica* 37 (2020): 67–86. https://doi.org/10.18778/0208-6107.37.06

Lang, Hans-Joachim, *Die Namen Der Nummern. Wie Es Gelang, Die 86 Opfer Eines NS-Verbrechens Zu Identifizieren* (Hamburg: Hoffmann und Campe, 2004).

Lang, Hans-Joachim, 'August Hirt and "Extraordinary Opportunities for Cadaver Delivery" to Anatomical Institutes in National Socialism: A Murderous Change in Paradigm', *Annals of Anatomy* 195 (2013): 373–80. https://doi.org/10.1016/j.aanat.2013.03.013

Lang, Hans-Joachim, Marquart, Lea, and Hildebrandt, Sabine, 'Biography of August Hirt', *Biographical database of the Reichsuniversität Straßburg at Rus-Med* (2022). Available at https://rus-med.unistra.fr/w/index.php/August_Hirt

Lautenschlager, Angelika, 'Grusswort', in *Entwicklungen und Perspektiven der Kinder- und Jugendmedizin 150 Jahre Pädiatrie in Heidelberg*, ed. Georg F. Hoffmann (Mainz: Kirchheim, 2010).

Le camp d'internement de Schirmeck (territoire de La Broque) = das Sicherungslager von Schirmeck-Vorbruck: témoignages (Essor, 1998).

Leeds, Norman E. and Kieffer, Stephen A., 'Evolution of Diagnostic Neuroradiology from 1904 to 1999', *Radiology* 217 (2000): 310. https://doi.org/10.1148/radiology.217.2.r00nv45309

Leniger, Markus, '"Heim ins Reich"? Das Amt XI und die Umsiedlerlager der Volksdeutschen Mittelstelle 1939–1945', in *Bürokratien: Initiative und Effizienz*, eds. Wolf Gruner and Armin Nolzen (Berlin: Assoziation A, 2001): 81–109.

Lennert, Thomas, 'Die Entwicklung der Berliner Pädiatrie', in *Exodus von Wissenschaften aus Berlin*, eds. W. Fischer, K. Hierholzer, M. Hubenstorf, P.T. Walther and R. Winau (Berlin: Forschungsbericht 7 der Akademie der Wissenschaften zu Berlin, 1994): 529–51. https://doi.org/10.1515/9783110883725-023

Leopoldina, German National Academy of Sciences. Mitgliedverzeichnis, Carl-Gottlieb Bennholdt-Thomsen, www.leopoldina.org/mitgliederverzeichnis/mitglieder/member/Member/show/carl-gottlieb-bennholdt-thomsen (accessed 23 June 2022).

Lévy, Jean-Marc, 'Les "Patrons" Successifs de La Clinique Infantile', *Histoire & Patrimoine Hospitalier: Mémoire de La Médecine à Strasbourg* 23 (2010): 14–29.

Ley, Astrid, *Zwangssteilisation und Ärzteschaft: Hintergründe und Ziele ärztlichen Handelns 1934–1945* (Frankfurt: Campus Verlag, 2004).

Lifton, Robert Jay, *The Nazi Doctors: Medical Killing and the Psychology of Genocide* (New York: Basic Books, 1986).

Lilienthal, Georg, *Der 'Lebensborn e.V.': Ein Instrument nationalsozialistischer Rassenpolitik* (Frankfurt: Fischer Verlag, 2003).

Maibaum, Thomas, *Die 'Führerschule der deutschen Ärzteschaft' Alt-Rehse Münster* (Ulm: Klemm + Oelschläg, 2011).

Mantz, Jean-Marie, 'Editorial', *Histoire & Patrimoine Hospitalier: Mémoire de La Médecine à Strasbourg* 23 (2010): 2–4.

Marx, Jens Thorsten, 'Die vertagten medizinischen Fakultäten zu Straßburg in ihren historischen, politischen, universitätsinstitutionellen und wissenschaftlichen Kontexten, 1538–1944', Med. Diss (Heidelberg, 2008).

Maurer, Catherine and Ripplingen, Gabriele, 'Destitute Children in Alsace from the Beginning of the Twentieth Century to the End of the 1930s: Orphan Care in Strasbourg, in between France and Germany', in *Borderland Studies Meets Child Studies: A European Encounter*, ed. Machteld Venken (New York/Frankfurt: Peter Lang, 2017): 40–63.

Mccrae, Niall, '"A Violent Thunderstorm": Cardiazol Treatment in British Mental Hospitals', *History of Psychiatry* 17.1 (2006): 70. https://doi.org/10.1177/0957154X06061723

Meyer, René, 'L'évacuation, une tragedie frontaliere', in *Alsace 1939–1945: la grande encyclopédie des années de guerre*, eds. Bernard Reumaux and Alfred Wahl (Strasbourg: La Nuée Bleue, 2009): 35–135.

Möhler, Rainer, 'Die Reichsuniversität Straßburg 1941–1944. Eine Nationalsozialistische Musteruniversität zwischen Wissenschaft, Volkstumspolitik, und Verbrechen', Habilitation (Universität Saarlandes, 2019).

Moser, Gabriele, 'Une science médicale normale sous l'occupation nationale- socialiste? Les thèses de la faculté de médecine de la Reichsuniversität Straßburg: état de la recherche, découvertes, perspectives de recherche', in *La faculté de médecine de la Reichsuniversität Straßburg et l'hôpital civil sous l'annexation de fait nationale-socialiste 1940–1945: Vie des cliniques au quotidien, experimentations humaines criminelles, collections medico-scientifiques, biographies des victims et du personnel de la faculté de médecine et préconations concernant les politiques mémorielles*, eds. Christian Bonah, Florian Schmalz, and Paul Weindling (Strasbourg: Presses universitaires de Strasbourg, 2022): 86–104.

Moser, Gabriele, Ärzte, Gesundheitswesen und Wohlfahrtsstaat. Zur Sozialgeschichte des ärztlichen Berufsstandes in Kaiserreich und Weimarer Republik (Freiburg im Breisgau: Centaurus Verlag, 2011).

Münch, Lea, '"Weil sich das Gerät als unentbehrliches Hilfsmittel … herausgestellt hat". Zur Einführung und Behandlungspraxis der Elektroschocktherapie an der Reichsuniversität Straßburg', in *La faculté de médecine de la Reichsuniversität Straßburg et l'hôpital civil sous l'annexation de fait nationale-socialiste 1940–1945: Vie des cliniques au quotidien, experimentations humaines criminelles, collections medico-scientifiques, biographies des victims et du personnel de la faculté de médecine et préconations concernant les politiques mémorielles*, eds. Christian Bonah, Florian Schmalz, and Paul Weindling (Strasbourg: Presses universitaires de Strasbourg, 2022): 65–72.

Münch, Lea, 'From Strasbourg to Hadamar: Nazi Psychiatry and Patient Biographies in Annexed Alsace (1941–1944)', unpublished lecture.

Neumaier, Dorothee, 'Das Lebensbornheim "Schwarzwald" in Nordrach 1942–1945', in *Vom Nationalsozialismus zur Besatzungsherrschaft: Fallstudien und Erinnerungen aus Mittel- und Südbaden*, eds. Heiko Haumann and Uwe Schellinger (Heidelberg: Ubstadt-Weiher, 2018): 83–101.

Neumaier, Dorothee, 'Die Zuzammenarbeit mit der Reichsuniversität Straßburg 1943 bis 1944', in *Das Lebensbornheim 'Schwarzwald' in Nordrach* (Baden-Baden: Tectum Verlag, 2017).

Nichols, Bradley J., 'Reclaimed for the Volk: Forced Migration and Assimilation in the Wartime Third Reich', in *A Transnational History of Forced Migrants in Europe: Unwilling Nomads in the Age of Two World Wars*, eds. Bastiaan Willems and Michał Adam Palacz (London: Bloomsbury, 2022): 165–79.

Nowak, Klara, Hess, Marga, *Ich Klage An: Tatsachen- und Erlebnisberichte der 'Euthanasie'-Geschädigten und Zwangssterilisierten* (Bund der Euthanasie geschädigten und Zwangssterilisierten, Detmold, 1989).

Obladen, Michael, 'Despising the Weak: Long Shadows of Infant Murder in Nazi Germany', *Archives of Disease in Childhood: Fetal and Neonatal Edition* 101 (2016): 190–94. https://doi.org/10.1136/archdischild-2015-309257

Olivier-Utard, Françoise, *Une université idéale?: histoire de l'Université de Strasbourg de 1919 à 1939* (Strasbourg: Presses universitaires de Strasbourg, 2015).

Osten, Philipp, Eckart, Wolfgang U., and Hoffmann, Georg F., 'Entwicklungen und Perspektiven der Kinder- und Jugendmedizin', in *Entwicklungen und Perspektiven der Kinder- und Jugendmedizin 150 Jahre Pädiatrie in Heidelberg*, eds. Georg F. Hoffmann (Mainz: Kirchheim, 2010): 19–29.

Oswald, Rolf, 'Recherche über SS-Verein "Lebensborn" aus Nordrach' (23 September 2015), Baden Online. www.bo.de/lokales/offenburg/recherche-ueber-ss-verein-lebensborn-aus-nordrach

Paul, Diane B. and Brosco, Jeffrey P., *The PKU Paradox: A Short History of a Genetic Disease* (Baltimore: Johns Hopkins University Press, 2013).

Pellegrino, Edmund D., 'The Nazi Doctors and Nuremberg: Some Moral Lessons Revisited', *Annals of Internal Medicine* 127.4 (15 August 1997): 307. https://doi.org/10.7326/0003-4819-127-4-199708150-00010

Pfeiffer, Jürgen, 'Phases in the Postwar German Reception of the "Euthanasia Program" (1939–1945) Involving the Killing of the Mentally Disabled and its Exploitation by Neuroscientists', *Journal of the History of the Neurosciences* 15.3 (2006): 210–44. https://doi.org/10.1080/09647040500503954

Pinwinkler, Alexander, 'Der Arzt als 'Führer der Volksgesundheit?' Wolfgang Lehmann (1904–1980) und das Institut für Rassenbiologie an der Reichsuniversität Straßbourg', *Revue d'Allemagne et des Pays de Langue Allemande* 43.3 (2011): 401–16.

Piotrowski, Bernhard, 'Die Rolle der "Reichsuniversitäten" in der Politik und Wissenschaft des hitlerfaschistischen Deutschlands', in *Universities During World War II. Materials of International Symposium Held at the Jagiellonian University on the 40th Anniversary of 'Sonderaktion Krakau', October 22–24, 1979*, eds. Joszef Buszko and Irena Paczyńska (Krakow: Nakładem Uniwersytetu Jagiellońskiego, 1984): 467–86.

Poore, Carol, 'Who Belongs? Disability and the German Nation in Postwar Literature and Film', *German Studies Review* 26 (2003): 21–42. https://doi.org/10.2307/1432900

Pressac, Jean-Claude, Klarsfeld, Serge, and Green-Krotki, Jan, *The Struthof Album: Study of the Gassing at Natzweiler-Struthof of 86 Jews Whose Bodies were to Constitute a Collection of Skeletons: A Photographic Document* (New York: The Beate Klarsfeld Foundation, 1985).

Ramet, Sabrina P., 'Nazi Germany, 1944–1945: Nonconformity as "Degeneration"', in *Nonconformity, Dissent, Opposition and Resistance in Germany, 1933–1990: The Freedom to Conform*, ed. Sabrina P. Ramet (Cham: Palgrave Macmillan, 2020): 15–86. https://doi.org/10.1007/978-3-030-55412-5_2

Reis, Shmuel P., Wald, Hedy S., and Weindling, Paul, 'The Holocaust, Medicine and Becoming a Physician: The Crucial Role of Education', *Israel Journal of Health Policy Research* 8 (2019): 1–5. https://doi.org/10.1186/s13584-019-0327-3

Riedweg, Eugène, *Strasbourg: ville occupée 1939–1945. La vie quotidienne dans la capitale de l'alsace durant la seconde guerre mondiale* (Éditions du Rhin, Steinbrunn-le-Haut, 1982).

Roelcke, Volker and Duckheim, Simon, 'Medizinische Dissertationen Aus Der Zeit Des Nationalsozialismus: Potential Eines Quellenbestands Und Erste Ergebnisse Zu "Alltag", Ethik Und Mentalität Der Universitären Medizinischen Forschung Bis (Und Ab) 1945', *Medizinhistorisches Journal* 49.3 (2014): 260–71.

Roelcke, Volker, Topp, Sascha, and Lepicard, Étienne, *Silence, Scapegoats and Self-Reflection: The Shadow of Nazi Medical Crimes on Medicine and Bioethics* (Göttingen: V&R Unipress, 2014).

Roelcke, Volker, 'Deutscher Sonderweg? Die eugenische Bewegung in europäischer Perspektive bis in die 1930er Jahre', in *Die Nationalsozialistische Euthanasie-Aktion T4 Und Ihre Opfer: Geschichte Und Ethische Konsequenzen Für Die Gegenwart*, eds. Petra Fuchs, Wolfgang U. Eckart, Christoph Mundt, Maike Rotzoll, Paul Richter, and Gerrit Hohendorf (Paderborn: Ferdinand Schoningh, 2010): 47–55. https://doi.org/10.30965/9783657765430_005

Roelcke, Volker, 'Medizinische Dissertationen Aus Der Zeit Des Nationalsozialismus: Potential Eines Quellenbestands Und Erste Ergebnisse Zu "Alltag", Ethik Und Mentalität Der Universitären Medizinischen Forschung Bis (Und Ab) 1945', *Medizinhistorisches Journal* (2014): 49.

Roelcke, Volker, 'Psychiatry During National Socialism: Historical Knowledge and Some Implications', *Neurology, Psychiatry and Brain Research* 22.2 (2016): 34–39. https://doi.org/10.1016/j.npbr.2016.01.006

Roelcke, Volker, 'The Use and Abuse of Medical Research Ethics: The German Richtlinien/Guidelines for Human Subject Research as an Instrument for the Protection of Research Subjects—and of Medical Science, ca.1931–1961/64', in *From Clinic to Concentration Camp: Reassessing Nazi Medical and Racial Research, 1933–1945*, ed. Paul Weindling (Milton Park: Routledge, 2017): 33–56. https://doi.org/10.4324/9781315583310-2

Rotzoll, Maike et al., 'The First National Socialist Extermination Crime: The T4 Program and Its Victims', *International Journal of Mental Health* 35.3 (2006): 17–29. https://doi.org/10.2753/IMH0020-7411350302

Rotzoll, Maike and Hohendorf, Geritt, 'Johann Duken und die Kinderklinik im Nationalsozialismus', in *Entwicklungen und Perspektiven der Kinder- und Jugendmedizin 150 Jahre Pädiatrie in Heidelberg*, ed. Georg F. Hoffmann (Mainz: Kirchheim, 2010): 86.

Rotzoll, Maike, Hohendorf, Gerrit, and Roelcke, Volker, 'Innovation und Vernichtung: Psychiatrische Forschung und "Euthanasie" an der Heidelberger Psychiatrischen Klinik 1939–1945', *Nervenarzt* 67 (1996): 935–946.

Rouquet, François, *Une épuration ordinaire, 1944–1949: petits et grands collaborateurs de l'administration française* (Paris: CNRS Editions, 2018).

Rzesnitzek, Lara and Lang, Sachsa, 'Electroshock Therapy in the Third Reich', *Medical History* 61.1 (2017): 66–88. https://doi.org/10.1017/mdh.2016.101

Sachse, Carole, 'What Research, to What End? The Rockefeller Foundation and the Max Planck Gesellschaft in the Early Cold War', *Central European History* 42 (2009), 97–141. https://doi.org/10.1017/S0008938909000041

Sauerteig, Lutz, 'Règles éthiques, droits des patients et ethos médical dans le cas d'essais médicamenteux (1892–1931)', in *La médecine expérimentale au tribunal: implications éthiques de quelques procès médicaux du XXe siècle européen*, eds. Christian Bonah, Volker Roelcke, and Étienne Lepicard (Pantin: Archives Contemporaine, 2003): 31–64.

Schäfer, D., 'Pädiatrische Netzwerke im "Dritten Reich" Helmut Seckel und seine Kollegen aus der Universitätskinderklinik Köln', *Monatsschrift für Kinderheilkunde* 165 (2017): 1102–1108. https://doi.org/10.1007/s00112-016-0195-7

Schaller, Helmut Wilhelm, *Die 'Reichsuniversität Posen' 1941–1945; Vorgeschichte, nationalsozialistische Gründung, Widerstand und polnischer Neubeginn* (Frankfurt: Peter Lang, 2010).

Schmaltz, Florian, 'Chemical Weapons Research on Soldiers and Concentration Camp Inmates in Nazi Germany', in *One Hundred Years of Chemical Warfare: Research, Deployment, Consequences*, eds. Bretislav Friedrich, Dieter Hoffmann, et al. (Berlin: Springer Open, 2017): 229–57. https://doi.org/10.1007/978-3-319-51664-6_13

Schmaltz, Florian, 'Les experiences au phosgène d'Otto Bickenbach', in *La faculté de médecine de la Reichsuniversität Straßburg et l'hôpital civil sous l'annexation de fait nationale-socialiste 1940–1945: Vie des cliniques au quotidien, experimentations humaines criminelles, collections medico-scientifiques, biographies des victims et du personnel de la faculté de médecine et préconations concernant les politiques mémorielles*, eds. Christian Bonah, Florian Schmalz, and Paul Weindling (Strasbourg: Presses universitaires de Strasbourg, 2022): 322–49.

Schmaltz, Florian, 'Biography of Otto Bickenbach', *Biographical database of the Reichsuniversität Straßburg at Rus-Med* (2022). Available at https://rus-med.unistra.fr/w/index.php/Otto_Bickenbach

Schmidt, Ulf, *Justice at Nuremberg: Leo Alexander and the Nazi Doctors' Trial* (New York: Palgrave Macmillan, 2004): 13.

Schmidtz-Köster, Dorothee, *Raubkind, Von der SS nach Deutschland verschleppt* (Augsburg: Weltbild, 2020).

Schmitz-Köster, Dorothee, *'Deutsche Mutter bist du bereit': Alltag im Lebensborn* (Augsburg: Weltbild, 2008).

Schmuhl, Hans-Walter, 'Reformpsychiatrie und Massenmord', in *Nationalsozialismus und Modernisierung*, eds. Rainer Zitelmann and Michael Prinz, 2nd edn (Darmstadt: Wiseenschaftliche Buchgesellschft, 1994): 239–66.

Schmuhl, Hans-Walter, 'Was heisst "Widerstand" gegen die NS-"Euthanasie"-Verbrechen?' *Historia hospitalium* 26 (2015): 237–55.

Schmuhl, Hans-Walter, *Rassenhygiene, Nationalsozialismus, Euthanasie. Von der Verhütung zur Vernichtung 'lebensunwerten Lebens' 1890–1945*, 2nd edn (Göttingen: V&R, 1992). https://doi.org/10.13109/9783666357374

Schöttler, Peter, 'La "Westforschung" Allemande Des Années 1930–1940: De La Odéensice à La Offensive Territoriale', in *Les Reichsuniversitäten de Strasbourg et de Poznan et Les Résistances Universitaires 1941–1944*, eds. Christian Baechler, François Igersheim, and Pierre Racine (Strasbourg: Presses de Strasbourg, 2005): 36–46.

Seidler, Eduard, 'Der Kinderarzt und "Euthanasie" -Gutachter Ernst Wentzler', *Monatsschrift für Kinderheilkunde* (2003): 151. https://doi.org/10.1007/s00112-003-0812-0

Seidler, Eduard, 'Die Kinderheilkunde und der Staat', *Monatsschrift für Kinderheilkunde* 143 (1995): 1184–91.

Seidler, Eduard, 'Die Schicksale jüdischer Kinderärzte im Nationalsozialismus', *Monatsschrift für Kinderheilkunde* 146 (1998): 744–53. https://doi.org/10.1007/s001120050316

Seidler, Eduard, *Ethics in Medicine: Historical Aspects of the Present Debate* (Sheffield: European Association for the History of Medicine and Health, 1996).

Seidler, Eduard, *Kinderarzte 1933–1945: entrechtet—geholfen—ermordet: Pediatricians—Victims of Persecution 1933–1945* (Bonn: Bouvier, 2000).

Seiler Vigorito, Sara, 'A Profile of Nazi Medicine: The Nazi Doctor, His Method and Goals', in *When Medicine Went Mad: Bioethics and the Holocaust*, ed. Arthur Caplan (Springer: New York, 1992): 9–13. https://doi.org/10.1007/978-1-4612-0413-8_2

Shalvey, Aisling, 'Career, Proximity to National Socialism, and Post War Reception of Dr Kurt Hofmeier, Director of the Children's Clinic at the Reichsuniversität Straßburg (1941–1944)', *Revue d'Allemagne* 54.1 (2022): 253-268.

Shalvey, Aisling, 'History of Paediatric Treatment in the Reichsuniversität Straßburg 1941-1944', PhD thesis (Université de Strasbourg, 2021).

Shalvey, Aisling, 'La clinique infantile, ses Médecins et ses patients', in *La faculté de médecine de la Reichsuniversität Straßburg et l'hôpital civil sous l'annexation de fait nationale-socialiste 1940–1945: Vie des cliniques au quotidien, experimentations humaines criminelles, collections medico-scientifiques, biographies des victims et du personnel de la faculté de médecine et préconations concernant les politiques mémorielles*, eds. Christian Bonah, Florian Schmalz, and Paul Weindling (Strasbourg: Presses universitaires de Strasbourg, 2022): 74.

Shalvey, Aisling, 'Little's Disease During National Socialism: A Comparative Case Study', *Medizinhistorisches Journal* 57.3 (2022): 260-246.

Sheffer, Edith, *Asperger's Children: The Origins of Autism in Nazi Vienna* (New York: W.W. Norton & Company, 2020).

Shields, L. and Bryan, B., 'The Effect of War on Children: The Children of Europe After World War II', *International Nursing Review, International Council of Nurses* 49.2 (2002): 87–98. https://doi.org/10.1046/j.1466-7657.2002.00110.x

Sibilia, Jean, 'Preface', in *Rapport final de la Commission Historique de la Reichsuniversität Straßburg* (Université de Strasbourg, Strasbourg 2022): 6–7.

Simonnet, Stéphane, Prime, Christophe, Levasseur, Claire, *Atlas de la seconde guerre mondiale: La France au combat: de la drôle de guerre à la Libération* (Éditions Autrement, Paris 2015).

Simunek, Michal, 'Getarnt—Verwischt—Vergessen. Die Lebensgänge von Prof. Dr. med. Luksch, Franz Xaver. von Prof. Dr. med. Carl Gottlieb Bennholdt-Thomsen im Kontext der auf dem Gebiet des "Protektorates Böhmen und Mähren" durchgeführten NS-Euthanasie', in *Universitäten und Hochschulen im Nationalsozialismus und in der frühen Nachkriegszeit. Gefälligkeitsübersetzung*, eds. Karen Bayer, Frank Sparing, and Wolfgang Woelk (Stuttgart: Steiner, 2004): 125–47.

Smith, Laura Jane, 'Taking the Children: Children, Childhood and Heritage Making', in *Children, Childhood and Cultural Heritage*, eds. Kate Darian-Smith and Carla Pascoe (London: Routledge, 2012).

Sofair, André N. and Kaldjian, Lauris C., 'Eugenic Sterilization and a Qualified Nazi Analogy: The United States and Germany, 1930–1945', *Annals of Internal Medicine* 132.4 (15 February 2000): 312. https://doi.org/10.7326/0003-4819-132-4-200002150-00010

Sollors, Werner, '"Everybody Gets Fragebogened Sooner or Later": The Denazification Questionnaire as Cultural Text', *German Life and Letters* 71.2 (1 April 2018): 139–53. https://doi.org/10.1111/glal.12188

Spoerer, Mark and Fleischhacker, Jochen, 'Forced Laborers in Nazi Germany: Categories, Numbers, and Survivors', *The Journal of Interdisciplinary History* 33.2 (2002): 182. https://doi.org/10.1162/00221950260208661

Steegman, Robert, *Le Camp de Natzweiler-Struthof* (Paris: Éditions du Seuil, 2009). https://doi.org/10.14375/NP.9782020956338

Steger, Florian, 'Günzburg State Hospital and the "Aktion T4": A Systematic Review', *Neurology, Psychiatry and Brain Research* (2016). https://doi.org/10.1016/j.npbr.2016.01.004

Steger, Florian, Andreas Görgl, Wolfgang Strube, Hans-Joachim Winckelmann, and Thomas Becker, 'Die "Aktion T4" und die Rolle der Heil- und Pflegeanstalt Günzburg', *Psychiatrische Praxis* 37.6 (2010): 300–305. https://doi.org/10.1055/s-0030-1248439

Stepe, Hilde, *Krankenpflege im Nationalsozialismus* (Frankfurt: Mabeuse Verlag, 2020).

Straßburg, Hans Michael, 'Prävention—Eine zentrale Aufgabe der Sozialpädiatrie', in *Entwicklungen und Perspektiven der Kinder- und Jugendmedizin 150 Jahre Pädiatrie in Heidelberg*, ed. Georg F. Hoffmann (Mainz: Kirchheim, 2010): 297–313.

Surawicz, Borys, 'Brief History of Cardiac Arrhythmias Since the End of the Nineteenth Century: Part I', *Journal of Cardiovascular Electrophysiology* 14.12 (December 2003): 1365–71. https://doi.org/10.1046/j.1540-8167.2003.03320.x

Thompson, Larry V., 'Lebensborn and the Eugenics Policy of the Reichsführer-SS', *Central European History* 4.1 (March 1971): 54–77. https://doi.org/10.1017/S0008938900000443

Toledano, Raphael, *Les expériences médicales du professeur Eugen Haagen de la Reichsuniversität Strassburg: faits, contexte et procès d'un médecin national-socialiste*: University of Strasbourg, MD Thesis (2010).

Topp, Sascha, '"Und jetzt nach Lambarene": Hermann Mai—Direktor der Universitätskinderklinik Münster (1943) 1950–1970', *Monatsschrift Kinderheilkunde* 164 (2016): 34–40.

Topp, Sascha, 'Shifting Cultures of Memory: The German Society of Pediatrics in Confrontation of is Nazi Past', in *Silence, Scapegoats, Self-Reflection: The Shadow of Nazi Medical Crimes on Medicine and Bioethics*, eds. Volker Roelcke, Sascha Topp, and Étienne Lepicard (Göttingen: V&R Unipress, 2014): 147-182. https://doi.org/10.14220/9783737003650.147

Turda, Marius, *Modernism and Eugenics* (Basingstoke: Palgrave Macmillan, 2011). https://doi.org/10.1057/9780230281332

van der Horst, Frank C.P. and van der Veer, René, 'Changing Attitudes Towards the Care of Children in Hospital: A New Assessment of the Influence of the Work of Bowlby and Robertson in the UK, 1940–1970', *Attachment & Human Development* 11.2 (1 March 2009): 119–42. https://doi.org/10.1080/14616730802503655

Uhlmann, Angelika and Winkelmann, Andreas, 'The Science Prior to the Crime: August Hirt's Career Before 1941', *Annals of Anatomy* 204 (2016): 118–26. https://doi.org/10.1016/j.aanat.2014.10.001

Venken, Machteld, 'Introduction', *Borderland Studies Meets Child Studies: A European Encounter* (Vienna: Peter Lang, 2017). https://doi.org/10.3726/b11559

Verneret, Anne-Ségolène, 'Nommer le conflit. Le cas de l'Alsace pendant son annexion de fait au Troisième Reich, 1940-1945', *Trajectoires. Travaux des jeunes chercheurs du CIERA* 5 (16 December 2011): 51. https://doi.org/10.4000/trajectoires.828

von Bueltzingsloewen, Isabelle, *L'Hécatombe des Fous; La Famine dans les Hôpitaux Psychiatriques Français sous l'Occupation* (Paris: Editions Flammarion, 2009).

von Cranach, Michael, 'Ethics in Psychiatry: The Lessons We Learn from Nazi Psychiatry', *European Archives of Psychiatry and Clinical Neuroscience* 260 (2010): 152–56. https://doi.org/10.1007/s00406-010-0158-2

Vonau, Jean-Laurent, *Le Gauleiter Wagner: le bourreau de l'Alsace* (Strasbourg: La Nuée Bleue, 2011).

Vitoux, Marie-Claire, 'Le Gau de Bade-Alsace (1940–1945)', in *Atlas historique d'Alsace*, www.atlas.historique.alsace.uha.fr (Université de Haute Alsace, 2012).

Wannell, Louise, 'Patients' Relatives and Psychiatric Doctors: Letter Writing in the York Retreat, 1875–1910', *Social History of Medicine* 20 (2007): 297–313. https://doi.org/10.1093/shm/hkm043

Wechsler, Patrick, *La Faculté de médecine de la 'Reichsuniversität Strassburg' (1941–1945) à l'heure nationale-socialiste*, PhD thesis (Freiburg im Breisgau, 2005).

Weinberger, Ruth Jolanda, *Fertility Experiments in Auschwitz-Birkenau: The Perpetrators and Their Victims* (Saarbrücken: Südwestdeutscher Verlag für Hochschulschriften, 2009).

Weindling, Paul, Czech, Herwig, and Druml, Christiane, 'From Scientific Exploitation to Individual Memorialization: Evolving Attitudes Towards Research on Nazi Victims' Bodies', *Bioethics* 35. 6 (2021): 508–17. https://doi.org/10.1111/bioe.12860

Weindling, Paul, Hohendorf, Gerrit, Hüntelmann, Axel, et al., 'The Problematic Legacy of Victim Specimens from the Nazi Era: Identifying the Persons Behind the Specimens at the Max Planck Institutes for Brain Research and of Psychiatry',

Journal of the History of the Neurosciences (18 October 2021): 1–22. https://doi.org/10.1080/0964704X.2021.1959185

Weindling, Paul, 'From Cradle to Barracks', in *Health, Race and German Politics Between National Unification and Nazism, 1870-1945*, ed. Paul Weindling (Cambridge: Cambridge University Press, 1993): 188–213.

Weindling, Paul, 'Painful and Sometimes Deadly Experiments which Nazi Doctors Carried Out on Children', *Acta Paediatri*ca (2022): 1–6. doi:10.1111/apa.16310

Weindling, Paul, 'The Extraordinary Career of the Virologist Eugen Haagen', *Infektion und Institution: Zur Wissenschaftsgeschichte des Robert Koch-Instituts im Nationalsozialismus*, eds. Marion Hulverscheidt and Anja Laukotter (Göttingen: Wallstein, 2009): 232–49.

Weindling, Paul, *Health, Race and German Politics Between National Unification and Nazism, 1870-1945* (Cambridge: Cambridge University Press, 1993).

Weirich, Angela and Hoffmann, Georg F., 'Von der privaten, überwiegend karitativen Kinderheilanstalt (1860) zur staatlichen Universitäts- kinderklinik Heidelberg (1923)', in *Entwicklungen und Perspektiven der Kinder- und Jugendmedizin 150 Jahre Pädiatrie in Heidelberg*, ed. Georg F. Hoffmann (Mainz: Kirchheim, 2010): 29–57.

Weiss, Sheila Faith, 'After the Fall: Political Whitewashing, Professional Posturing, and Personal Refashioning in the Postwar Career of Otmar Freiherr von Verschuer', *Isis* 101.4 (December 2010): 722–58. https://doi.org/10.1086/657474

Weiss, Sheila Faith, 'Human Genetics and Politics as Mutually Beneficial Resources: The Case of the Kaiser Wilhelm Institute for Anthropology, Human Heredity and Eugenics During the Third Reich', *Journal of the History of Biology* 39 (2006): 41–88. https://doi.org/10.1007/s10739-005-6532-7

Werner, Leonie, 'Medizinstudierende an der "Reichsuniversität" Straßburg (1941–1944)', Master's thesis (University of Freiburg, 2019).

Wiesel, Elie, 'Without Conscience', *New England Journal of Medicine* 352 (2005): 1511–13, https://doi.org/10.1056/NEJMp058069

Woniak, Katarzyna, 'Polen als Patienten Während der NS-Zwangsarbeit', *Acta Universitatis Lodziensis. Folia Philosophica. Ethica—Aesthetica—Practica* 37 (2020): 51–66. https://doi.org/10.18778/0208-6107.37.05

Zambito Marsala, S., Gioulis, M. and Pistacchi, M., 'Cerebrospinal Fluid and Lumbar Puncture: The Story of a Necessary Procedure in the History of Medicine', *History of Neurology* 36 (2015): 1011–15. https://doi.org/10.1007/s10072-015-2104-6

Ziegler, Herbert F., 'Fight Against the Empty Cradle: Nazi Prenatal Policies and the SS-Führerkorps', *Historical Social Research/Historische Sozialforschung* 38 (April 1986): 25–40.

Notes

1. Introduction

1. Marie-Claire Vitoux, 'Le Gau de Bade-Alsace (1940–1945)', in *Atlas historique d'Alsace*, www.atlas.historique.alsace.uha.fr (Université de Haute Alsace, 2012).
2. Karl Baedeker, *Das Elsass, Strassburg und die Vogesen. Reisehandbuch* (Leipzig: Karl Baedeker, 1942).
3. Jean Sibilia, 'Preface', in *Rapport final de la Commission Historique de la Reichsuniversität Straßburg* (2022): 6–7.
4. Alexandra Bacopoulos-Viau and Aude Fauvel, 'The Patients Turn: Roy Porter and Psychiatry's Tales Thirty Years On', *Medical History* 60 (2016): 1–18.
5. Hans-Heinz Eulner, 'Kinderheilkunde', in *Die Entwicklung der medizinischen Spezialfächer an den Universitäten des deutschen Sprachgebietes*, ed. Hans-Heinz Eulner (Stuttgart: Ferdinand Enke Verlag, 1970): 202–21.
6. This speciality was contested as children were often seen as smaller versions of adults, and so initially it was not considered necessary. However, due to the prevalence of certain diseases in childhood, the speciality of paediatrics emerged in relation to public health measures. This will be discussed in greater detail in Chapter 3. This is sometimes spelled policlinic, often in French sources, but as this book deals largely with German sources, the German spelling is retained.
7. Paul Weindling, 'From Cradle to Barracks', in *Health, Race and German Politics Between National Unification and Nazism, 1870–1945*, ed. Paul Weindling (Cambridge: Cambridge University Press, 1993): 188–213.
8. Some examples that discuss paediatric care in comparable hospital settings include Edward Ross Dickinson, *The Politics of German Child Welfare from the Empire to the Federal Republic* (1996), Georg F. Hoffmann, *Entwicklungen und Perspektiven der Kinder- und Jugendmedizin 150 Jahre Pädiatrie in Heidelberg* (2010), Eduard Seidler, *Kinderarzte 1933–1945: entrechtet—geholfen—ermordet* (2000), and Thomas Beddies, *'Du hast die Pflicht, gesund zu sein'. Der Gesundheitsdienst der Hitler-Jugend 1933–1945* (2010), among others.
9. AVES: 1 FI 132 40—Retour des réfugiés alsaciens en gare de Strasbourg, 1940. Photographed by Hellmuth Struckmeyer-Wolff.
10. Aisling Shalvey, 'History of Paediatric Treatment in the Reichsuniversität Straßburg 1941–1944', PhD thesis (Université de Strasbourg, 2021).

11. David F. Crew, 'Alltagsgeschichte: A New Social History "From Below"?' *Central European History* 22 (1989): 394–407.
12. C.R. King, 'The Historiography of Medical History: From Great Men to Archaeology', *Bulletin of the New York Academy of Medicine* 67 (1991): 407–28.
13. René Meyer, 'L'évacuation, une tragedie frontaliere', in *Alsace 1939–1945. La grande encyclopédie des années de guerre*, eds. Bernard Reumaux and Alfred Wahl (Strasbourg: La Nuée Bleue, 2009): 35–135.
14. Ibid.
15. Ute Benz and Wolfgang Benz, *Sozialisation und Traumatisierung: Kinder in der Zeit des Nationalsozialismus* (Frankfurt: Fischer Taschenbuch, 1998): 131.
16. Machteld Venken, 'Introduction', in *Borderland Studies Meets Child Studies: A European Encounter* (Vienna: Peter Lang, 2017): 1–34.
17. René Meyer, 'L'évacuation, une tragedie frontaliere', in *Alsace 1939–1945. La grande encyclopedie des années de guerre*: 56.
18. Olivier Forcade, Mathieu Dubois, and Johannes Grossmann, *Exils intérieurs: les évacuations à la frontière franco-allemande (1939–1940)* (Paris: Presse universitaires Paris Sorbonne, 2017): 46.
19. Jens Thorsten Marx, 'Die vertagten medizinischen Fakultäten zu Straßburg in ihren historischen, politischen, universitätsinstitutionellen und wissenschaftlichen Kontexten, 1538–1944', Med. Diss (Heidelberg, 2008): 271.
20. René Meyer, 'L'évacuation, une tragedie frontaliere', in *Alsace 1939–1945. La grande encyclopedie des années de guerre*: 100.
21. Ibid.
22. Bradley J. Nichols, 'Reclaimed for the Volk: Forced Migration and Assimilation in the Wartime Third Reich', in *A Transnational History of Forced Migrants in Europe: Unwilling Nomads in the Age of Two World Wars*, eds. Bastiaan Willems and Michał Adam Palacz (Bloomsbury: London, 2022): 168.
23. Ibid.: 169.
24. Ibid.: 169.
25. René Meyer, 'L'évacuation, une tragedie frontaliere', in *Alsace 1939–1945. La grande encyclopedie des années de guerre*: 116.
26. Jean-Laurent Vonau, *Le Gauleiter Wagner: le bourreau de l'Alsace* (Strasbourg: La Nuée Bleue, 2011): 196.
27. Jean-Nöel Grandhomme, 'La "mise Au Pas" (Gleichschaltung) de l'Alsace-Moselle En 1940–1942', *Revue d'Allemagne et Des Pays de Langue Allemande* 46.2 (July 2014): 443–65.
28. AVES. 1 FI 132 40—Retour des réfugiés Alsaciens en gare de Strasbourg, 1940. Photograph by Hellmuth Struckmeyer-Wolff.
29. It is important to note that although this was the case with some of the population, others felt very strongly French, while others felt a sense of independence and regional belonging to Alsace, with its own language and culture. Therefore, any discussions of desire to return to Strasbourg on a population level will leave out a considerable degree of nuance on the personal level. For an example of the personal difficulties experienced, and the plurality of identity and how this impacted medical careers in Strasbourg, consult Christian Bonah, Thomas Beddies, Susanne Michl, and Frank Jung, *Zwangsversetzt—Vom Elsass an Die Berliner Charité: Die Aufzeichnungen Des Chirurgen Adolphe Jung, 1940–1945* (Berlin: Schwabe Verlag, 2019).

30. Julie Kalman, 'Presence and Absence of the Shoah in Strasbourg: A Regional Narrative', *Journal of Contemporary History* 52.2 (2017): 229–49.
31. Bradley J. Nichols, 'Reclaimed for the Volk: Forced Migration and Assimilation in the Wartime Third Reich', in *A Transnational History of Forced Migrants in Europe: Unwilling Nomads in the Age of Two World Wars*, eds. Bastiaan Willems and Michał Adam Palacz (Bloomsbury: London, 2022): 165.
32. Ibid.
33. Jean-Nöel Grandhomme, 'La "mise Au Pas" (Gleichschaltung) de l'Alsace-Moselle En 1940–1942': 443–65.
34. Anne-Ségolène Verneret, 'Nommer le conflit. Le cas de l'Alsace pendant son annexion de fait au Troisième Reich, 1940–1945', *Trajectoires. Travaux des jeunes chercheurs du CIERA* 5 (16 December 2011), http://journals.openedition.org/trajectoires/828.
35. Ibid.
36. Ernest Lachmann, 'Anatomist of Infamy: August Hirt', *Bulletin of the History of Medicine* 51 (1977): 594–602.
37. Ibid.: 598.
38. Hans-Joachim Lang, *Die Namen Der Nummern. Wie Es Gelang, Die 86 Opfer Eines NS-Verbrechens Zu Identifizieren* (Hamburg: Hoffmann und Campe, 2004).
39. François Rouquet, *Une épuration ordinaire, 1944–1949: petits et grands collaborateurs de l'administration française* (Paris: CNRS Editions, 2018): 257. Refer to the map of the city at the beginning of this book for further examples.
40. ADBR. 1558 W 52167. René Mehl.
41. Catherine Maurer and Gabriele Ripplingen, 'Destitute Children in Alsace from the Beginning of the Twentieth Century to the End of the 1930s: Orphan Care in Strasbourg, in between France and Germany', in *Borderland Studies Meets Child Studies: A European Encounter*, ed. Machteld Venken (New York/Frankfurt: Peter Lang, 2017): 40–63.
42. Julien Fuchs, 'Youth Movements in Alsace and the Issue of National Identity, 1918–1970', in *Borderland Studies Meets Child Studies: A European Encounter*, ed. Machteld Venken (New York/Frankfurt: Peter Lang, 2017): 85–114.
43. Christian Bonah and Lea Münch, 'La Medizinische Klinik II (Médicale A): vie quotidienne et patients', in *La faculté de médecine de la Reichsuniversität Straßburg et l'hôpital civil sous l'annexation de fait nationale-socialiste 1940–1945: Vie des cliniques au quotidien, experimentations humaines criminelles, collections medico-scientifiques, biographies des victims et du personnel de la faculté de médecine et préconations concernant les politiques mémorielles*, eds. Christian Bonah, Florian Schmalz, and Paul Weindling (Strasbourg: Presses universitaires de Strasbourg, 2022): 81–115.
44. Anne-Ségolène Verneret, 'Nommer le conflit. Le cas de l'Alsace pendant son annexion de fait au Troisième Reich, 1940–1945', *Trajectoires. Travaux des jeunes chercheurs du CIERA* 5 (16 December 2011): 51, http://journals.openedition.org/trajectoires/828.
45. Hellmuth Will, 'Auftreten von Nervenerkrankungen bei Kindern im Zugangsgebiet der Universitätskinderklinik Strassburg', Diss. Med. (1943): 6.
46. Edith Schneider, 'Fingerleistenuntersuchungen Bei Strassburger Schulkindern', Diss. Med. (1944).
47. Machteld Venken, 'Introduction', in *Borderland Studies Meets Child Studies: A European Encounter* (Vienna: Peter Lang, 2017): 29.

48. Christian Bonah and Lea Münch, 'La Medizinische Klinik II (Médicale A): vie quotidienne et patients', in *La faculté de médecine de la Reichsuniversität Straßburg et l'hôpital civil sous l'annexation de fait nationale-socialiste 1940–1945* (2022): 31.
49. Aisling Shalvey, 'La clinique infantile, ses Médecins et ses patients', in *La faculté de médecine de la Reichsuniversität Straßburg et l'hôpital civil sous l'annexation de fait nationale-socialiste 1940–1945* (2022): 74.
50. 1558 W 229 16473 Apffel, Charles. Archives Départementales du Bas-Rhin, Strasbourg.
51. Christian Bonah and Lea Münch, 'La Medizinische Klinik II (Médicale A): vie quotidienne et patients', in *La faculté de médecine de la Reichsuniversität Straßburg et l'hôpital civil sous l'annexation de fait nationale-socialiste 1940–1945* (2022): 81–115.
52. Bernhard Piotrowski, 'Die Rolle der "Reichsuniversitäten" in der Politik und Wissenschaft des hitlerfaschistischen Deutschlands', in *Universities During World War II: Materials of International Symposium Held at the Jagiellonian University on the 40th Anniversary of 'Sonderaktion Krakau', October 22–24, 1979*, eds. Joszef Buszko and Irena Paczyńska (Krakow: Nakładem Uniwersytetu Jagiellońskiego, 1984): 467–86.
53. Helmut Wilhelm Schaller, *Die 'Reichsuniversität Posen' 1941–1945; Vorgeschichte, nationalsozialistische Gründung, Widerstand und polnischer Neubeginn* (Frankfurt: Peter Lang, 2010): 152.
54. Peter Schöttler, 'La "Westforschung" Allemande Des Années 1930–1940: De La Odéensice à La Offensive Territoriale', in *Les Reichsuniversitäten de Strasbourg et de Poznan et Les Résistances Universitaires 1941–1944*, eds. Christian Baechler, François Igersheim, and Pierre Racine (Strasbourg: Presses de Strasbourg, 2005): 36–46.
55. Tania Elias, 'La Cérémonie Inaugurale De La Reichsuniversität De Strasbourg (1941)', *Revue d'Allemagne et Des Pays de Langue Allemande* 43.3 (July 2011): 341–61.
56. Jacques Héran, ed., *Histoire de la médecine à Strasbourg* (Strasbourg: La Nuée Bleue, 1997): 346.
57. Tania Elias, 'La Cérémonie Inaugurale De La Reichsuniversität De Strasbourg (1941)': 341–61.
58. Helmut Wilhelm Schaller, *Die 'Reichsuniversität Posen' 1941–1945; Vorgeschichte, nationalsozialistische Gründung, Widerstand und polnischer Neubeginn*: 22.
59. Ibid.: 31. Propaganda poster urging the newly arrived population to speak German, available at BNU: NIM35806. 'Elsässer, sprecht Euere deutsche Muttersprache!' 1940, Strasbourg.
60. AVES. 1 FI 139 11. Inauguration de la 'Reichsuniversität Straßburg', 23 Novembre 1941. Photographed by Charles Spehner.
61. Robert Heinrich Wagner (1895–1946) was the head of the government in Alsace and Baden. For further information on his time in office as Gauleiter, see https://stadtlexikon.karlsruhe.de/index.php/De:Lexikon:bio-0064.
62. Tania Elias, 'La Cérémonie Inaugurale de la Reichsuniversität De Strasbourg (1941)': 341–61.
63. Ibid.
64. Reichsuniversität Straßburg, *Personal-und Vorlesungsverzeichnis* (Straßburg: Heintz Verlag, 1941–1944).
65. The number of courses available in racial biology increased from only one course in 1941/42: 23, to four in 1944: 61. Consult Vorlesungsverzeichnissen for further details.

66. Jacques Héran, *Histoire de la médecine à Strasbourg*: 586.
67. Examples provided in Chapter 2, concerning the staff of the paediatric clinic, René Mehl 1558 W 52167. ADBR.
68. Ota Konrad, 'Die Geisteswissenschaften an der Prager Universität (1938/9–1945)', in *Universitäten und Hochschulen im Nationalsozialismus und in der frühen Nachkriegszeit. Gefälligkeitsübersetzung*, eds. Karen Bayer, Frank Sparing, and Wolfgang Woelk (Stuttgart: Steiner, 2004): 219–49.
69. Michal Simunek, 'Getarnt—Verwischt—Vergessen. Die Lebensgänge von Prof. Dr. med. Franz Xaver Luksch und von Prof. Dr. med. Carl Gottlieb Bennholdt-Thomsen im Kontext der auf dem Gebiet des "Protektorates Böhmen und Mähren" durchgeführten NS-Euthanasie', in *Universitäten und Hochschulen im Nationalsozialismus und in der frühen Nachkriegszeit. Gefälligkeitsübersetzung*: 125–47.
70. Ernst Klee, *Das Personenlexikon zum Third Reich* (Frankfurt: Fischer Taschenbuch, 2007), 38.
71. Sascha Topp, 'Shifting Cultures of Memory: The German Society of Pediatrics in Confrontation of its Nazi Past', in *Silence, Scapegoats, Self-Reflection: The Shadow of Nazi Medical Crimes on Medicine and Bioethics*, eds. Volker Roelcke, Sascha Topp, Étienne Lepicard (Göttingen: V&R Unipress, 2014): 162.
72. Michal Simunek, 'Getarnt—Verwischt—Vergessen. Die Lebensgänge von Prof. Dr. med. Franz Xaver Luksch und von Prof. Dr. med. Carl Gottlieb Bennholdt-Thomsen im Kontext der auf dem Gebiet des "Protektorates Böhmen und Mähren" durchgeführten NS-Euthanasie', in *Universitäten und Hochschulen im Nationalsozialismus und in der frühen Nachkriegszeit. Gefälligkeitsübersetzung*: 125.
73. www.leopoldina.org/mitgliederverzeichnis/mitglieder/member/Member/show/carl-gottlieb-bennholdt-thomsen
74. Ernst Klee, *Das Personenlexikon zum Dritten Reich* (Frankfurt: Fischer Taschenbuch, 2007): 38.
75. Sascha Topp, '"Und jetzt nach Lambarene" Hermann Mai—Direktor der Universitätskinderklinik Münster (1943) 1950–1970', *Monatsschrift Kinderheilkunde* (164): 34–40.
76. Deutsche Gesellschaft für Kinder-und Jugendmedizin e.V. Die Stiftung für internationale Kindergesundheit der DGKJ (vormals 'Hermann-Mai-Stiftung'), available at www.dgkj.de/unsere-arbeit/projekte-fuer-die-kindergesundheit/stiftung-fuer-internationale-kindergesundheit/die-stiftung-fuer-internationale-kindergesundheit-der-dgkj.
77. Bundesarztkammer, Träger der Paracelsus-Medaille, available at www.bundesaerztekammer.de/page.asp?his=0.2.1825.1830.
78. Sascha Topp, '"Und jetzt nach Lambarene" Hermann Mai—Direktor der Universitätskinderklinik Münster (1943) 1950–1970', *Monatsschrift Kinderheilkunde* (164): 34–40..
79. For a more in-depth biographical account of Hirt, see Hans-Joachim Lang, Lea Marquart, and Sabine Hildebrandt, 'Biography of August Hirt', in *Biographical Database of the Reichsuniversität Straßburg at Rus-Med* (2022). Available at https://rus-med.unistra.fr/w/index.php/August_Hirt; for a biography of Bickenbach, see Florian Schmaltz, 'Biography of Otto Bickenbach', in *Biographical Database of the Reichsuniversität Straßburg at Rus-Med* (2022). Available at https://rus-med.unistra.fr/w/index.php/Otto_Bickenbach.

80. Angelika Uhlmann and Andreas Winkelmann, 'The Science Prior to the Crime: August Hirt's Career Before 1941', *Annals of Anatomy* 204 (2016): 118–26.
81. Hans-Joachim Lang, 'August Hirt and "Extraordinary Opportunities for Cadaver Delivery" to Anatomical Institutes in National Socialism: A Murderous Change in Paradigm', *Annals of Anatomy* 195 (2013): 373–80.
82. Hans-Joachim Lang, *Die Namen Der Nummern. Wie Es gelang, Die 86 Opfer Eines NS-Verbrechens Zu identifizieren* (Hamburg: Hoffmann und Campe, 2004): 220.
83. Florian Schmaltz, 'Chemical Weapons Research on Soldiers and Concentration Camp Inmates in Nazi Germany', in *One Hundred Years of Chemical Warfare: Research, Deployment, Consequences*, eds. Bretislav Friedrich, Dieter Hoffmann, et al. (Berlin: Springer Open, 2017): 229–57.
84. Ibid.
85. Florian Schmaltz, 'Les experiences au phosgène d'Otto Bickenbach', in *La faculté de médecine de la Reichsuniversität Straßburg et l'hôpital civil sous l'annexation de fait nationale-socialiste 1940–1945* (2022): 322–49.
86. Florian Schmaltz, 'Chemical Weapons Research on Soldiers and Concentration Camp Inmates in Nazi Germany', in *One Hundred Years of Chemical Warfare: Research, Deployment, Consequences*: 229–57.
87. Jean-Claude Pressac, Serge Klarsfeld, and Jan Green-Krotki, *The Struthof Album: Study of the Gassing at Natzweiler-Struthof of 86 Jews Whose Bodies Were to Constitute a Collection of Skeletons: A Photographic Document* (New York: The Beate Klarsfeld Foundation, 1985): 6.
88. Christian Bonah and Florian Schmaltz, 'From Witness to Indictee: Eugen Haagen and His Court Hearings from the Nuremberg Medical Trial (1946–47) to the Struthof Medical Trials (1952–54)', in *From Clinic to Concentration Camp: Reassessing Nazi Medical and Racial Research, 1933–1945*, ed. Paul Weindling (London: Routledge, 2017): 293–315; Paul Weindling, 'The Extraordinary Career of the Virologist Eugen Haagen', in *Infektion und Institution: Zur Wissenschaftsgeschichte des Robert Koch-Instituts im Nationalsozialismus*, eds. Marion Hulverscheidt and Anja Laukotter (Göttingen: Wallstein, 2009): 232–49.
89. Ibid.: 232–49.
90. Raphael Toledano, *Les expériences médicales du professeur Eugen Haagen de la Reichsuniversität Strassburg: faits, contexte et procès d'un médecin national-socialiste*: University of Strasbourg, MD Thesis (2010). 40; Christian Bonah and Florian Schmaltz, 'From Nuremberg to Helsinki: The Preparation of the Declaration of Helsinki in the Light of the Prosecution of Medical War Crimes at the Struthof Medical Trials, France 1952–1954', in *Human Research Ethics and the Helsinki Declaration*, eds. Ulf Schmidt and Andreas Frewer (Oxford: Oxford University Press, 2019): 293–315.
91. Robert Steegman, *Le Camp de Natzweiler-Struthof* (Paris: Éditions du Seuil, 2009): 350.
92. Raphael Toledano, *Les expériences médicales du professeur Eugen Haagen de la Reichsuniversität Strassburg: faits, contexte et procès d'un médecin national-socialiste*: 35. For a detailed list of victims of these experiments, please consult 'Victims of Biomedical Research under NS. Collaborative Database of Medical Victims', Research Centre Leopoldina, German National Academy of Sciences, Halle, Germany.
93. Christian Bonah and Florian Schmaltz, 'The Reception of the Nuremberg Code and Its Impact on Medical Ethics in France: 1947–1954', *Wiener Klinische Wochenschrift* 130 (2018): 199–202.

94. Christian Bonah and Florian Schmaltz, 'From Nuremberg to Helsinki: The Preparation of the Declaration of Helsinki in the Light of the Prosecution of Medical War Crimes at the Struthof Medical Trials, France 1952–1954': 293–315.
95. While it is difficult to make such a distinct differentiation between 'criminal' and 'normal' in a university founded on the principles of National Socialism, for the purposes of this thesis, it is taken to mean that normal research is aligned with what was of research interest in an international context in this era and was not similar to research that was prosecuted in the postwar era due to ethical violations. Consult Chapter 5, on medical theses, for a further breakdown from the University of Gießen on what can be considered Nazi research and what was standard research.
96. Christian Bonah, Thomas Beddies, Susanne Michl, and Frank Jung, *Zwangsversetzt—Vom Elsass an Die Berliner Charite: Die Aufzeichnungen Des Chirurgen Adolphe Jung, 1940-1945* (Berlin: Schwabe Verlag): (2019).

2. Staff of the Children's Clinic of the Reichsuniversität Straßburg

1. Adalbert Czerny, 'Straßburgs neue Kinderklinik', *JB Kinderheilkunde* 73 (1911): 1–8.
2. Hans-Heinz Eulner, *Die Entwicklung der medizinischen Spezialfächer an den Universitäten des deutschen Sprachgebietes* (Stuttgart: Ferdinand Enke Verlag, 1970): 202.
3. Eduard Seidler, *Kinderarzte 1933–1945: entrechtet—geholfen—ermordet: Pediatricians—victims of persecution 1933–1945* (Bonn: Bouvier, 2000): 69; D. Schäfer, 'Pädiatrische Netzwerke im "Dritten Reich" Helmut Seckel und seine Kollegen aus der Universitätskinderklinik Köln', *Monatsschrift für Kinderheilkunde* 165 (2017): 1102–1108.
4. Edward Ross Dickinson, *The Politics of German Child Welfare from the Empire to the Federal Republic* (Cambridge, MA: Harvard University Press, 1996): 62.
5. Paul Weindling, *Health, Race and German Politics Between National Unification and Nazism, 1870–1945* (Cambridge: Cambridge University Press, 1993): 188.
6. Hans-Heinz Eulner, 'Kinderheilkunde', in *Die Entwicklung der medizinischen Spezialfächer an den Universitäten des deutschen Sprachgebietes* (Stuttgart: Ferdinand Enke Verlag, 1970): 202–22.
7. Philipp Osten, Wolfgang U. Eckart, and Georg F. Hoffmann, 'Entwicklungen und Perspektiven der Kinder- und Jugendmedizin', in *Entwicklungen und Perspektiven der Kinder- und Jugendmedizin 150 Jahre Pädiatrie in Heidelberg*, ed. Georg F. Hoffmann (Mainz: Kirchheim, 2010): 19–29.
8. Angela Weirich and Georg F. Hoffmann, 'Von der privaten, überwiegend karitativen Kinderheilanstalt (1860) zur staatlichen Universitäts- Kinderklinik Heidelberg (1923)', in *Entwicklungen und Perspektiven der Kinder- und Jugendmedizin 150 Jahre Pädiatrie in Heidelberg*: 29–57.
9. Angelika Lautenschlager, 'Grussworte', in *Entwicklungen und Perspektiven der Kinder- und Jugendmedizin 150 Jahre Pädiatrie in Heidelberg*: 15.
10. Hans Michael Straßburg, 'Prävention—Eine zentrale Aufgabe der Sozialpädiatrie', in *Entwicklungen und Perspektiven der Kinder- und Jugendmedizin 150 Jahre Pädiatrie in Heidelberg*: 297–313.
11. Paul Weindling, *Health, Race and German Politics Between National Unification and Nazism, 1870–1945*: 189. The German birth rate in this era was not the lowest in Europe,

and other countries were similarly concerned with a reduction in birth rate, but this illustrates the degree of concern about the decreasing family size in Germany at the time.

12. Edward Ross Dickinson, *The Politics of German Child Welfare from the Empire to the Federal Republic*: 55, 78.
13. Laura Jane Smith, 'Taking the Children: Children, Childhood and Heritage Making', in *Children, Childhood and Cultural Heritage*, eds. Kate Darian-Smith and Carla Pascoe (London: Routledge, 2012): 113.
14. Michael Buddrus, 'HJ im Kampf um ein gesundes Volk. Die "Gesundheitsführung der deutschen Jugend" und die HJ-Medizinalorganisation', in *Totale Erziehung für den totalen Krieg: Hitlerjugend und nationalsozialistische Jugendpolitik* (Berlin/Boston: De Gruyter, 2003): 903.
15. Edward Ross Dickinson, *The Politics of German Child Welfare from the Empire to the Federal Republic*: 143.
16. Eduard Seidler, *Ethics in Medicine: Historical Aspects of the Present Debate* (Sheffield: European Association for the History of Medicine and Health, 1996): 11.
17. Paul Rohmer, *La Clinique Infantile et l'Enseignant de la Pédiatrie à Strasbourg* (Strasbourg: Les Editions Universitaires, 1931): 2.
18. Hans-Heinz Eulner, 'Kinderheilkunde': 202–221.
19. Adalbert Czerny, 'Straßburgs neue Kinderklinik', *JB-Kinderheilkunde* 73 (1911): 1–8.
20. John Eldon Craig, *A Mission for German Learning: The University of Strasbourg and Alsatian Society 1870–1918*. PhD thesis (Ann Arbor, 1977): 340.
21. Hans-Heinz Eulner, 'Kinderheilkunde': 202–221.
22. Adalbert Czerny, 'Straßburgs neue Kinderklinik': 1–8.
23. Jean-Marie Mantz, 'Editorial', *Histoire & Patrimoine Hospitalier: Mémoire de La Médecine à Strasbourg* 23 (2010): 2–4.
24. Adalbert Czerny, 'Straßburgs neue Kinderklinik': 1–8.
25. I. Greenhalgh and A. R. Butler, 'Sanatoria Revisited: Sunlight and Health', *The Journal of the Royal College of Physicians of Edinburgh* 47.3 (1 September 2017): 276–80.
26. Françoise Olivier-Utard, *Une université idéale? Histoire de l'Université de Strasbourg de 1919 à 1939* (Strasbourg: Presses universitaires de Strasbourg, 2015): 223.
27. Adalbert Czerny, 'Straßburgs neue Kinderklinik': 1–8.
28. Jean-Marc Lévy, 'Les "Patrons" Successifs de La Clinique Infantile', *Histoire & Patrimoine Hospitalier: Mémoire de La Médecine à Strasbourg* 23 (2010): 14–29.
29. Ibid.
30. ADBR, 126 AL 37, n°4. While Med A and Med B, as well as Surgery A and Surgery B cumulatively comprised a higher bed count, the medical wards and surgical wards were counted as two separate entities through designation as A and B. The children's clinic was classified as one single clinic, thus making it the largest.
31. ADBR. 126AL77 E. Letter, 13 March 1942, concerning Dr Steinmaurer, Kinder und Säuglingspflegeschule Strassburg Medizinalwesen.
32. Ibid.
33. AVES. 7AH 358 inventory lists.
34. 'KL-Natzweiler and the Faculty of Medicine of the Reichsuniversität Straßburg: interconnecting stories'—exhibition at Centre européen du résistant déporté Natzweiler-Struthof, May 2022–February 2023.

35. For a more detailed biography of Kurt Hofmeier, consult Aisling Shalvey, 'Career, Proximity to National Socialism, and Post War Reception of Dr Kurt Hofmeier, Director of the Children's Clinic at the Reichsuniversität Straßburg (1941–1944)', *Revue d'Allemagne* 54.1 (2022): 253-268.
36. UAH. Lebenslauf Dr Hofmeier, Personalakten der Dozent Dr Kurt Hofmeier Medizinische Fakultät (Geschlossen 1938–1941).
37. Rainer Möhler, *Die Reichsuniversität Straßburg 1941–1944. Eine Nationalsozialistische Musteruniversität zwischen Wissenschaft, Volkstumspolitik, und Verbrechen*: 20.
38. Ibid.: 624.
39. Detlev Humann, 'Alte Kämpfer in der neuen Zeit. Die sonderbare Arbeitsvermittlung für NS-Parteigänger nach 1933', *Vierteljahrschrift für Sozial- und Wirtschaftsgeschichte* 98.2 (2011): 173–94.
40. UAH. Lebenslauf Dr Hofmeier, Personalakten der Dozent Dr Kurt Hofmeier Medizinische Fakultät (Geschlossen 1938–1941).
41. Anrich an Schmidt, Bonn, 2 August 1940: NL Anrich 111/437, cited in Rainer Möhler, 'Die Reichsuniversität Straßburg 1941–1944. Eine Nationalsozialistische Musteruniversität zwischen Wissenschaft, Volkstumspolitik, und Verbrechen', Habilitation Universität Saarlandes (2019): 512.
42. Thomas Lennert, 'Die Entwicklung der Berliner Pädiatrie', in *Exodus von Wissenschaften aus Berlin*, eds. W. Fischer, K. Hierholzer, M. Hubenstorf, P. T. Walther and R. Winau (Berlin: Forschungsbericht 7 der Akademie der Wissenschaften zu Berlin, 1994): 529–51; Edward Ross Dickinson, *The Politics of German Child Welfare from the Empire to the Federal Republic*: 57.
43. UAH. Letter, 23 September 1941, from Dr Hofmeier, Personalakten der Dozent Dr Kurt Hofmeier Medizinische Fakultät (Geschlossen 1938–1941).
44. UAH. Letter, 26 February 1938, from Dr Lenz concerning Dr Hofmeier, Personalakten der Dozent Dr Kurt Hofmeier Medizinische Fakultät (Geschlossen 1938–1941).
45. Kurt Hofmeier, *Die Bedeutung der Erbanlage für die Kinderheilkunde*: Vorwort (not paginated).
46. Kurt Hofmeier, *Die Bedeutung der Erbanlage für die Kinderheilkunde*: 73.
47. Michael Obladen, 'Despising the Weak: Long Shadows of Infant Murder in Nazi Germany', *Archives of Disease in Childhood: Fetal and Neonatal Edition* 101 (2016): 190–94.
48. For further information, consult Hans-Walter Schmuhl, *Rassenhygiene, Nationalsozialismus, Euthanasie. Von der Verhütung zur Vernichtung 'lebensunwerten Lebens' 1890–1945*, 2nd edn (Göttingen: V&R, 1992).
49. Kurt Hofmeier, *Die Bedeutung der Erbanlage für die Kinderheilkunde*: 174.
50. Edith Sheffer, *Asperger's Children: The Origins of Autism in Nazi Vienna*: 108; Eduard Seidler, 'Die Kinderheilkunde und der Staat', *Monatsschrift für Kinderheilkunde* 143 (1995): 1184–91.
51. Kurt Hofmeier, *Körperliche und geistige Erziehung der Kinder und Jugendlichen* (Stuttgart: Ferdinand Enke Verlag, 1939): 10.
52. ADHVS, Collection René Burgun, Album de photographies, 'Führerschule der deutschen Ärzteschaft Alt-Rehse', 1941, in Erinnerung an den Lehrgang 2/41 für Ärzte vom 13. März bis 5. April 1941 in Alt-Rehse. Signé, Oberstarzt.

53. Thomas Maibaum, *Die 'Führerschule der deutschen Ärzteschaft' Alt-Rehse* (Münster: Klemm + Oelschläg, 2011).
54. ADHVS, Collection René Burgun, Album de photographies, 'Führerschule der deutschen Ärzteschaft Alt-Rehse', 1941, in Erinnerung an den Lehrgang 2/41 für Ärzte vom 13. März bis 5. April 1941 in Alt-Rehse. Signé, Oberstarzt.
55. Patrick Wechsler, *La Faculté de Médecine*: 132. Cited in Dorothee Neumaier, 'Die Zuzammenarbeit mit der Reichsuniversität Straßburg 1943 bis 1944', in *Das Lebensbornheim 'Schwarzwald' in Nordrach* (Baden-Baden: Tectum Verlag, 2017): 319–30.
56. Ibid.
57. ADBR. 1558 W 77322. Hans Jörg Steinmaurer Personalfragebogen, NSDAP number 1.611.493, joined 26 April 1933.
58. Hans Jörg Steinmaurer, 'Nachweis von Freiem Diphtherietoxin im Patientenblut', *Medizinische Klinik* 41 (1939).
59. A habilitation is an extra qualification in Germany which is required to lecture in a university or to become head of a department or a professor. It requires a postdoctoral thesis of original research in the individual's subject area.
60. Edith Sheffer, *Asperger's Children: The Origins of Autism in Nazi Vienna*: 108. Eduard Seidler, 'Die Kinderheilkunde und der Staat', *Monatsschrift für Kinderheilkunde* 143 (1995): 1184–91.
61. AT-UAW/MED PA 502; Steinmaurer, Hans Jörg Medizinische Personalakten, letter, 5 April 1940.
62. ADBR. 1558 W 77322. Antrag auf Einstellung eines Assistenten, 5 February 1942, Leiter der Dozentenschaft Prof. Anrich, 'In politischer und charakterlicher Beziehung keine Bedenken'.
63. AT-UAW/MED PA 502; Steinmaurer, Hans Jörg Medizinische Personalakten.
64. ADBR. 1558 W 77322. Letter from Reichsminister für Wissenschaft Erziehung und Volksbildung 23 March 1942.
65. ADBR. 1558 W 77322. Letter from Der Kurator der Universität Straßburg, 24 July 1941.
66. Christian Bonah and Lea Münch, 'La Medizinische Klinik II (Médicale A): vie quotidienne et patients', in *La faculté de médecine de la Reichsuniversität Straßburg et l'hôpital civil sous l'annexation de fait nationale-socialiste 1940–1945* (2022).
67. Personal-und Vorlesungsverzeichnis der Reichsuniversität Straßburg, Winter-Semester, 1941–1942 (Henitz Verlag: Straßburg, 1941): 24.
68. Personal-und Vorlesungsverzeichnis der Reichsuniversität Straßburg, Sommer-Semester, 1942 (Henitz Verlag: Straßburg, 1942): 50.
69. Personal-und Vorlesungsverzeichnis der Reichsuniversität Straßburg. Sommer-Semester, 1943 (Henitz Verlag: Straßburg, 1943): 63.
70. Personal-und Vorlesungsverzeichnis der Reichsuniversität Straßburg. Winter-Semester, 1943–1944 (Henitz Verlag: Straßburg, 1943): 37.
71. ADBR. 1558 W 7877757. Politische Beurteilung der Dr Karl Willer, 26 March 1942.
72. Ibid.
73. ADBR. 1558 W 7877757. Letter from Kreispersonalamt der NSDAP Straßburg, 22 May 1942.
74. Ibid.

75. ADBR. 1558 W 7877757. Letter from Dekan den Medizinischen Fakultät Straßburg to Chef der Zivilverwaltung Straßburg, 26 August 1942.
76. Michael Buddrus, 'HJ im Kampf um ein gesundes Volk. Die "Gesundheitsführung der deutschen Jugend" und die HJ-Medizinalorganisation', in *Totale Erziehung für den totalen Krieg: Hitlerjugend und nationalsozialistische Jugendpolitik*, ed. Michael Buddrus (Berlin: De Gruyter, 2015): 910.
77. ADBR. 1558 W 52167. Letter from Kreisleitung der NSDAP, 12 August 1941, René Mehl.
78. ADBR. 1558 W 52167. Letter from Rektor der Medizinisches Fakultät Reichsuniversität Strassburg, 17 September 1941, René Mehl.
79. ADBR. 1558 W 52167. Letter from NSDAP, 14 October 1943, René Mehl.
80. Ibid.
81. Historique, www.diaconesses.fr/qui-sommes-nous/historique.
82. Sophie Ehret, 'Entre rupture et entente avec la ville: la congrégation des Soeurs de la Charité de Strasbourg de 1914 à 1945', MA Diss. (Université de Strasbourg, 2003): 194–97.
83. Ibid.
84. AVES. 7AH120. DRK-Schwestern.
85. Information on the history of the German Red Cross available at www.drk.de/das-drk/geschichte/das-drk- von-den-anfaengen-bis-heute/1930/1937.
86. 'Gesetz über das Deutsche Rote Kreuz', 9 December 1937.
87. Information on the history of the German Red Cross available at www.drk.de/das-drk/geschichte/das-drk- von-den-anfaengen-bis-heute/1930/1937.
88. Hilde Stepe, *Krankenpflege im Nationalsozialismus* (Frankfurt: Mabeuse Verlag, 2020).
89. Ibid.: 109.
90. C. Wood, 'A Training of Nurses for Sick Children', *Nursing Record* 1.36 (1888): 507–10.
91. AVES. 7AH120. DRK-Schwestern.
92. ADBR. 126AL77 B. Medizinalwesen Prüfung der Säuglings und Kleinkinderpflegerinnen, 20 January 1942, Liste der Schülerinnen, and 11 April 1944, Liste der Schülerinnen.
93. Adalbert Czerny refers to the presence of the Poliklinik in his work in 1911, and the same Poliklinik was still in use up to the Reichsuniversität era. Not to be conflated with the general poliklinik of the Reichsuniversität hospital, as this did not cater to children. From here, the children's poliklinik as a section of the children's clinic will be referred to as 'the Poliklinik'.
94. Further information on outpatient capacity is discussed in Chapter 3.
95. NIM18720. Diene Deinem Volk. Komm als Schwester in die NSV. Arbeit. Verantwortlich: NSDAP, Gauleitung Baden, Amt für Volkswohlfahrt, Abt. Propaganda. Available at the BNU. Estimated publication date 1941.
96. Paul Rohmer, *La Clinique Infantile et l'Enseignant de la Pédiatrie à Strasbourg*: 8.
97. These consultations are covered in more detail in Hilde Stepe, *Krankenpflege im Nationalsozialismus* (Frankfurt: Mabeuse Verlag, 2020).
98. Hilde Stepe, *Krankenpflege im Nationalsozialismus*: 109.
99. AHUS. Case of Hedwig H., 1942 (case number 341/42): Admission chart, 15 May 1942.
100. AVES. 7AH486. Letter of Dr Hofmeier concerning breast milk bank in the Kinderklinik.

101. Melissa Kravetz, *Women Doctors in Weimar and Nazi Germany: Maternalism, Eugenics, and Professional Identity*: 18.
102. ADBR. 126AL77 A. Strasbourg 18 June 1941; Chef der Zivilverwaltung im Elsass, Richtlinien für Säuglingsschwestern in der nachgehenden Säuglingsfürsorge (vorbeugende Familienhilfe), Ordnung des Säuglings- und Kinderpflege Berufs im Elsass.
103. Ibid.
104. ADBR. 126AL77 B. Medizinalwesen Prüfung der Säuglings und Kleinkinderpflegerinnen.
105. Melissa Kravetz, *Women Doctors in Weimar and Nazi Germany: Maternalism, Eugenics, and Professional Identity*: 206.
106. Edward Ross Dickinson, *The Politics of German Child Welfare from the Empire to the Federal Republic*: 62.
107. Melissa Kravetz, *Women Doctors in Weimar and Nazi Germany: Maternalism, Eugenics, and Professional Identity*: 185. Referencing Eckhardt and Feldweg, *Die Frauenmilchsammelstellen* (1944): 14.
108. BNU. NIM18718. Gesund geworden durch Frauenmilch: Mutter gib deinen Milchüberfluss an die Frauenmilchsammelstelle der NSV in der Kinderklinik der Reichsuniversität Strassburg.
109. ADBR. 142AL436. Unterricht und Erziehung Universität Heidelberg, NSDAP letter to Oberstadtskommissar Stadtichsgesundheitsamt, 1 December 1942.
110. ADBR. 126AL77 A. 14 September 1941 Verordnung zu Ordnung des Säuglings und Kinderpflegeberufs im Elsass.
111. AVES. 7AH120. DRK-Schwestern.
112. ADBR. 126AL77 E. Kinder und Saüglingspflegeschule Straßburg Medizinalwesen. Säuglings-und Kinderpflege' Eröffnung einer Schule an der Kinderklinik der Reichsuniversität Straßburg, *Strassburger Neueste Nachrichten*, 22 November 1941.
113. Kate Docking, 'Medical Misconduct: The Nurses of Ravensbrück Concentration Camp, 1939–1945', *UK Association for the History of Nursing* 8.1 (2020): not paginated.
114. ADBR. 126AL77 E. Kinder und Saüglingspflegeschule Straßburg Medizinalwesen. Säuglings-und Kinderpflege' Eröffnung einer Schule an der Kinderklinik der Reichsuniversität Straßburg, *Strassburger Neueste Nachrichten*, 22 November 1941.
115. Ibid.
116. AVES. 7AH120. DRK-Schwestern.
117. ADBR. 126AL77 F. 11 April 1944, letter from Uni Kinderklinik Oberin Reiter to Chef der Zivilverwaltung Dr Sprauer concerning the exam results of nursing students, Notdienstverpflichtung der Säuglings u Kinderschwestern Schülerinnen der Lehranstalt bei der Universität Kinderklinik in Straßburg.
118. Georg Lilienthal, *Der 'Lebensborn e.V.': Ein Instrument nationalsozialistischer Rassenpolitik* (Frankfurt: Fischer Verlag, 2003): 28.
119. Larry V. Thompson, 'Lebensborn and the Eugenics Policy of the Reichsführer-SS', *Central European History* 4.1 (March 1971): 54–77.
120. ITS. 4.1.0/ 82452169. 100% breastfeeding rate noted in letter from Dr Kiehl, 15 July 1943.
121. Herbert F. Ziegler, 'Fight Against the Empty Cradle: Nazi Prenatal Policies and the SS-Führerkorps', *Historical Social Research / Historische Sozialforschung* 38 (April 1986): 25–40.

122. ITS. 4.1.0/82466612. Extensive menu cards from 1942 to 1944 indicate no change in quantity or quality of food, despite the circumstances of rationing with the progression of war. Speisezettel, menus of the Lebensborn home 'Schwarzwald'.
123. Ines Hopfer, *Geraubte Identität Die gewaltsame 'Eindeutschung' von polnischen Kindern in der NS-Zeit* (Vienna: Bohlau Verlag, 2010): 62.
124. Kurt Hofmeier, 'Erbwissenschaft und Adoption; Die Bedeutung von Krankhaften Erbanlagen und Erbkrankheiten bei Adoptiveltern und Adoptivkindern', *Gesundheitsführung* 6 (1942): 160–68.
125. Herbert F. Ziegler, 'Fight Against the Empty Cradle: Nazi Prenatal Policies and the SS-Fuhrerkorps': 25–40.
126. ITS. 4.1.0/82449011. Fernschrieben über Reichsvereinigung der Juden in Deutschland—Heilanstalt der Rothschild'schen Stiftung in Nordrach/Baden.
127. Rolf Oswald, Recherche über SS-Verein 'Lebensborn' aus Nordrach (23 September 2015) Baden Online. www.bo.de/lokales/offenburg/recherche-ueber-ss-verein-lebensborn-aus-nordrach.
128. Dorothee Neumaier, 'Das Lebensbornheim "Schwarzwald" in Nordrach 1942–1945', in *Vom Nationalsozialismus zur Besatzungsherrschaft: Fallstudien und Erinnerungen aus Mittel- und Südbaden*, eds. Heiko Haumann and Uwe Schellinger (Heidelberg: Ubstadt-Weiher, 2018): 83–101.
129. Ibid.
130. Dorothee Neumaier, 'Die Zusammenarbeit mit der Reichsuniversität Straßburg 1943 bis 1944', in *Das Lebensbornheim "Schwarzwald" in Nordrach* (Baden-Baden: Tectum Verlag, 2017).
131. ITS. 4.1.0/82450597. Letter from Hofmeier to Ebner, 28 May 1943.
132. Ibid.
133. ITS. 4.1.0/82452131. Letter from Ebner to Bissing, 1 June 1943.
134. ITS. 4.1.0/82452190. Aktenvermerk Ebners, 13 November 1943.
135. ITS. 4.1.0/82452169. Kiehl to Ebner, Kurzer Bericht, 15 July 1943.
136. Ibid.
137. ITS. 4.1.0/82452192. Letter from Kiehl to Ebner, 7 December 1943.
138. ITS. 4.1.0/82452169. Kiehl to Ebner, Kurzer Bericht, 15 July 1943.
139. ITS. 4.1.0/82452192. Letter from Kiehl to Dr Ebner, 7 December 1943.
140. Dorothee Schmidtz-Köster, *Raubkind, Von der SS nach Deutschland verschleppt* (Augsburg: Weltbild, 2020): 53.
141. Correspondence and other documents concerning the birth of abnormal children, 4.1.0 / 82451648 ITS.
142. Letter from 30 March 1942 to Dr Schwab confirming Dr Gasser's diagnosis of psychologically underdeveloped. Correspondence and other documents concerning the birth of abnormal children, 4.1.0 / 82451648 ITS. It is not clear how they determined this 'underdevelopment', as she was an infant.
143. Letter from Dr Schwab in Lebensbornheim Wienerwald to SS Oberführer Dr Ebner on 8 April 1942 concerning Brigitte Schmidt. Correspondence and other documents concerning the birth of abnormal children, 4.1.0 / 82451649 ITS.
144. Brigitte Schmidt, victim ID. 8420, 'Victims of Biomedical Research under NS' Database.
145. Michael Buddrus, *Totale Erziehung für den totalen Krieg: Hitlerjugend und nationalsozialistische Jugendpolitik* (Berlin/Boston: De Gruyter, 2003): 903.

146. Christian Bonah and Lea Münch, 'La Medizinische Klinik II (Médicale A): vie quotidienne et patients', in *La faculté de médecine de la Reichsuniversität Straßburg et l'hôpital civil sous l'annexation de fait nationale-socialiste 1940–1945*: 81–115.
147. For lists of further experiments conducted in this era, consult 'Victims of Biomedical Research under NS. Collaborative Database of Medical Victims', Research Centre Leopoldina, German National Academy of Sciences, Halle, Germany.

3. Paediatric Treatment at the Children's Clinic of the Reichsuniversität Straßburg

1. Kurt Hofmeier, *Die Bedeutung der Erbanlage für die Kinderheilkunde* (Stuttgart: Ferdinand Enke Verlag, 1938): 174.
2. Flora Graefe, *Arbeitskraft, Patient, Objekt; Zwangsarbeiter in der Gießener Universitätsmedizin zwischen 1939 und 1945* (Frankfurt/New York: Campus Verlag, 2011); Isabelle von Bueltzingsloewen, *L'Hécatombe des Fous; La Famine dans les Hôpitaux Psychiatriques Français sous l'Occupation* (Paris: Editions Flammarion, 2009).
3. Hilde Stepe, *Krankenpflege im Nationalsozialismus* (Frankfurt: Mabeuse Verlag, 2020).
4. For further information about economics and healthcare in Germany in the nineteenth and twentieth centuries, please consult Gabriele Moser, *Ärzte, Gesundheitswesen und Wohlfahrtsstaat. Zur Sozialgeschichte des* ärztlichen *Berufsstandes in Kaiserreich und Weimarer Republik* (Freiburg im Breisgau: Centaurus Verlag, 2011).
5. LA-BW. GLA. Holdings 235, no. 29990. Letter from the Directorate of the Institute for Experimental Cancer Research to the Ministry of Culture and Education from 26 April 1940.
6. Ibid.
7. AHUS. Case of Francine L., 1943 (case number 1638/43).
8. AHUS. Ibid.
9. AHUS. Case number 1638/43. Letter, 24 September 1943, from Professor Hofmeier to Dr Mommsen in Metz concerning Professor Zukschwerdt's decision on surgery. Case of Francine L., 1943.
10. Hofmeier published extensively on this topic both prior to his appointment as clinic director in Strasbourg and during his time there; some examples are: Kurt Hofmeier 'die Ernährung des Kleinkindes', *Deutsche Medizinische Wochenschrift* (1939) and Kurt Hofmeier and F. Holz 'Über die Wirkung von Fischleberöl Konzentrat (vitamin d3) auf die Rachitis des Kindes', *Deutsche Medizinische Wochenschrift* (1941).
11. AHUS. Case of Francine L., 1943 (case number 1638/43).
12. AHUS. Ibid. Letter from Mrs L. to Dr Hofmeier, 20 November 1943.
13. AHUS. Ibid.
14. Aisling Shalvey, 'Little's Disease During National Socialism: A Comparative Case Study', *Medizinhistorisches Journal* 57.3 (2022): 260-246.
15. Volker Roelcke, 'Psychiatry During National Socialism: Historical Knowledge and Some Implications', *Neurology, Psychiatry and Brain Research* (2016).
16. Ibid.
17. Jürgen Pfeiffer, 'Phases in the Postwar German Reception of the "Euthanasia Program" (1939–1945) Involving the Killing of the Mentally Disabled and its Exploitation by Neuroscientists', *Journal of the History of the Neurosciences* 15.3 (2006): 210–44.

18. For further statistical analysis, please consult the appendices.
19. 1 FI 132 7—Retour des réfugiés alsaciens, convoi ferroviaire, 1940, photographed by Struckmeyer-Wolff. Available at AVES.
20. AHUS. Case of Ernst Z. (case number 1270/41) 1942, Dr Levy referral note, 2 February 1942.
21. AHUS. Ibid, X-ray department test results, 4 February 1942.
22. AHUS. Ibid, Dr Hofmeier note to Dr Levy, 7 March 1942.
23. AHUS. Case of Irmgard D., 1943 (case number 3100/43), admission record.
24. Dorothee Schmitz-Köster, *'Deutsche Mutter bist du bereit": Alltag im Lebensborn* (Augsburg: Weltbild, 2008): 41.
25. Ibid.: 38. Note that this emphasis on number of children born as a marker of status was an important concept in Alsace as well as in Germany; Margaret Andersen, 'Kinderreicher Familien or familles nombreuses? French pronatalism in Alsace', *French History* 34 (2020).
26. AHUS. Case of Wida K., 1942 (case number 336/42).
27. Isabel Heinemann, *'Rasse, Siedlung, deutsches Blut': Das Rasse- und Siedlungshauptamt der SS und die rassenpolitische Neuordnung Europas* (Göttingen: Wallstein, 2003): 314; Maria Fiebrandt, *Auslese für die Siedlergesellschaft Die Einbeziehung Volksdeutscher in die NS-Erbgesundheitspolitik im Kontext der Umsiedlungen 1939–1945* (Göttingen: Vandenhoeck & Ruprecht Verlag, 2014): 28.
28. AHUS. Case of Johann B., 1941 (case number 590/41), admission record.
29. Florian Steger, 'Günzburg State Hospital and the "Aktion T4": A Systematic Review', *Neurology, Psychiatry and Brain Research*, 2016.
30. AHUS. Case of Johann B., 1941 (case number 590/41). Letter from Dr Hofmeier to Dr Hans, 9 October 1941.
31. AHUS. Case of Johann B., 1941 (case number 590/41), admission record. 'Der Zustand ist ganz unverändert', 'Krankheit: geistig ruckheit'.
32. Florian Steger, 'Günzburg State Hospital and the "Aktion T4": A Systematic Review', *Neurology, Psychiatry and Brain Research*, 2016.
33. Consult appendices for further statistics.
34. AHUS. Case of Margarete O., 1944 (case number 865/44).
35. *Les Hospices Civils de Strasbourg*, Les Grands Hospices Français, vol 1. (Strasbourg: Edari, 1932): not paginated.
36. AHUS. Ibid. Staatliche Medizinal Untersuchungsanstalt.
37. Thomas Abraham, *Polio: The Odyssey of Eradication* (London: Hurst & Co., 2018): 115.
38. Adalbert Czerny, 'Straßburgs neue Kinderklinik': 1–8.
39. AHUS. Case of Margarete O., 1944 (case number 865/44).
40. Borys Surawicz, 'Brief History of Cardiac Arrhythmias Since the End of the Nineteenth Century: Part I', *Journal of Cardiovascular Electrophysiology* 14.12 (December 2003): 1365–71.
41. AHUS. Case of Klaus D., 1943 (case number 659/43).
42. AHUS. Ibid. Letter from the Poliklinik to Kinderklinik.
43. Christian Bonah, '"The Strophanthin Question": Early Scientific Marketing of Cardiac Drugs in Two National Markets (France and Germany, 1900–1930)', *History and Technology* 26 (2013): 135–52.
44. AHUS. Case of Klaus D., 1943 (case number 659/43).

45. While the term Kinderreiche preceded National Socialism, due to the focus on increasing the population, this is significant. Margaret Andersen, 'Kinderreicher Familien or familles nombreuses? French pronatalism in Alsace': 63–81.
46. AHUS. Case of Peter G., 1942 (case number 411/42), referral letter from Dr Albert Bury, 23 May 1943.
47. AHUS. Ibid.
48. Sheila Faith Weiss, 'Human Genetics and Politics as Mutually Beneficial Resources: The Case of the Kaiser Wilhelm Institute for Anthropology, Human Heredity and Eugenics During the Third Reich', *Journal of the History of Biology* 39 (2006): 41–88. https://doi.org/10.1007/s10739-005-6532-7
49. Otmar Freiherr von Verschuer, 'Twin Research from the Time of Francis Galton to the Present Day', *Proceedings of the Royal Society of London* (1939): 62–81.
50. Ruth Jolanda Weinberger, *Fertility Experiments in Auschwitz-Birkenau: The Perpetrators and Their Victims* (Saarbrücken: Südwestdeutscher Verlag für Hochschulschriften, 2009): 236.
51. See Ruth Jolanda Weinberger, *Fertility Experiments in Auschwitz-Birkenau: The Perpetrators and Their Victims* (2009), as well as for further information on the experiments. Consult the database, 'Victims of Biomedical Research under NS. Collaborative Database of Medical Victims', at the Research Centre Leopoldina, German National Academy of Sciences, for victim profiles, numbers, and individual experiment information.
52. For further information on the racial hygiene department, consult Alexander Pinwinkler. 'Der Arzt als "Führer der Volksgesundheit?" Wolfgang Lehmann (1904–1980) und das Institut für Rassenbiologie an der Reichsuniversität Straßbourg', *Revue d'Allemagne et des Pays de Langue Allemande* 43.3 (2011): 401–416.
53. Otto Dahms, 'Poliomyelitis Bei Zwillingen', Diss. Med. (1944). For examples of the racial hygiene department assessment forms included in his thesis, consult appendices.
54. It appears that this thesis is a direct conclusion, or at least a follow-up study, from Hofmeier's work entitled 'Poliomyelitis von cerebralen typ bei eineiigen Zwillingen', in *Zeitschrift der Menschlichen Vererbung und Konstitutionslehre* (1938), which was co-authored with Dinckler in the Charlottenburg maternity and children's hospital in Berlin. In this article, he looks at monozygotic twins versus dizygotic twins in contracting poliomyelitis.
55. Ibid., case of Marlene and Irmgard.
56. Otto Dahms, 'Poliomyelitis Bei Zwillingen', Diss. Med. Bundesarchiv Berlin, R 76 IV/29/, Case 2, Brigitte and Christiana.
57. For a further history of lumbar puncture as a diagnostic test, and possible side effects of the procedure, consult S. Zambito Marsala, M. Gioulis, and M. Pistacchi, 'Cerebrospinal Fluid and Lumbar Puncture: The Story of a Necessary Procedure in the History of Medicine', *History of Neurology* 36 (2015): 1011–15. https://doi.org/10.1007/s10072-015-2104-6
58. Case of Monika T., 1943 (case number 2436/43), and Helga T., 1943 (case number 2437/43).
59. Case of Helga T., 1943 (case number 2437/43); letter from Maria T., on 23 February 1943.
60. Paul Weindling, 'Painful and Sometimes Deadly Experiments which Nazi Doctors Carried Out on Children', *Acta Paediatrica* (2022): 1–6. doi:10.1111/apa.16310

61. Kurt Hofmeier and K. Dinckler, 'Poliomyelitis vom zerebralen Typ bei einiigen Zwillingen', *Zeitschrift für menschliche Vererbung und Konstitütions Lehre* 22 (1938): 224–37.
62. Ibid.
63. Ibid.
64. Jean-Nöel Grandhomme, 'La "mise Au Pas" (Gleichschaltung) de l'Alsace-Moselle En 1940–1942', *Revue d'Allemagne et Des Pays de Langue Allemande* 46.2 (July 2014): 443–65. For the advertising of savings banks, 'Tradition bewahren, Bei der Sparkasse sparen', Stadtsparkasse Strassburg, Thomasplatz 9, 1941. Bibliothèque nationale et universitaire de Strasbourg, NIM18747.
65. Ute Benz and Wolfgang Benz, *Sozialisation und Traumatisierung: Kinder in der Zeit des Nationalsozialismus*: 20; Dominik Figiel, 'The Experience of the Hitler Youth: Boys in National-Socialism', *The Journal of Education, Culture, and Society* 5.2 (2014): 112–25.
66. Geneviève Humbert, 'Capter la Jeunesse', in *Alsace 1939–1945. La grande encyclopedie des années de guerre*, eds. Bernard Reumaux and Alfred Wahl (Strasbourg: La Nueé Bleue, 2009): 577–91.
67. Geneviève Humbert, 'Capter la Jeunesse', in *Alsace 1939–1945. La grande encyclopedie des années de guerre*, eds. Bernard Reumaux and Alfred Wahl (Strasbourg: La Nueé Bleue, 2009): 587.
68. Sabrina P. Ramet, 'Nazi Germany, 1944–1945: Nonconformity as "Degeneration"', in *Nonconformity, Dissent, Opposition and Resistance in Germany, 1933–1990: The Freedom to Conform*, ed. Sabrina P. Ramet (Cham: Palgrave Macmillan, 2020): 15–86.
69. AFMS. Hellmuth Will, 'Auftreten von Nervenerkrankungen Bei Kindern Im Zugangsgebiet Der Universitätskinderklinik Strassburg', Diss. Med. (1943).
70. ADBR 1 FI 135 24—Réception des jeunesses hitlériennes par le Gauleiter Robert Wagner, place Broglie en présence du Dr Robert Ernst (no date).
71. Kurt Hofmeier, 'Über die erbliche Bedingtheit infektiöser Erkrankungen des Nervensystems', *Monatsschrift für Kinderheilkunde* 75 (1938): not paginated.
72. AFMS. Hellmuth Will, 'Auftreten von Nervenerkrankungen Bei Kindern im Zugangsgebiet der Universitätskinderklinik Straßburg', Diss. Med. (1943): 7.
73. AFMS. Werner Hesseling, 'Sterblichkeit und Todesursachen an der Straßburger Universitätskinderklinik vom 1.1.1941 bis 31.12.1942', Diss. Med. (1944): 19.
74. Kurt Hofmeier, 'Erbwissenschaft und Adoption; Die Bedeutung von Krankhaften Erbanlagen und Erbkrankheiten bei Adoptiveltern und Adoptivkindern': 160–68.
75. Ibid.
76. Daniel J. Kevles, *In the Name of Eugenics: Genetics and the Uses of Human Heredity* (Cambridge, MA: Harvard University Press, 2004): 117.
77. AHUS. Case of Karl Heinz B., 1943 (case number 725/43), admission record.
78. AHUS. Ibid. Observations.
79. AHUS. Ibid. Staatliche Medizinal-Untersuchungsanstalt examinations.
80. AHUS. Ibid. Röntgenabteilung observations, 2 August 1943.
81. Maike Rotzoll, Gerrit Hohendorf, Volker Roelcke, 'Innovation und Vernichtung: Psychiatrische Forschung und "Euthanasie" an der Heidelberger Psychiatrischen Klinik 1939–1945', *Nervenarzt* 67 (1996): 935–46.
82. Consult Appendix 6.
83. AHUS. 7AH120. DRK-Schwestern.
84. AHUS. Case of Irene E., 1943 (case number 452/43).
85. Ibid.

86. NLM. 9504906. James Robertson, *A Two Year Old Goes to Hospital*, Robertson Films (1952).
87. Frank C. P. van der Horst and René van der Veer, 'Changing Attitudes Towards the Care of Children in Hospital: A New Assessment of the Influence of the Work of Bowlby and Robertson in the UK, 1940–1970', *Attachment & Human Development* 11.2 (1 March 2009): 119–42. https://doi.org/10.1080/14616730802503655
88. ADHVS Psych. Case of Andreas N. (K27/520). AHUS. Case of Erich M. (657/43).
89. ADHVS. Case of Erich M. (657/43), letter from Karoline M. on 24 June 1943 requesting a visit to her grandson. ADHVS Psych. Case of Andreas N. (K27/520). Letter from Alfons N. on 15 November 1942 requesting a visit to his son.
90. As Bradley J. Nichols states, social class played a significant role in how the resettled and Germanized populations were received, and what sort of social care systems they had access to, including hospital services. Consult Bradley J. Nichols, 'Reclaimed for the Volk: Forced Migration and Assimilation in the Wartime Third Reich', in *A Transnational History of Forced Migrants in Europe: Unwilling Nomads in the Age of Two World Wars*, eds. Bastiaan Willems and Michał Adam Palacz (London: Bloomsbury, 2022): 165–79 for further details.
91. Günther K., victim number 8751, available at Victims of Biomedical Research under National Socialism, https://ns-medical-victims.org/nmv_view_victim?ID_victim=8751.
92. Waltraud Haüpl, *Die ermordeten Kinder vom Spiegelgrund: Gedenkdokumentation für die Opfer der NS-Kindereuthanasie in Wien* (Vienna: Bohlau Verlag, 2006): 256–58.
93. Günther K., victim number 8751, available at Victims of Biomedical Research under National Socialism, https://ns-medical-victims.org/nmv_view_victim?ID_victim=8751.
94. Michael Jeremy Jolley, 'A Social History of Paediatric Nursing 1920–1970', PhD thesis (University of Hull, 2003):11.
95. AHUS. Case of Francine L., 1943 (case number 1638/43).
96. Pam Barnes, 'Thirty Years of Play in Hospital', *International Journal of Early Childhood* 27.1 (1 March 1995): 48. https://doi.org/10.1007/BF03178105
97. AVES. Letter from A. Reiter Oberin, March 1943.
98. AHUS. Case of Francine L., 1943 (case number 1638/43).
99. AHUS. Case of Ulof H., 1944 (case number 559/44); patient chart, observations, 30 June 1944.
100. Herwig Czech, 'Hans Asperger, National Socialism, and "Race Hygiene" in Nazi-Era Vienna', *Molecular Autism* 9 (19 April 2018): 29. https://doi.org/10.1186/s13229-018-0208-6
101. ADHVS Path. Case number 514/43 of a three-year-old child admitted to Surgical Clinic 2 for bomb injuries in 1943 but did not survive. Pathology Record Books.

4. Paediatric Patients in Psychiatric Care

1. Michael von Cranach, 'Ethics in Psychiatry: The Lessons We Learn from Nazi Psychiatry', *European Archives of Psychiatry and Clinical Neuroscience* 260 (2010): 152–56.
2. AVES. 7AH47 *Direktion Generale Krisenmaßnahmen Bergung und Rückführung aus den Bergungsgebieten.* For further information on the psychiatric clinic in general, in

particular treatment of adult patients, and biographies of the former heads of department and staff of the clinic, consult Lea Münch, '"Weil sich das Gerät als unentbehrliches Hilfsmittel … herausgestellt hat." Zur Einführung und Behandlungspraxis der Elektroschocktherapie an der Reichsuniversität Straßburg', in *La faculté de médecine de la Reichsuniversität Straßburg et l'hôpital civil sous l'annexation de fait nationale-socialiste 1940–1945: Vie des cliniques au quotidien, experimentations humaines criminelles, collections medico-scientifiques, biographies des victims et du personnel de la faculté de médecine et préconations concernant les politiques mémorielles* (2022): 65–72.

3. Thirty-five boxes of psychiatric files from 1941 to 1944 (the period of German occupation) at the archives of the Département d'Histoire des sciences de la Vie et de la Santé at the University of Strasbourg, with approximately eighty-six files per box, resulting in an estimated 3,010 cases in the psychiatric clinic treated during German occupation.
4. Patrick Wechsler, *La Faculté de médecine de la 'Reichsuniversität Strassburg' (1941–1945) à l'heure nationale-socialiste*: 103.
5. Ernst Klee, *Das Personenlexikon zum Dritten Reich: Wer war was vor und nach 1945*, Bostroem August entry (Frankfurt: Fischer Verlag, 2005): 67.
6. Patrick Wechsler, *La Faculté de médecine de la 'Reichsuniversität Strassburg'* (1991): 103.
7. Ibid.
8. BArch. R9361-VIII Kartei / 3590565 NSDAP Zentralkartei, Bostroem, August.
9. Patrick Wechsler, *La Faculté de médecine de la 'Reichsuniversität Strassburg'* (1991), publications list: 104.
10. Ibid.: 238.
11. Ibid.: 100.
12. Ernst Klee, *Das Personenlexikon zum Dritten Reich: Wer war was vor und nach 1945*, Jensch Nikolaus entry (Frankfurt: Fischer Verlag, 2005): 286.
13. Nikolaus Jensch, *Untersuchungen an Entmannten Sittlichkeitsverbrechern. Sammlung psychiatrischer und neurologischer Einzeldarstellungen* (Leipzig: Thieme, 1944).
14. ADHVS Psych. Case of Susanna D., 1943 (case number K27/170); letter, 7 May 1943, from Kork recommending Dr Bostroem for her treatment, and thus she is transferred to Strasbourg.
15. AVES. 7AH90. Ärztliche Betreuung. Letter from Dr Bostroem to Dr Stein on 25 January 1944.
16. AVES. Ibid.
17. For further discussion, consult the closing chapter on the postwar era and evacuation.
18. ADBR. 126AL77 F. 14 April 1944, letter from Dr Hofmeier to chef der Zivilverwaltung, concering the transfer of the children's clinic to Stephansfeld, Notdienstverpflichtung des Säuglings u. Kinderschwester Schülerinnen der Lehranstalt bei der Universität Kinderklinik in Straßburg.
19. AVES. 7AH90. Ärztliche Betreuung. Dr Stein letter, 26 January 1944.
20. For further information on the Knauer case, which was a catalyst for the euthanasia programme, consult Udo Benzenhofer. As a preface to the Knauer case, consult further literature on the Meltzer survey; Ewald Meltzer, *Das Problem der Abkürzung 'lebensunwerten Lebens'* (The Problem of Shortening 'Life Unworthy of Life') (C. Marhold, Halle, 1925). The Meltzer survey is referenced in student research in Strasbourg which discussed the survey, and asked student doctors if they agreed

with it (see Johanna Wehrung, *Erläuterungen zum Euthanasie Problem auf Grund einer ruckfrage bei Frauen*, Med. Diss. (Reichsuniversität Straßburg, 1944)). And further information can be found in Binding and Hoche's book, which influenced the adoption of so-called euthanasia: Karl Binding and Alfred Hoche, *Die Freigabe der Vernichtung lebensunwerten Lebens: ihr Maß und ihre Form* (Leipzig: Meiner, 1920).

21. Volker Roelcke, 'Deutscher Sonderweg? Die eugenische Bewegung in europäischer Perspektive bis in die 1930er Jahre', in *Die Nationalsozialistische Euthanasie-Aktion T 4 Und Ihre Opfer: Geschichte Und Ethische Konsequenzen Für Die Gegenwart*, eds. Petra Fuchs, Wolfgang U. Eckart, Christoph Mundt, Maike Rotzoll, Paul Richter, and Gerrit Hohendorf (Paderborn: Ferdinand Schoningh, 2010): 47–55.
22. Gerrit Hohendorf, '"Death as a Release from Suffering": The History and Ethics of Assisted Dying in Germany Since the End of the 19th Century', *Neurology, Psychiatry, and Brain Research* 22.2 (2016): 56–62.
23. Ibid.
24. Edith Sheffer, *Asperger's Children: The Origins of Autism in Nazi Vienna*: 101.
25. Maike Rotzoll et al., 'The First National Socialist Extermination Crime: The T4 Program and Its Victims', *International Journal of Mental Health* 35.3 (2006): 17–29.
26. Florian Steger, 'Günzburg State Hospital and the "Aktion T4": A Systematic Review', *Neurology, Psychiatry and Brain Research* 22.2 (2016): 40–45.
27. Herwig Czech, 'Von der "Aktion T4" zur "dezentralen Euthanasie" Die niederösterreichischen Heil- und Pflegeanstalten Gugging, Mauer-Öhling und Ybbs', in *Fanatiker, Pflichterfüller, Widerständige*, eds. Dokumentationsarchiv des österreichischen Widerstandes (Vienna, 2016): 219–66. www.doew.at
28. Hans-Walter Schmuhl, 'Was heißt "Widerstand" gegen die NS-"Euthanasie"-Verbrechen?' *Historia Hospitalium* 26 (2015): 237–55 .
29. Klara Nowak, *Ich klage An: Tatsachen- und Erlebnisberichte der 'Euthanasie'-Geschädigten und Zwangssterilisierten* (Detmold, 1989). For a further discussion on representations of 'mercy killing', including a debate on *Ich klage An*, consult Carol Poore, 'Who Belongs? Disability and the German Nation in Postwar Literature and Film', *German Studies Review* 26 (2003), 21–42.
30. Tanja Maria Kipfelsperger, *Die Associationsanstalt Schönbrunn und der Nationalsozialismus die Konfrontation einer katholischen Pflegeanstalt mit Zwangssterilisierung, NS-'Euthanasie'-Maßnahmen und 'Klostersturm'* (Munich: Utz Verlag, 2021): 18–19.
31. Heinz Faulstich, *Hungersterben in der Psychiatrie 1914–1949 mit einer Topographie der NS-Psychiatrie* (Freiburg im Breisgau: Lambertus, 1998): 25.
32. Gerrit Hohendorf, 'Die Selektion der Opfer zwischen rassenhygienischer "Ausmerze", ökonomischer Brauchbarkeit und medizinischem Erlösungsideal', in *Die Nationalsozialistische Euthanasie-Aktion T4 Und Ihre Opfer: Geschichte Und Ethische Konsequenzen Für Die Gegenwart*, eds. Petra Fuchs, Wolfgang U. Eckart, Christoph Mundt, Maike Rotzoll, Paul Richter, and Gerrit Hohendorf (Paderborn: Ferdinand Schoningh, 2010): 310–24.
33. Volker Roelcke, 'Psychiatry During National Socialism: Historical Knowledge and Some Implications', *Neurology, Psychiatry and Brain Research* 22.2 (2016): 34–39.
34. For further information, consult Astrid Ley, *Zwangssterilisation und Ärzteschaft: Hintergründe und Ziele ärztlichen Handelns 1934–1945* (Frankfurt: Campus Verlag, 2004).
35. Hilde Stepe, *Krankenpflege im Nationalsozialismus* (Frankfurt: Mabeuse Verlag, 2020).

36. Maike Rotzoll, Gerrit Hohendorf, and Volker Roelcke, 'Innovation und Vernichtung: Psychiatrische Forschung und "Euthanasie" an der Heidelberger Psychiatrischen Klinik 1939–1945', *Nervenarzt* 67 (1996): 935–46.
37. Original title: Reichsausschuss zur wissenschaftlichen Erfassung erb- und anlagebedingter schwerer Leiden. There was a strong distinction between curable and incurable, which influenced the degree of therapeutic optimism and treatment provided. Consult Jürgen Pfeiffer, 'Phases in the Postwar German Reception of the "Euthanasia Program" (1939–1945) Involving the Killing of the Mentally Disabled and its Exploitation by Neuroscientists', *Journal of the History of the Neurosciences* 15.3 (2006): 210–44, for further information on the distinction between curable and incurable over time in German psychiatry.
38. Robert Jay Lifton, *The Nazi Doctors: Medical Killing and the Psychology of Genocide* (New York: Basic Books, 1986): 52.
39. ADHVS Psych. Case of Ludwig F., 1944 (case number unknown).
40. ADHVS Psych. Case of Melitta S. (case number K27/873), case of Sydenham's chorea, and the cases of Robert M. (case number K27/428) and Herbert H. (case number K27/420), both with a sudden onset fatal encephalitis.
41. Maike Rotzoll and Geritt Hohendorf, 'Johann Duken und die Kinderklinik im Nationalsozialismus', in *Entwicklungen und Perspektiven der Kinder- und Jugendmedizin 150 Jahre Pädiatrie in Heidelberg*, ed. Georg F. Hoffmann (Mainz: Kirchheim, 2010): 86.
42. Florian Steger, 'Günzburg State Hospital and the "Aktion T4": A Systematic Review', *Neurology, Psychiatry and Brain Research* 22.2 (2016): 40–45.
43. Paul Weindling, Gerrit Hohendorf, Axel Hüntelmann, et al., 'The Problematic Legacy of Victim Specimens from the Nazi Era: Identifying the Persons Behind the Specimens at the Max Planck Institutes for Brain Research and of Psychiatry', *Journal of the History of the Neurosciences* (18 October 2021): 1–22.
44. ADHVS Psych. Case of Melitta S. (case number K27/873), admission file.
45. ADHVS Psych. Ibid. 8 February 1944 letter from Die Lehrerinnen KLV Lager Klingenthal.
46. ADHVS Psych. Ibid. Patient observations.
47. ADHVS Psych. Ibid. 22 February 1944, letter from Dr Jensch to the Hitler Jugend Gesundheitsabteilung Straßburg.
48. ADHVS Psych. Ibid. Staatliche Medizinal-Untersuchungsanstalt examination, 10 February 1944.
49. ADHVS Psych. Ibid. Patient chart.
50. ADHVS Psych. Ibid. 15 February 1944, letter from Dr Frank to Dr Jensch.
51. ADHVS Psych. Ibid. 3 March 1944, letter from Dr Jensch to Dr Holscher.
52. Michael von Cranach, 'Ethics in Psychiatry: The Lessons We Learn from Nazi Psychiatry', *European Archives of Psychiatry and Clinical Neuroscience* 260 (2010): 152–56.
53. AVES. 7AH90. Ärztliche Betreuung. Another possible reason is the less than ideal situation of children being treated at an adult psychiatric facility; letter from Dr Bostroem to Dr Stein on 25 January 1944.
54. ADHVS Psych. Case of Susanna D., 1943 (case number K27/170), 8 May 1943, letter from Mr D. to Dr Bostroem.
55. ADHVS Psych. Ibid.
56. ADHVS Psych. Ibid. 7 May 1943, referral letter from Kork Heil-und Pflegeanstalt.

57. Louise Wannell, 'Patients' Relatives and Psychiatric Doctors: Letter Writing in the York Retreat, 1875–1910', *Social History of Medicine* 20 (2007): 297–313.
58. ADHVS Psych. Case of Susanna D., 1943 (case number K27/170), admission form.
59. ADHVS Psych. Ibid. 7 May 1943, referral letter from Kork Heil-und Pflegeanstalt.
60. ADHVS Psych. Ibid. 1 June 1943, letter from Graz medical centre detailing her previous treatment.
61. Ivar Asbjørn Følling 'Über Ausscheidung von Phenylbrenztraubensäure in den Harn als Stoffwechselanomalie in Verbindung: mit Imbezillität', *Hoppe-Seyler's Zeitschrift für physiologische Chemie* 227.1–4 (1934): 169–81.
62. Diane B. Paul and Jeffrey P. Brosco, *The PKU Paradox: A Short History of a Genetic Disease* (Baltimore: Johns Hopkins University Press, 2013): 64.
63. ADHVS Psych. Case of Susanna D., 1943 (case number K27/170), 1 June 1943, letter from Graz medical centre detailing Dr Berzaczy's perceptions of her medical condition.
64. ADHVS Psych. Case of Karl F., 1942 (case number K27/519), 9 March 1942, letter from Mr and Mrs F. requesting the admission of their child to Stephansfeld.
65. ADHVS Psych. Ibid. Admission file.
66. ADHVS Psych. Ibid. 16 March 1942, letter from Dr Burckel.
67. ADHVS Psych. Ibid. Patient observation file.
68. ADHVS Psych. Ibid. 12 March 1942, telegram from Dr Frey to Mr F., agreeing with his decision to send his son to Stephansfeld.
69. ADHVS Psych. Ibid. 9 March 1942, letter from Mr F. to the psychiatric clinic in Strasbourg.
70. Paul Weindling, Herwig Czech, and Christiane Druml, 'From Scientific Exploitation to Individual Memorialization: Evolving Attitudes Towards Research on Nazi Victims' Bodies', *Bioethics* 35.6 (2021): 508– 17.
71. Lutz Kaelber, 'Child Murder in Nazi Germany: The Memory of Nazi Medical Crimes and Commemoration of "Children's Euthanasia" Victims at Two Facilities (Eichberg, Kalmenhof)', *Societies* (2012): 157–94.
72. Ibid.
73. AEPSANS. Case of Karl F. 355, 1942, admission file to Stephansfeld Heil-und Pflegeanstalt.
74. AEPSANS. Ibid. Letter from the director of Stephansfeld Heil-und Pflegeanstalt, 27 March 1942. Original quote: 'Sie erhalten hiermit ausnahmsweise die Erlaubnis mit ihren beiden Söhnen den kranken Karl einmal an einem Sonntag im Monat zu besuchen. Sie wollen diesen schreiben dem Anstaltsporter als Ausweis vorlegen.'
75. AEPSANS. Ibid. Letter from the F. family to Stephansfeld Heil-und Pflegeanstalt on 2 June 1942.
76. AEPSANS. Ibid. Letter from Stephansfeld Heil-und Pflegeanstalt to Emil F., 6 June 1942.
77. AEPSANS. Ibid. Release form signed 30 July 1942 from Stephansfeld Heil-und Pflegeanstalt.
78. Consult the introduction for a full explanation of the problematic nature of the categorization of Alsatian as a nationality, and the factors that influence the determination of German nationality in this era.
79. For a full explanation of nationality politics, please consult the introduction.

80. ADHVS Psych. Case of Emilie G., 1942 (case number K27/481).
81. ADHVS Psych. Case of Emilie G., 1942 (case number K27/481).
82. ADHVS Psych. Ibid. 25 March 1942, Staatliche Medizinal-Untersuchungsanstalt examinations.
83. Norman E. Leeds and Stephen A. Kieffer, 'Evolution of Diagnostic Neuroradiology from 1904 to 1999', *Radiology* 217 (2000): 310.
84. Mariam Ishaque, David J. Wallace, and Ramesh Grandhi, 'Pneumoencephalography in the Workup of Neuropsychiatric Illnesses: A Historical Perspective', *Neurosurgical Focus* 43 (2017): 2.
85. ADHVS Psych. Ibid. 21 March 1942, pneumoencephalography consent form.
86. ADHVS Psych. Ibid. 25 March 1942, Röntgenabteilung examinations.
87. ADHVS Psych. Ibid. 25 March 1942, patient observations.
88. ADHVS Psych. Ibid. 3 March 1942, patient observations.
89. For further information on this case, and the important distinction of regions in diagnosis and treatment during the Nazi era, consult Aisling Shalvey, 'Little's Disease During National Socialism: A Comparative Case Study', *Medizinhistorisches Journal* 57.3 (2022): 260-246.
90. ADHVS Psych. Case of Watzlaff Z., 1944 (case number K27/951), admission form.
91. ADHVS Psych. Ibid.
92. AN. BB30/1797. 10 March, Goldberg court 1 case VIII , 5308, in Procès de Germanisation VIII 1948.
93. Markus Leniger, '"Heim ins Reich"? Das Amt XI und die Umsiedlerlager der Volksdeutschen Mittelstelle 1939–1945', in *Bürokratien: Initiative und Effizienz*, eds. Wolf Gruner and Armin Nolzen (Berlin: Assoziation A., 2001): 81–109.
94. ADHVS Psych. Case of Watzlaff Z., 1944 (case number K27/951), 16 September 1944, letter from SS Hauptsturmfuhrer.
95. ADHVS Psych. Case of Watzlaff Z., 1944 (case number K27/951), Zeugnis der Ortspolizeibehörde.
96. ADHVS Psych. Ibid. Admission form.
97. ADHVS Psych. Ibid. 16 September 1944, letter from SS Hauptsturmfuhrer concerning the 'naturalization process'.
98. ADHVS Psych. Ibid. 21 March 1944, letter from psychiatric clinic Strasbourg.
99. Maria Fiebrandt, *Auslese für die Siedlergesellschaft Die Einbeziehung Volksdeutscher in die NS-Erbgesundheitspolitik im Kontext der Umsiedlungen 1939–1945*: 216.
100. Lara Rzesnitzek and Sascha Lang, 'Electroshock Therapy in the Third Reich', *Medical History* 61.1 (2017): 66–88.
101. Schweizerische Gesellschaft für Psychiatrie, 'Bericht über die wissenschaftlichen Verhandlungen auf der 89 Versammlung der Schweizerischen Gesellschaft für Psychiatrie in Münsingen b. Bern am 29–31 Mai 1937', *Schweizer Archiv für Neurologie und Psychiatrie* 39 (suppl.) (1937): 1–240.
102. A.M. Wyllie, 'Treatment of Mental Disorders by Cardiazol', *Glasgow Medical Journal* 129 (1938): 269–79.
103. Insulin shock therapy also fell out of favour during the Second World War, in part due to the shortage of insulin, so alternative methods were favoured, such as cardiazol and electroshock. Niall Mccrae, '"A Violent Thunderstorm": Cardiazol Treatment in British Mental Hospitals', *History of Psychiatry* 17.1 (2006): 70.

104. Lea Münch, '"Weil sich das Gerät als unentbehrliches Hilfsmittel ... herausgestellt hat." Zur Einführung und Behandlungspraxis der Elektroschocktherapie an der RUS', in *Commission Historique Report 2021* (in press).
105. AFMS. Rudolf Gross, 'Gedanknißstörungen bei der Schockbehandlung das manisch-depressiven Formenkreises', Diss. Med. (1944): 19.
106. ADHVS Psych. Case of Georg E., 1942 (case number K27/269), admission file.
107. ADHVS Psych. Ibid. Patient observations.
108. Diminishing ability or willingness to work, as well as physical strength, among other factors, was often an indication of selection of a patient for 'euthanasia'. Florian Steger, Andreas Görgl, Wolfgang Strube, Hans-Joachim Winckelmann, and Thomas Becker, 'Die "Aktion T4" und die Rolle der Heil- und Pflegeanstalt Günzburg', *Psychiatrische Praxis* 37.6 (2010): 300–305.

    ADHVS Psych. Ibid. 1 August 1942, letter from Städtisches Krankenhaus Metz.
109. ADHVS Psych. Ibid. Electroconvulsive therapy record.
110. ADHVS Psych. Ibid. 4 July 1942, patient observations.
111. ADHVS Psych. Ibid. 15 September 1942, patient observations.
112. ADHVS Psych. Ibid. Patient medical chart.
113. ADHVS Psych. Case of Georg E., 1942, electroshock chart 1.
114. ADHVS Psych. Ibid. 27 March 1943, letter from the psychiatric clinic in Strasbourg.
115. Thomas Beddies, *Die Patienten der Wittenauer Heilstätten in Berlin 1919–1960* (Husum: Matthiesen, 1999): 162; Corwin Boake, 'From the Binet Simon to the Wechsler Bellevue: Tracing the History of Intelligence Testing', *Journal of Clinical and Experimental Neuropsychology* 24.3 (2002): 383–405. For a full list of questions provided in Binet Bobertag Norden intelligence testing, please consult Appendix 4 for a copy of a test carried out in the Reichsuniversität Straßburg psychiatric clinic.
116. Kurt Hofmeier, *Die Bedeutung der Erbanlage für die Kinderheilkunde*: 8.
117. Ibid.: 173. A Hilfschule was an institutional school setting with an alternative curriculum for those considered to be of lower intelligence to the extent that they could not participate in mainstream schooling.
118. Valentine Hoffbeck, 'De l'arriéré Au Malade Héréditaire: Histoire de La Prise En Charge et Des Représentations Du Handicap Mental En France et Allemagne (1890–1934)', PhD thesis (University of Strasbourg, 2016): 383.
119. Ibid.
120. Hans-Walter Schmuhl, 'Reformpsychiatrie und Massenmord', in *Nationalsozialismus und Modernisierung*, eds. Rainer Zitelmann and Michael Prinz, 2nd edn (Darmstadt: Wissenschaftliche Buchgesellschft, 1994): 239–66. See also Steger (2016).
121. See Appendix 4, illustrating an example of the intelligence testing used in the psychiatric clinic of Reichsuniversität Straßburg. Original quotes:

    Wieviel tage hat das Jahr?
    Wieviel Stunde hat der Tag?
    Wie heißt die Hauptstadt von Frankreich?
    Wer War Bismarck?
122. Ibid. Original quote:

    Was heißt das: Hunger ist die beste Kost?
123. Ibid. Original quotes:

    Bilden Sie einen Satz mit folgenden Worten: Soldat, Krieg, Vaterland.

Welche Feinde hatten wir im Weltkriege?

See Appendix 4, illustrating an example of the intelligence testing used in the psychiatric clinic of Reichsuniversität Straßburg.

124. A.F. Tredgold, *Mental Deficiency (Amentia)* (New York: William Wood and Company, 1920): 388.
125. For further information on the ideological nature of intelligence testing, consult Valentine Hoffbeck, 'De l'arriéré Au Malade Héréditaire: Histoire de La Prise En Charge et Des Représentations Du Handicap Mental En France et Allemagne (1890–1934)', PhD thesis (University of Strasbourg, 2016): 458.
126. ADHVS Psych. Case of Renatus T., 1944 (case number K26/260). Original quote: 'Körperlicher Befund: Zarter blasser Junge, Sommersprossen.'
127. ADHVS Psych. Ibid. Aktenauszug über Renatus T.
128. ADHVS Psych. Ibid. Aktenauszug über Renatus T. Original quote: 'Sei sehr grob und brutal mit ihm.'
129. ADHVS Psych. Ibid.
130. ADHVS Psych. Ibid. Original quote: 'Zusammenfassung: aus asozialer Familie stammender, von der Mutter unzureichend versorgter 10 jähriger Junge der durch einen Mangel an Intelligenz auffällig [...] geworden ist [...] Aufnahme nach Stephansfeld.'
131. Greg Eghigian, 'A Drifting Concept for an Unruly Menace: A History of Psychopathy in Germany', *Isis* 106.2 (2015): 283–309.
132. ADHVS Psych. Case of Renatus T., 1944 (case number K26/260). Befund.
133. ADHVS Psych. Ibid. Aktenauszug. It is unclear who conducted the home visit on which they base their comments.
134. ADHVS Psych. Case of Renatus T., 1944 (case number K26/260); Psychisches verhalten observations.
135. ADHVS Psych. Ibid.
136. ADHVS Psych. Ibid.
137. Michael S. Bryant, *Confronting the 'Good Death': Nazi Euthanasia on Trial, 1945–1953* (Boulder, CO: University Press of Colorado, 2005): 135.
138. ADHVS Psych. Case of Josef L., 1942 (case number K27/491), admission file.
139. ADHVS Psych. Ibid.
140. ADHVS Psych. Ibid. 21 October 1942, letter from the Hals Nasen Ohren Klinik from Dr Hagdorn.
141. ADHVS Psych. Ibid. Drawings.
142. ADHVS Psych. Ibid. 21 October 1942, patient observation notes.
143. ADHVS Psych. Ibid. Drawings.
144. ADHVS Psych. Ibid.
145. ADHVS Psych. Ibid. Drawings.
146. ADHVS Psych. Case of Johann H., 1943 (case number K27/508), admission file.
147. ADHVS Psych. Ibid. Patient observations.
148. ADHVS Psych. Ibid.
149. ADHVS Psych. Ibid. Ärztliches Zeugnis.
150. Lutz Kaelber, 'Child Murder in Nazi Germany: The Memory of Nazi Medical Crimes and Commemoration of "Children's Euthanasia" Victims at Two Facilities (Eichberg, Kalmenhof)': 157–94.
151. ADHVS Psych. Case of Johann H., 1943 (case number K27/508).

152. ADHVS Psych. Ibid. 21 September 1943, Staatliche Medizinal-Untersuchungsanstalt examinations.
153. ADHVS Psych. Ibid. 20 October 1943, letter from Dr Bostroem to Wehrbezirkskommando Hagenau.
154. ADHVS Psych. Case of Susanna D., 1943 (case number K27/170), 7 May 1943, referral letter from Kork Heil-und Pflegeanstalt.
155. As Lara Rzesnitzek and Sachsa Lang note, the process of informed consent differed between regions, institutions, and even individual clinics. Therefore, the process of written informed consent as present for child patients in Strasbourg should not be considered the standard. Consult 'Electroshock Therapy in the Third Reich' *Medical History* 61.1 (2017): 66–88.
156. Norman E. Leeds and Stephen A. Kieffer, 'Evolution of Diagnostic Neuroradiology from 1904 to 1999', *Radiology* 217 (2000): 310.
157. ADHVS Psych. Case of Andreas N., 1942 (case number K27/520), 15 November 1942, letter from Mr Alfons N. requesting to visit his son.
158. Lea Münch, 'From Strasbourg to Hadamar: Nazi Psychiatry and Patient Biographies in Annexed Alsace (1941–1944)', unpublished lecture.
159. Volker Roelcke, 'Psychiatry During National Socialism: Historical Knowledge and Some Implications', *Neurology, Psychiatry and Brain Research* 22.2 (2016): 34–39.

5. Medical Research and Student Theses on Paediatrics

1. Florian Bruns and Tessa Chelouche, 'Lectures on Inhumanity: Teaching Medical Ethics in German Medical Schools Under Nazism', *Annals of Internal Medicine* 166.8 (18 April 2017): 591. https://doi.org/10.7326/M16-2758
2. Elie Wiesel, 'Without Conscience', *New England Journal of Medicine* 352 (2005): 1511–13. https://doi.org/10.1056/NEJMp058069
3. BIAB. SZT6310684. Opening of the Reichsuniversität Straßburg, 1941 (28 November 1941), photographed by Scherl.
4. Volker Roelcke and Simon Duckheim, 'Medizinische Dissertationen Aus Der Zeit Des Nationalsozialismus: Potential Eines Quellenbestands Und Erste Ergebnisse Zu "Alltag", Ethik Und Mentalität Der Universitären Medizinischen Forschung Bis (Und Ab) 1945', *Medizinhistorisches Journal* 49.3 (2014): 260–71.
5. 'Richtlinien für neuartige Heilbehandlung und für die Vornahme wissenschaftlicher Versuche am Menschen', *Deutsche Medizinische Wochenschrift* 57.12 (1931): 509.
6. Christian Bonah, Étienne Lepicard, and Volker Roelcke, *La médecine expérimentale au tribunal: implications éthiques de quelques procès médicaux du XXe siècle européen* (Paris: Éd. des Archives contemporaines, 2003): introduction.
7. Volker Roelcke, Sascha Topp, and Étienne Lepicard, *Silence, Scapegoats and Self-Reflection: The Shadow of Nazi Medical Crimes on Medicine and Bioethics* (Göttingen: V&R Unipress, 2014): 64.
8. 'Richtlinien für neuartige Heilbehandlung und für die Vornahme wissenschaftlicher Versuche am Menschen.'
9. Volker Roelcke, 'The Use and Abuse of Medical Research Ethics: The German Richtlinien/Guidelines for Human Subject Research as an Instrument for the

Protection of Research Subjects—and of Medical Science, ca.1931–1961/64', in *From Clinic to Concentration Camp: Reassessing Nazi Medical and Racial Research, 1933–1945*, ed. Paul Weindling (Milton Park: Routledge, 2017): 33–56.

10. Ulf Schmidt, *Justice at Nuremberg: Leo Alexander and the Nazi Doctors' Trial* (New York: Palgrave Macmillan, 2004): 13.
11. 'Richtlinien für neuartige Heilbehandlung und für die Vornahme wissenschaftlicher Versuche am Menschen.'
12. *Carly Seyfarth, Der Ärzte-Knigge: über den Umgang mit Kranken und* über *Pflichten, Kunst und Dienst der Krankenhausärzte* (Leipzig: Georg Thieme, 1938): introduction.
13. Volker Roelcke, 'The Use and Abuse of Medical Research Ethics: The German Richtlinien/Guidelines for Human Subject Research as an Instrument for the Protection of Research Subjects—and of Medical Science, ca. 1931–1961/64': 33–56.
14. Volker Roelcke, 'Medizinische Dissertationen Aus Der Zeit Des Nationalsozialismus: Potential Eines Quellenbestands Und Erste Ergebnisse Zu "Alltag", Ethik Und Mentalität Der Universitären Medizinischen Forschung Bis (Und Ab) 1945', *Medizinhistorisches Journal* (2014): 49.
15. ADHVS Psych. Case of Emilie G., 1942 (case number K27/481); consent form signed by her father for the procedure of a pneumoencephalography on 21 March 1942.
16. Carole Sachse, 'What Research, to What End? The Rockefeller Foundation and the Max Planck Gesellschaft in the Early Cold War', *Central European History* 42 (2009): 97–141.
17. Ibid.
18. André N. Sofair and Lauris C. Kaldjian, 'Eugenic Sterilization and a Qualified Nazi Analogy: The United States and Germany, 1930–1945', *Annals of Internal Medicine* 132.4 (15 February 2000): 312. https://doi.org/10.7326/0003-4819-132-4-200002150-00010
19. Henry E Sigerist, *Einführung in die Medizin* (Leipzig: G. Thieme, 1931): 390.
20. Rudolf Ramm, Ärztliche *Rechts- und Standeskunde. Der Arzt als Gesundheitserzieher* (Berlin: De Gruyter, 1942); Karl Binding and Alfred Hoche, *Die Freigabe der Vernichtung lebensunwerten Lebens, ihr Maß und ihre Form* (Leipzig: F. Meiner, 1922).
21. Lutz Sauerteig, 'Règles éthiques, droits des patients et ethos médical dans le cas d'essais médicamenteux (1892- 1931)', in *La médecine expérimentale au tribunal: implications éthiques de quelques procès médicaux du XXe siècle européen*, eds. Christian Bonah, Volker Roelcke, and Étienne Lepicard (Pantin: Archives Contemporaine, 2003): 31–64.
22. Florian Bruns and Tessa Chelouche, 'Lectures on Inhumanity: Teaching Medical Ethics in German Medical Schools Under Nazism': 591.
23. Edmund D. Pellegrino, 'The Nazi Doctors and Nuremberg: Some Moral Lessons Revisited', *Annals of Internal Medicine* 127.4 (15 August 1997): 307. https://doi.org/10.7326/0003-4819-127-4-199708150-00010
24. Shmuel P. Reis, Hedy S. Wald, and Paul Weindling, 'The Holocaust, Medicine and Becoming a Physician: The Crucial Role of Education', *Israel Journal of Health Policy Research* 8 (2019): 1–5.
25. Alessandra Colaianni, 'A Long Shadow: Nazi Doctors, Moral Vulnerability and Contemporary Medical Culture', *Journal of Medical Ethics* 38.7 (1 July 2012): 435–38.

26. Shmuel P. Reis, Hedy S. Wald, and Paul Weindling, 'The Holocaust, Medicine and Becoming a Physician: The Crucial Role of Education': 1–5.
27. Noting that experimentation is necessary and that banning it was not the aim of the Lübeck trial or the Nuremberg trial, see Christian Bonah, 'Le drame de Lübeck: la vaccination BCG, le "procès Calmette" et les Richtlinen de 1931', in *La médecine expérimentale au tribunal: implications éthiques de quelques procès médicaux du XXe siècle européen*, eds. Christian Bonah, Volker Roelcke, and Étienne Lepicard (Pantin: Archives Contemporaine, 2003): 65–94.
28. Sue Black, *All that Remains: A Life in Death* (London: Penguin, 2019): 119.
29. Alessandra Colaianni, 'A Long Shadow: Nazi Doctors, Moral Vulnerability and Contemporary Medical Culture', *Journal of Medical Ethics* 38.7 (1 July 2012): 435–38.
30. ADHVS, RUS Collection, Prüfungsunterlagen Dissertationen 1–242.
31. Dritte Anordnung zur Wiedereinführung der Muttersprache vom 18 August 1940, *Verordnungsblatt des Chefs der Zivilverwaltung im Elsaß 1940*, n° 1 / 24 August 1940, 2.
32. Leonie Werner, 'Medizinstudierende an der "Reichsuniversität" Straßburg (1941–1944)', Master's thesis (University of Freiburg, 2019).
33. Deutsche Bücherei (dir.), *Jahresverzeichnis der deutschen Hochschulschriften 1943* (59 Jahrgang) (Leipzig, 1962): 431 (A. Hartmann, G. Möckel), and Hermann Voss, 'Die Medizinische Fakultät der Reichsuniversität Posen', *Deutsches Ärzteblatt* 72.31 (1942): 356–57.
34. Gabriele Moser, 'Une science médicale normale sous l'occupation nationale-socialiste? Les thèses de la faculté de médecine de la Reichsuniversität Straßburg: état de la recherche, découvertes, perspectives de recherche', in *Rapport final de la Commission Historique de la Reichsuniversität Straßburg* (2022): 86–104.
35. Robert M. Zollinger, Francois H.K. Reynolds, George F. Jeffcot, and Hans Schlumberger, *Medical, Dental and Veterinary Education and Practice in Germany as Reflected by the Universities of Leipzig, Jena, Halle and Erlangen* (Washington, DC, 1945), http://hdl.handle.net/2027/umn.31951d03595646d
36. BArch. R76 IV 46. Concerning the reconstruction of the psychiatric clinic Reichsuniversität Straßburg, rebuilding costs, 1944.
37. Rainer Möhler, 'Die Reichsuniversität Straßburg 1941–1944. Eine Nationalsozialistische Musteruniversität zwischen Wissenschaft, Volkstumspolitik, und Verbrechen': 520.
38. Ibid.: 668.
39. BNU. NIM18815. Männer des Elsass, Eine Mission für die gesamte Kulturwelt. Elsässische Männer, Der Platz der Jugend ist an der Front des stählernen Helms. Strasbourg, 1941.
40. For further information on women studying medicine in German universities, consult Melissa Kravetz, *Women Doctors in Weimar and Nazi Germany: Maternalism, Eugenics, and Professional Identity* (Toronto: University of Toronto Press, 2019).
41. Robert M. Zollinger et al., *Medical, Dental and Veterinary Education and Practice in Germany*: 21.
42. D. Schäfer, 'Pädiatrische Netzwerke im "Dritten Reich": Helmut Seckel und seine Kollegen aus der Universitätskinderklinik Köln', *Monatsschrift Kinderheilkunde: Zeitschrift für Kinder- und Jugendmedizin* 165.12 (2017): 1102–1108.

43. AFMS. Hans-Joachim Gawantka, 'Die Bedeutung krankhafter Erbanlagen und Erbkrankheiten bei Adoptiveltern und Adoptivkindern', Diss. Med. (1943)
44. Ibid.: 1.
45. Ibid.: 13.
46. Ibid.: 12.
47. Ibid.: 30.
48. AFMS. Doktorprüfung als Hans-Joachim Gawantka.
49. AFMS. Wolfgang Wendel, 'Zwei Fälle von jugendlicher Poikilodermie im lothringischen InzuchtgebietRimlingen', Diss. Med. (1945).
50. Ibid.: 12. Referring to M. Sydney Thomson, 'Poikiloderma Congenitale', *British Journal of Dermatology* 48 (1936): 221–34.
51. Ibid.: 15.
52. Ibid.: 25.
53. Ibid.: 26.
54. Ibid.: 29. The original German emphasizes this consanguinity as evidence of 'degeneration' of the population in the area.
55. Ibid.: 29.
56. Ibid.: 29.
57. Ibid.: 33.
58. Ibid.: 35.
59. Ibid.: 35.
60. Ibid.: 799.
61. AFMS. Rosemarie von der Decken, 'Hand-Schüller-Christian'sche Erkrankung bei zweieiigen Zwillingen', Diss. Med. (1942).
62. Ibid.: 5.
63. Ibid.: 14.
64. Rosemarie von der Decken, 'Hand-Schüller-Christian'sche Erkrankung bei zweieiigen Zwillingen', *Archiv für Kinderheilkunde* (1943).
65. Hans Forssman and Brita Rudberg, 'Study of Consanguinity in Twenty-one Cases of Hand-Schüller-Christian Disease (Systemic Reticuloendothelial Granuloma)', *Acta Medica Scandinavica* 168. 5–6 (12 January 1960): 427–29. https://doi.org/10.1111/j.0954-6820.1960.tb06673.x
66. Rosemarie von der Decken, 'Hand-Schuller-Christian'sche Erkrankung bei zweieiigen Zwillingen', *Archiv für Kinderheilkunde* (1943).
67. AFMS. Referat über die Dissertationsarbeit Rosemarie von der Decken, 31 August 1943.
68. AFMS. Edith Schneider, 'Fingerleistenuntersuchungen Bei Straßburger Schulkindern' Diss. Med. (1944).
69. Ibid.: 1.
70. Ibid.: 2.
71. Ibid.: 5–7, table 2.
72. Jens Kolata et al., 'In Fleischhackers Händen: Wissenschaft, Politik und das 20. Jahrhundert' diese Publikation erscheint anlässlich der Ausstellung 'In Fleischhackers Händen. Tübinger Rassenforscher in Łódź 1940–1942' im Schloss Hohentübingen (24 April bis 28. Juni 2015) (Tübingen: Museum der Universität Tübingen, 2015).

73. AFMS. Johanna Wehrung, 'Erläuterungen zum Euthanasie-Problem aufgrund einer Rückfrage bei Frauen', Diss. Med. (1944).
74. Karl Binding and Alfred Hoche, *Die Freigabe der Vernichtung lebensunwerten Lebens, ihr Maß und ihre Form* (Leipzig: F. Meiner, 1920).
75. Johanna Wehrung, 'Erläuterungen zum Euthanasie-Problem aufgrund einer Rückfrage bei Frauen': 19.
76. Ibid.: 1.
77. Ibid.: 13.
78. Ibid.: 12.
79. AFMS. Karl Robert Bacher, 'Zum Euthanasieproblem', Diss. Med. (1943).
80. Ewald Meltzer, *Das Problem der Abkürzung Lebensunswerten Lebens* (C. Marhold, Halle, 1925).
81. Gerrit Hohendorf, '"Death as a Release from Suffering": The History and Ethics of Assisted Dying in Germany Since the End of the 19th Century', *Neurology, Psychiatry, and Brain Research* 22.2 (2016): 56–62.
82. AFMS. Johanna Wehrung, 'Erläuterungen zum Euthanasie-Problem aufgrund einer Rückfrage bei Frauen': 15.
83. Marius Turda, *Modernism and Eugenics* (Basingstoke: Palgrave Macmillan, 2011): 2.
84. Sara Seiler Vigorito, 'A Profile of Nazi Medicine: The Nazi Doctor, His Method and Goals', in *When Medicine Went Mad: Bioethics and the Holocaust*, ed. Arthur Caplan (New York: Springer, 1992): 9–13.
85. Christian Bonah and Florian Schmaltz, 'The Reception of the Nuremberg Code and Its Impact on Medical Ethics in France: 1947–1954': 199–202.
86. Sabine Hildebrandt, *The Anatomy of Murder: Ethical Transgressions and Anatomical Science During the Third Reich* (New York/Oxford: Berghahn Books, 2016): 267.

6. Paediatric Patients at the Internal Medicine Clinic

1. Flora Graefe and Volker Roelcke, 'Zwangsarbeiter in der Medizin—Zivile "Fremdarbeiter" als Arbeitskräfte und Patienten am Universitätsklinikum Gießen im Zweiten Weltkrieg', in *Die Medizinische Fakultät der Universität Gießen 1607 bis 2007. Band I IDie Medizinische Fakultät der Universität Gießen im Nationalsozialismus und in der Nachkriegszeit: Personen und Institutionen, Umbrüche und Kontinuitäten*, ed. Sigrid Oehler-Klein (Gießen: Franz Steiner Verlag, 2007): 381.
2. Thomas Beddies, *'Du hast die Pflicht, gesund zu sein!': der Gesundheitsdienst der Hitler-Jugend 1933–1945* (Berlin: BeBra Verlag, 2010): 10–14.
3. For further information on the statistics of the clinic, consult the appendices.
4. Consult Chapter 3 for further information on the structure of the clinic.
5. AHUS. Case of Günther F., 1943 (case number 9/2201).
6. AHUS. Case of Günther F., 1943 (case number 9/2201).
7. AHUS. Case of Günther F., 1943, Short Pathology Record (dissection number 613).
8. AHUS. Case of Georgine S., 1943 (case number 9/2130).
9. AHUS. Case of Georgine S., 1943, Dr Klinge pathology referral letter, 20 January 1943 (pathology case number 169/43).

10. AHUS. Case of Georgine S., 1943, Dr Klinge pathology referral letter, 20 January 1943 (pathology case number 169/43).
11. AHUS. Case of Luise S., 1944 (case number 9/3547).
12. AHUS. Case of Luise S., 1944 (case number 9/3547).
13. Tami Davis Biddle, 'British and American Approaches to Strategic Bombing: Their Origins and Implementation in the World War II Combined Bomber Offensive', *Journal of Strategic Studies* 18 (1995): 91–144. https://doi.org/10.1080/01402399508437581
14. L. Shields and B. Bryan, 'The Effect of War on Children: The Children of Europe after World War II', *International Nursing Review, International Council of Nurses* 49.2 (2002): 87–98.
15. AHUS. Case of Luise S., 1944 (case number 9/3547).
16. AHUS. Case of Dieter H., 1944 (case number 9/1208).
17. 1 FI 103 129—Ruelle des Trois-Gâteaux vers l'église Sainte-Madeleine après le bombardement aérien du 11 août 1944 (1944). Available at the Archives de la Ville et de l'Eurometropole.
18. Katarzyna Woniak, 'Polen als Patienten Während der NS-Zwangsarbeit', *Acta Universitatis Lodziensis. Folia Philosophica. Ethica—Aesthetica—Practica* 37 (2020): 51–66. https://doi.org/10.18778/0208-6107.37.05
19. Wojciech Kwieciński, 'Medizinische Versorgung polnischer Zwangsarbeiter in der Region Bielefeld', *Acta Universitatis Lodziensis. Folia Philosophica. Ethica—Aesthetica—Practica* 37 (2020): 67–86.
20. Gelinada Grinchenko and Marta D. Olynyk, 'The Ostarbeiter of Nazi Germany in Soviet and Post-Soviet Ukrainian Historical Memory', *Canadian Slavonic Papers* 54 (2012): 3–4, 401–26. DOI: 10.1080/00085006.2012.11092715
21. Christian Bonah and Lea Münch, 'La Medizinische Klinik II (Médicale A): vie quotidienne et patients', in *La faculté de médecine de la Reichsuniversität Straßburg et l'hôpital civil sous l'annexation de fait nationale-socialiste 1940–1945*: 108.
22. Eva Hallama, 'Between the Projection of Danger, Objectification, and Exploitation: Medical Examination of Polish Civilian Forced Labourers Before their Deportation into the German Reich', *Acta Universitatis Lodziensis. Folia Philosophica. Ethica—Aesthetica—Practica* 37 (2020): 35–50. https://doi.org/10.18778/0208-6107.37.04
23. Grinchenko, Gelinada, 'Forced Labour in Nazi Germany in the Interviews of Former Child Ostarbeiters', in *Reclaiming the Personal: Oral History in Post-Socialist Europe*, eds. Natalia Khanenko-Friesen and Gelinada Grinchenko (Toronto: University of Toronto Press, 2017): 176–204. https://doi.org/10.3138/9781442625235-010
24. Christian Bonah and Lea Münch, 'La Medizinische Klinik II (Médicale A): vie quotidienne et patients', in *La faculté de médecine de la Reichsuniversität Straßburg et l'hôpital civil sous l'annexation de fait nationale-socialiste 1940–1945*: 108. Referencing the document 'Courrier du commissaire au plan quadrriennal plenipotentiare a la main-douvre du 16 octobre 1942 a l'attention a de MM. Les presidents des Arbeitsamter regionaux'.
25. Katarzyna Woniak, 'Polen als Patienten Während der NS-Zwangsarbeit', *Acta Universitatis Lodziensis. Folia Philosophica. Ethica—Aesthetica—Practica* 37 (2020): 51–66. https://doi.org/10.18778/0208-6107.37.05
26. For further information on this decree and the impact on medical care, consult Christian Bonah and Lea Münch, 'La Medizinische Klinik II (Médicale A): vie quotidienne et patients', in *La faculté de médecine de la Reichsuniversität Straßburg et l'hôpital civil sous l'annexation de fait nationale-socialiste 1940–1945*: 109.

27. Wojciech Kwieciński, 'Medizinische Versorgung polnischer Zwangsarbeiter in der Region Bielefeld', *Acta Universitatis Lodziensis. Folia Philosophica. Ethica—Aesthetica—Practica* 37 (2020): 67–86.
28. AHUS. Case of Michal G, 1944 (case number 9/3327).
29. Flora Graefe and Volker Roelcke, 'Zwangsarbeiter in der Medizin—Zivile "Fremdarbeiter" als Arbeitskräfte und Patienten am Universitätsklinikum Gießen im Zweiten Weltkrieg', in *Die Medizinische Fakultät der Universität Gießen 1607 bis 2007. Band I Die Medizinische Fakultät der Universität Gießen im Nationalsozialismus und in der Nachkriegszeit: Personen und Institutionen, Umbrüche und Kontinuitäten*, ed. Sigrid Oehler-Klein (Gießen: Franz Steiner Verlag, 2007): 391.
30. AHUS. Case of Michal G., 1944 (case number 9/3327), referral for outpatient care from ear, nose, and throat clinic on 16 February 1944.
31. Katarzyna Woniak, 'Polen als Patienten Während der NS-Zwangsarbeit', *Acta Universitatis Lodziensis. Folia Philosophica. Ethica—Aesthetica—Practica* 37 (2020): 51–66. https://doi.org/10.18778/0208-6107.37.05
32. AHUS. Case of Iwan P., 1944 (case number 9/3344).
33. AHUS. Case of Iwan P., 1944 (case number 9/3344), 7 March 1944, release letter from Dr Dietz.
34. AHUS. Case of Wassily D., 1943 (case number 9/418).
35. Mark Spoerer, Jochen Fleischhacker, 'Forced Laborers in Nazi Germany: Categories, Numbers, and Survivors', *The Journal of Interdisciplinary History* 33.2 (2002): 182.
36. AHUS. Case of Wassily D., 1943 (case number 9/418).
37. AHUS. Case of Wassily D., 1943 (case number 9/418).
38. AHUS. Case of Katherine S., 1943 (case number /43).
39. Ibid.
40. AHUS. Case of Katherine S., 1943 (case number 9/483).
41. Katarzyna Woniak, 'Polen als Patienten Während der NS-Zwangsarbeit', *Acta Universitatis Lodziensis. Folia Philosophica. Ethica—Aesthetica—Practica* 37 (2020): 51–66. https://doi.org/10.18778/0208-6107.37.05
42. For further information on menstrual disturbances in forced labourers, consult Sabine Hildebrandt, 'The Women on Stieve's List: Victims of National Socialism Whose Bodies Were Used for Anatomical Research', *Clinical Anatomy* 26.1 (2013): 3–21. https://doi.org/10.1002/ca.22195
43. AHUS. Case of Katherine S,, 1943 (case number 9/483).
44. Consult ADHVS Psych. Case of Johann H., 1943 (case number K27/508), for further details of paediatric patients' awareness of the Gestapo, and the staff dismissal of these concerns as paranoia.
45. Service Regional Police Judiciaire, ADBR, 1095 W 17 2391: not paginated.
46. For further information on the internment camp of Schirmeck, consult *Le camp d'internement de Schirmeck (territoire de La Broque) = das Sicherungslager von Schirmeck-Vorbruck: témoignages* (Essor, 1998).
47. 126AL77 B Medizinalwesen Prüfung der Säuglings und Kleinkinderpflegerinnen, 2 July 1942, letter stating that Georgette Sittler has quit the nursing school with no prior notice.
48. Service Regional Police Judiciaire, ADBR, 1095 W 17 2391. Testimony of Gabriele Krebs, 18 December 1945.
49. Service Regional Police Judiciaire, ADBR, 1095 W 17 2391.

50. Service Regional Police Judiciaire, ADBR, 1095 W 17 2391. Testimony of Gabriele Krebs, 18 December 1945.
51. Service Regional Police Judiciaire, ADBR, 1095 W 17 2391. Testimony of Emilie Richert, 18 December 1945.
52. Account of the evacuation of Strasbourg, Dr Kurt Hofmeier, available at Bundesarchiv Berlin, R 76 IV 27.
53. BArch. R 76 IV 27. Account of the evacuation of Strasbourg, Dr Kurt Hofmeier.
54. Ibid.
55. ADBR. 126AL77 F. Letter from Oberin Reiter to Chef der Zivilverwaltung with exams planned for fifty students in 1945 and thirty-five students in 1946. Notdienstverpflichtung der Säuglings u Kinderschwestern Schülerinnen der Lehranstalt bei der Universität Kinderklinik in Straßburg.
56. Stéphane Simonnet and Christophe Prime, *Atlas de la seconde guerre mondiale: La France au combat: de la drôle de guerre à la Libération* (2015).
57. 'Histoire / Général Franz Vaterrodt / Condamné à Mort Pour La Reddition de Strasbourg—Les DNA Archives', accessed 5 September 2019, http://sitemap.dna.fr/articles/201003/13/condamne-mort-pour-la-reddition-de-strasbourg,strasbourg,000006351.php
58. Account of the evacuation of Strasbourg, Dr Kurt Hofmeier, available at Bundesarchiv Berlin, R 76 IV 27.
59. Rainer Möhler, *Die Reichsuniversität Straßburg 1941–1944. Eine Nationalsozialistische Musteruniversität zwischen Wissenschaft, Volkstumspolitik, und Verbrechen*, Diss. Phil. (Universität Saarlandes, 2019): 761.
60. Antony Beevor, *Ardennes 1944: Hitler's Last Gamble* (London: Viking, 2015).
61. Rainer Möhler, *Die Reichsuniversität Straßburg 1941–1944. Eine Nationalsozialistische Musteruniversität zwischen Wissenschaft, Volkstumspolitik, und Verbrechen*: 761.
62. Account of the evacuation of Strasbourg, Dr Kurt Hofmeier, available at Bundesarchiv Berlin, R 76 IV 27.
63. Rainer Möhler, *Die Reichsuniversität Straßburg 1941–1944. Eine Nationalsozialistische Musteruniversität zwischen Wissenschaft, Volkstumspolitik, und Verbrechen*, Diss. Phil. (Universität Saarlandes, 2019): 761.
64. Account of the evacuation of Strasbourg, Dr Kurt Hofmeier, available at Bundesarchiv Berlin, R 76 IV 27.
65. Ibid.
66. Ibid.
67. Eight hundred and sixty-nine, to be exact, as they were recovered from the routine destruction of the clinic to make room for the new hospital wing in 1989.

7. Final Days of the Reichsuniversität Straßburg

1. Kurt Hofmeier, *Erbwissenschaft und Adoption*: 163.
2. Dr Elena Alexandraviciene was the least senior doctor in the children's clinic, as she had only begun working there in 1944. This is possibly why she was chosen to stay behind.
3. Rainer Möhler, *Die Reichsuniversität Straßburg 1941–1944. Eine Nationalsozialistische Musteruniversität zwischen Wissenschaft, Volkstumspolitik, und Verbrechen*, Diss. Phil. (Universität Saarlandes, 2019): 761.

4. BIAB. SAI188962900022217 Liberation de l'Alsace, 1944, René Saint Paul.
5. Ibid.
6. Fritz Klinge, *Der Sektionskurs und was dazu gehört. Auch zur Zusammenarbeit des Pathologen mit dem Arzt* (Stuttgart: Georg Thieme Verlag, 1948).
7. Verena Buser, 'Child Survivors and Displaced Children in the Aftermath Studies. An Overview', in *Freilegungen: Rebuilding Lives—Child Survivors and DP Children in the Aftermath of the Holocaust and Forced Labor* (Göttingen: Wallstein, Bad Arolsen International Tracing Service, 2017): 27–40.
8. Boaz Cohen, 'Research on Child Holocaust Survivors and Displaced Persons: Goals and Challenges', in *Freilegungen: Rebuilding Lives—Child Survivors and DP Children in the Aftermath of the Holocaust and Forced Labor* (Göttingen: Wallstein, Bad Arolsen International Tracing Service, 2017).
9. Boaz Cohen and Rita Horvath, 'Young Witnesses in the DP Camps: Children's Holocaust Testimony in Context', *Journal of Modern Jewish Studies* 11.1 (2012): 103–25.
10. Photographs of some forced labourers can be found in Eugène Riedweg, *Strasbourg: ville occupée 1939–1945. La vie quotidienne dans la capitale de l'alsace durant la seconde guerre mondiale* (Steinbrunn-le-haut, 1982): 154.
11. Rainer Möhler, 'Die Reichsuniversität Straßburg 1941–1944. Eine Nationalsozialistische Musteruniversität zwischen Wissenschaft, Volkstumspolitik, und Verbrechen': 811.
12. Denis Durand De Bousingen, 'La Clinique Infantile de l'Hôpital Civil (1910–1989). Une Réalisation Modèle Au Service Des Enfants Malades', *Histoire & Patrimoine Hospitalier: Mémoire de La Médecine à Strasbourg* 23 (2010): 4–11.
13. Jean-Marc Lévy, 'Les "Patrons" Successifs de La Clinique Infantile': 14–29.
14. 'Strasbourg: un "Nouvel Hôpital Civil"', *Le Figaro*, 31 March 2008.
15. AVES. 1 FI 144 7. Place de l'Hôpital, entrée principale des hospices civiles (1941).
16. LA-BW StAS. Wü 13 T 2 Nr. 2133/014. Dr Kurt Hofmeier Entnazifizierung.
17. Corine Defrance and Frank Hüther, 'Un nouveau personel pour une nouvel université ? Les défis du recrutement des enseignants à Mayence, 1945–1949', in *La Allemagne et la denazification Allemagne après 1945*, eds. Sébastien Cahuffour, Corine Defrance, Stefan Martens, and Marie-Bénédicte Vincent (Brussels: Peter Lang, 2019): 45–64.
18. LA-BW StAS. Wü 13T2133. Denazification of Dr Kurt Hofmeier.
19. Kurt Hofmeier, 'Fragekasten', *Deutsche Medizinische Wochenschrift* 79 Jahrgang (1949): 589–90.
20. Wilhelm Hagen, Hans Thomae, and Anna Ronge, *10 Jahre Nachkriegskinder* (München: J.A. Barth, 1962); Carl Coerper and Anneliese Coerper, *Deutsche Nachkriegskinder: Methoden und erste Ergebnisse der deutschen Längsschnittuntersuchungen über die körperliche und seelische Entwicklung im Schulkindalter* (Stuttgart: G. Thieme, 1954).
21. Kurt Hofmeier, Werner Schwidder, and Friedrich Müller, *Alles über dein Kind: Auskunfts- und Nachschlagewerk nach Altersstufen über die körperliche und seelische Entwicklung, Pflege und Erziehung des Kindes für alle Eltern, Lehrer und Erzieher* (Bielefeld: Gieseking, 1970).
22. *Stuttgarter Nachrichten*, 10 September 1971.
23. *Stuttgarter Zeitung*, 4 September 1989.
24. Werner Sollors, '"Everybody Gets Fragebogened Sooner or Later": The Denazification Questionnaire as Cultural Text', *German Life and Letters* 71.2 (1 April 2018): 139–53. https://doi.org/10.1111/glal.12188

25. Sheila Faith Weiss, 'After the Fall: Political Whitewashing, Professional Posturing, and Personal Refashioning in the Postwar Career of Otmar Freiherr von Verschuer', *Isis* 101.4 (December 2010): 722–58.
26. For a full list of Hofmeier's publications, consult the appendices.
27. Thomas Lennert, 'Die Entwicklung der Berliner Pädiatrie': 529–51.
28. Ibid., referring to a review of the Kaiserin Auguste Viktoria Haus in 1939 where Hofmeier explains his position on Leo Langstein.
29. Eduard Seidler, 'Die Schicksale jüdischer Kinderärzte im Nationalsozialismus', *Monatsschrift für Kinderheilkunde* 146 (1998): 744–53.
30. Rainer Möhler, *Die Reichsuniversität Straßburg 1941–1944. Eine Nationalsozialistische Musteruniversität zwischen Wissenschaft, Volkstumspolitik, und Verbrechen*: 811.
31. Cathy Caruth, 'The Body's Testimony: Dramatic Witness in the Eichmann Trial', *Paragraph* 40.3 (2017): 259–78.

Index

References to figures appear in *italic* type; those in **bold** type refer to tables; and the letter 'n' indicates an endnote.

H

I

J

K

L

M

R

S

Y

Z

CPSIA information can be obtained
at www.ICGtesting.com
Printed in the USA
JSHW022137130723
44337JS00001BA/3

9 781804 130896